Perfect
Weight

JORDAN RUBIN

with Bernard Bulwer, MD

SILOAM
A STRANG COMPANY

Most STRANG COMMUNICATIONS/CHARISMA HOUSE/SILOAM/FRONTLINE/REALMS/EXCEL BOOKS products are available at special quantity discounts for bulk purchase for sales promotions, premiums, fund-raising, and educational needs. For details, write Strang Communications/Charisma House/Siloam/FrontLine/Realms/Excel Books, 600 Rinehart Road, Lake Mary, Florida 32746, or telephone (407) 333-0600.

PERFECT WEIGHT CANADA by Jordan Rubin with Bernard Bulwer, MD
Published by Siloam
A Strang Company
600 Rinehart Road
Lake Mary, Florida 32746
www.siloam.com

Unless otherwise noted, all Scripture quotations are from the New King James Version of the Bible. Copyright © 1979, 1980, 1982 by Thomas Nelson, Inc., publishers. Used by permission.

Scripture quotations marked NLT are from the Holy Bible, New Living Translation, copyright © 1996. Used by permission of Tyndale Cover Designer: Bill Johnson

International Standard Book Number: 978-1-59979-324-5
The Library of Congress has catalogued the previous edition as follows:
Library of Congress Cataloging-in-Publication Data
Rubin, Jordan.
  Perfect weight Canada / Jordan Rubin. -- 1st ed.
     p. cm.
  Includes bibliographical references and index.
  ISBN 978-1-59979-263-7
  1. Weight loss--Canada. 2. Obesity--Canada--Prevention. 3. Nutrition--Canada. I. Title.
RM222.2.R816 2008
614.5'939800971--dc22
                                        2007039974

Neither the publisher nor the author is engaged in rendering professional advice or services to the individual reader. The ideas, procedures, and suggestions in this book are not intended as a substitute for consulting with your physician. All matters regarding your health require medical supervision. Neither the author nor the publisher shall be liable or responsible for any loss or damage allegedly arising from any information or suggestion in this book.

The recipes in this book are to be followed exactly as written. The publisher is not responsible for your specific health or allergy needs that may require medical supervision. The publisher is not responsible for any adverse reactions to the recipes contained in this book.

While the author has made every effort to provide accurate telephone numbers and Internet addresses at the time of publication, neither the publisher nor the author assumes any responsibility for errors or for changes that occur after publication.

08 09 10 11 12 — 987654321
Printed in the United States of America

Contents

A Note to the Reader

I LIVE IN South Florida, and following the American Thanksgiving in late November, it isn't difficult to notice the traffic jam on Interstate 95 as flocks of Canadian snowbirds arrive in their gleaming motor homes to winter in the Sunshine State.

Listen, I've been to Winnipeg when it resembled an icicle—"Winterpeg" is how I heard the locals describe their city—so I understand the seasonal migration to warmer climes. As for myself, I've made several trips to Canada to speak at health events and in churches, and I've loved interacting with Canadians on each occasion. I remember visiting a farm outside Toronto where I addressed a group of local farmers about a concept called "sustainable agriculture" and how their high-quality whole foods could improve the health of Toronto-area residents as well as Canadians in every province.

Another interesting trip happened the time I flew to Vancouver, British Columbia, to attend and present at the Canadian Natural Products Expo during the midst of the SARS health crisis in April 2003. At that time, an outbreak of SARS in Toronto had occurred, which lead the World Health Organization to issue a travel warning that prompted Canadian authorities to strictly monitor the arrival of international travelers. At the Vancouver customs, I'll never forget the sight of hundreds of passengers—mostly Asians flying in from the Far East—wearing white protective masks as they stood in line to enter your country.

My most enjoyable meal on the trip happened at one of the best Japanese restaurants in Vancouver. The sushi was phenomenal, the wasabi wasn't green because it wasn't artificially coloured, and the pickled ginger was more beige than pink. What really caught my attention, though, was the wild-caught salmon, whose flavourful meat was as red as a fire truck.

When I conducted a health seminar in Vancouver, I found the audience to be very friendly to my message on health and wellness. One question I get asked whenever I'm in Canada is whether I think Canadians are healthier and more health conscious than Americans. The answer is yes, but not by much. I think Canadians are facing the same health challenges found elsewhere in the world from eating lousy meals on the go, not getting enough exercise or sleep, and dealing with overabundant amounts of stress and toxins.

Let's face it: Canadians eat pretty much the same junk that Americans do. You have McDonald's and Pizza Huts and Taco Bells and your homegrown Tim Hortons. Winnipeg has the highest per capita consumption of 7-Eleven Slurpees than anywhere in North America.[1] You can buy the same high-sugar, high-salt, and low-nutrition "convenience" foods in your supermarkets as Americans can. I'm sure that your long, harsh winters are conducive to staying inside, where the temptation to snack on sweets is strong and the opportunity to exercise is scant.

The wheat fields of Manitoba may be the world's breadbasket, but much of that wheat undergoes the same "enriching" process that American wheat undergoes. After the harvest, machines strip the wheat stalks of germs and bran, which contain vitamins and fibre. Flour mills rinse the wheat with various chemical bleaches, and the result is the transformation of healthy foods that have been on families' tables for centuries—usually in the form of bread, pasta, or baked goods—into one of the most highly allergenic, difficult-to-digest substances.

But don't get me started. The book you're about to read, *Perfect Weight Canada*, is releasing at the same time as a book geared toward your cousins to the south: *Perfect Weight America*. You will notice that much of *Perfect Weight Canada* refers to a health initiative that my team and I began in Toledo, Ohio, called "Healthy Toledo." I think what happened in Toledo over the course of an eleven-week pilot program applies north of the 49th parallel as well. Toledo is only eighty-five kilometres southwest of Windsor, Ontario, and I think the results that ordinary people have achieved in Toledo can be experienced by millions of Canadians.

I believe Canadians can lead the way in North America and show Americans a thing or two about living healthy and achieving your perfect weight. All it takes is following the health principles behind *Perfect Weight Canada*.

You know, people often ask me when it's too late to begin this health program. *Am I too overweight...too unhealthy...too old?*

My answer is that the only way you can start *Perfect Weight Canada* too late is if you wait until tomorrow.

Your journey to extraordinary health begins today.

The Perfect Weight Canada Campaign

"WELCOME TO TOLEDO, Ohio."

I gripped the firm handshake belonging to Mayor Carleton "Carty" Finkbeiner as he waved me into his blue-carpeted office perched on the twenty-second floor high above the muddy Maumee River and Toledo's hardscrabble downtown district. The casually dressed mayor, wearing a long-sleeved lemon dress shirt, khaki pants, and penny loafers, escorted me to a cozy corner where three team jerseys—stencilled with FINKBEINER on the back—were pinned on the wall, including one from one of my favourite team names in baseball, the Toledo Mud Hens.

On this Monday afternoon in early April, the elected leader of Ohio's fourth largest city had carved out precious time from his jam-packed schedule to see me and Tony Scott, a local pastor who facilitated the meeting. Their paths had crossed in Toledo civic circles for twenty years, but I had a feeling that Pastor Tony cashed in a few chips to arrange a face-to-face with the mayor.

The topic on the table was health—actually, the lousy health of Toledans. This heavily blue-collar city, where Jeep vehicles have rolled off the assembly line since 1941, may bill itself as the "crossroads of America" since the metropolis lies at the busy intersection of Interstate 90 and Interstate 75, but the collective health of its 300,000 citizens was at a junction point as well. A month before our meeting, *Men's Health* magazine had ranked Toledo ninety-eighth out of the one hundred best and worst U.S. cities for men after crunching numbers in twenty-four categories, including life-and-death data on cancer, heart disease, and strokes.[1] *Men's Health* also ran a "sweat check," looking at how often, how long, and how intensely men exercise, but from what I saw in Toledo, pubs and sports bars far outnumbered fitness centres. The joke around town was that the only heavy lifting Toledo guys did following work was raising a cold longneck after a long day on the factory floor.

And lighting up. Toledo has the highest adult smoking rate in the United States—31 percent—according to a city-by-city study of tobacco use released by the Centers for Disease Control. "We're a blue-collar town," explained Arnie Elzey, a Toledo bar owner. "People enjoy sitting down with a beer and smoking a cigarette. It's Toledo. It's not California."[2]

With its basement ranking, Hizzoner appeared quite interested to hear about the launch of a "Healthy Toledo" initiative that I had led at Pastor Tony's church the previous evening—an eleven-week pilot program for the Perfect Weight America campaign. "We had around one hundred fifty folks sign up," I reported. "We're going to conduct objective health screenings before and after so that we can scientifically quantify the improvement in their health."

The energetic mayor slapped his thigh. "That's great, because I'm a fanatic on diet and exercise," he said. "I follow the South Beach Diet, not because it's the best, but I had to do something about what I was eating. You see, I had quadruple bypass heart surgery three years ago at the Cleveland Clinic, and let me tell you, that was a wake-up call. I'm also taking Zocor to get my cholesterol levels down."

I regarded the slender, healthy-looking, sixty-eight-year-old mayor, who I later learned carried 167 pounds on his five-foot, nine-inch frame. "We're hoping for positive results," I explained, "just like the encouraging news we've heard from the Joe Arrington Cancer Center in Lubbock, Texas, where one hundred employees followed a similar program to Healthy Toledo. One of the early results is that the number of sick days dropped 65 percent in a designated time period."

The mayor whistled. "The average Toledo person is not living a healthy life," he said. "If your program can drop the cost of health care and sick days, think of what that could do to get a Fortune 500 company to move here."

I smiled at the Fortune 500 reference. Pastor Tony's church, The Church on Strayer, had moved into an empty 120,000-square-foot building two years ago—a sprawling grey-and-beige brick structure planted in a leafy, campus-like setting. Before The Church on Strayer congregation moved in, the showcase property had been the corporate headquarters of a Fortune 500 company until the business enterprise pulled up stakes and moved out of Toledo. Could the Glass City's spiralling employee health costs have been an issue?

Mayor Finkbeiner snapped me back to the present. "Tony says you've written some books," the mayor offered to keep the conversation moving along.

I was about to describe *The Maker's Diet* and the Great Physician's Rx series when Pastor Tony interjected.

"They're great books, mayor," he said. "You have to take a look at them. Tell you what: I'll drop off a half-dozen copies for you and your staff tomorrow morning by nine o'clock."

"I'd like that," said the mayor, who turned the discussion back to the nuts and bolts of the Healthy Toledo pilot program. Our meeting, which was supposed to last ten minutes, stretched to a half hour, which I thought was a great indicator of Mayor Carty's interest in what we were attempting to do. I explained how we were trying to help Toledo families get healthier through an eleven-week lifestyle program that involved a comprehensive, individualized eating plan, a nutritional supplement protocol, an easy-to-follow exercise program, ways to reduce stress and get more rest, and ideas to improve emotional and spiritual health. While the Perfect Weight America program would span sixteen weeks, I informed the mayor that we had shortened the duration of Healthy Toledo to eleven weeks in order to share the results with the Toledo community at Freedom Fest, a part Fourth of July celebration and part health fair to be held at The Church on Strayer on the Saturday night before the Fourth of July.

The mayor clasped his hands in appreciation and stood, signalling the end of our meeting. He wished me all the best, and while Mayor Finkbeiner didn't offer me the proverbial key to the city before leaving his office, I sensed his unqualified support. "If there's anything I can do you—make a phone call, open a door—just let me know," he said.

I thanked the mayor for placing such importance on the health of his constituents, especially in the face of Toledo's unflattering health statistics. "I think you'll be pleased with the final results eleven weeks from now."

The mayor nodded his understanding. "What you're doing is great," Mayor Carty declared as he escorted us out of his expansive office. "Good luck to you."

Launch Time

The collective health of Toledans probably doesn't compare very well to the sunny citizens of Richmond, British Columbia, which was named the healthiest city in Canada by Statistics Canada.[3] But someplace had to be the first stop in the "Perfect Weight" campaign, which I hope you'll join whether you live in Vancouver, British Columbia, St. John's, Newfoundland, or points in between. (In case you're wondering, I'll share the results of the Healthy Toledo campaign in chapter 13, "Holy Toledo! The Results Are In...")

If you're looking to change your diet, change your life, and change your world, then you've come to the right place. *Perfect Weight Canada* is all about giving you the directions you need to make a U-turn in life and get headed in the right direction. Maybe it's been years since you've woken up feeling refreshed or since you attacked the day with some spring in your step. Maybe your life has revolved around innumerable visits to the family doctor and expensive specialists who struggle to find out what's "wrong" with you. Maybe you gulp down powerful drugs to fight off the ravages of hypertension, type 2 diabetes, heartburn, and a host of other ailments—and wonder if the side effects aren't worse than the disease.

If this sounds like your life, then following the health recommendations set forth in *Perfect Weight Canada* will hand you the tools to transform yourself in ways you never thought possible. A great place to start would be visiting www .PerfectWeightCanada.com and taking your health assessment.

PerfectWeightCanada.com is an online resource that will serve as your personal Perfect Weight coach. After you log in and fill out a questionnaire, you'll receive a detailed, individualized daily health and wellness plan that covers diet, supplementation, exercise, cleansing and detoxification, and stress management. Once you have this plan in hand, you will have practical tools to reach your perfect weight.

Later in this book, in chapter 7, you will find a four-phase Perfect Weight Eating

Plan that will tell what foods you should and should not consume during the sixteen-week program. Or, if you prefer, I highly recommend taking advantage of our free customized program available online at www.PerfectWeightCanada.com.

When you complete your health assessment questionnaire, you will become part of an online community with access to multiple tools to keep you on track: daily reminders, an online journal, shopping lists, recipes, exercise charts and demonstrations, and an individualized daily diet and exercise plan. When this diagnostic is in place, you'll have a road map that you can follow, step-by-step, to enjoy the optimal health and wellness that you haven't experienced for years or perhaps decades.

You will learn what to eat, when to eat it, how to cheat right, which foods can add fat, and which foods can help it disappear. You will discover which foods make you hungrier and which foods keep you feeling full. You will be reminded about the importance of staying hydrated, how to integrate strategic snacking, and how adding superior supplements to your daily regimen will give you that extra edge. You will also experience the Perfect Cleanse, an innovative cleansing and detoxification program that you should do seasonally in January, April, July, and October.

An integral part of Perfect Weight Canada is a groundbreaking fitness plan I call FIT—Functional Interval Training. In just twenty minutes you'll strengthen your heart and lungs, build muscle, and ignite your body's fat-burning furnace so you can scorch fat during and after your workout.

In addition, you will learn how to create a toxin-free home to prevent harmful chemical poisons from storing in your fat cells—which will become fewer by the day when you follow this program. You will learn how to put on the Perfect Weight Canada helmet of success to squash all your weight-loss saboteurs. You will be equipped to reduce stress and create the life you've always dreamed of. You will learn the underlying secret to transforming your physical appearance and self-esteem as well as ways to improve the health of family and friends around you.

Check Out the Perfect Weight Canada Web Site—Right Away!

Don't wait another minute: visit www.PerfectWeightCanada.com right now. Your individualized Perfect Weight Canada health and wellness plan will be created following your online health assessment questionnaire. With the tapping of a few keys, you will tell us about your height, weight, and age; how your body reacts to certain foods; your "food mood" connection; your sleeping patterns; your fitness profile; your exposure to environmental toxins; and your global footprint. This online diagnostic, which uses a proprietary formula for assessing your current state of health, will provide you with a comprehensive sixteen-week battle plan to help you win the battle of the bulge and rid your body of killer fat.

The cost is free for a twelve-month subscription; simply go to the Web site and type in PWC as your access code. A one-year membership to the Perfect Weight Canada online program is valued at more than $240 Canadian.

What's Different About Perfect Weight Canada?

Please know that *Perfect Weight Canada* is not just another diet book. You won't shake off 22 pounds in a hurry like singer Beyoncé Knowles did before playing the role of Deena in the hit film *Dreamgirls*. Beyoncé lost all that weight after embarking on a crash diet that consisted of drinking a mixture of water, cayenne pepper, and maple syrup—and starving herself of regular food. When the supermarket tabloids splashed photos of her newly svelte figure, shoppers made a dash for the maple syrup on aisle 4.[4]

While Beyoncé's "maple syrup diet" may be one of the more outlandish fads to capture attention in recent years, her story is an instructive reminder that millions of Americans are on the lookout for the "next big thing" to lose weight swiftly as well as effortlessly. Fad diets make up a tidy chunk of a multibillion-dollar weight-loss industry in North America that churns out books, CDs, DVDs, shakes, bars, pills, supplements, gym equipment, and infomercials for everything from the latest weight-burning shakes and slimming supplements to bun trainers and ab sculptors. Yet as anyone who's suffered through a crash diet will tell you, weight quickly lost is weight destined to return. Nearly none of these diets can be sustained because these food-restrictive regimes do not deliver a variety of well-rounded, nutritious foods necessary for good health. Nor do they speak to the mental, emotional, and spiritual health of individuals, which is just as important as physical well-being.

Perfect Weight Canada addresses all four legs of this stool, which is why this well-rounded program holds its own with many of the diet and exercise books vying for attention on your nation's bookshelves. *Perfect Weight Canada* outlines a new lifestyle based on holistic principles that focus on the whole person: physical, mental, emotional, and spiritual. This approach is more in line with the etymology of the word *diet*, which originated from the Greek word *diaita*, meaning "life, lifestyle, way of living."

You're going to be better off jumping in all the way—making a complete lifestyle change—than poking your toes around the edges of the pool. According to a recent study published in the *Archives of Internal Medicine*, smoking, drinking, eating junk food, and getting no exercise are all risk factors for poor health, but tackling all these habits *at the same time* is better than dealing with them one by one in a sequential fashion.[5]

So, if you weigh too much, get tired too easily, live a sedentary lifestyle, or deal with high blood pressure, high cholesterol, and high anxiety, the fact that you're holding this book, *Perfect Weight Canada*, tells me that regaining your health is a top priority. You're sick and tired of being sick and tired.

I'm confident that *Perfect Weight Canada* will be a great resource for you. You will have to change your American mind-set, though, the one that's dialed into instant gratification. Instead, you'll have to take personal responsibility for the shape you're in.

Once you do that, you must stop listening to yourself. Your nimble mind, which is the essence of your will and determination, loves to capture negative thoughts and spin them around like liquid sugar and pink dye in a cotton candy machine to whip up a confection of doubt and hesitation. Toss those negative thoughts in the trash. Don't listen when your agile mind coughs up one rationalization after another against making a major course correction in life. Shut down your excuse making because at the end of the day, that's all they are—excuses, such as:

- "I'm too busy."
- "I'm too fat."
- "I don't have the energy."
- "I've got kids."
- "I've got parents to take care of."
- "I'm going on vacation."
- "It costs too much to join a fitness club."
- "I can't get motivated."
- "I don't have the money."
- "Nothing's ever worked before."

The Perfect Weight program calls for an attitude adjustment—fast. *The most important attitude you can have is this: I'm following the Perfect Weight Canada program for my health and for those who count on me. The more I put into it, the more I will receive from it. If I give this my best effort, then I can expect the best results.*

Perfect Weight Canada follows the steady route to successful weight management and a lifetime of extraordinary health. Sure, you'll probably lose a few pounds right away, but the point is that you won't reach your perfect weight in two weeks. You'll certainly be a lot closer, however, after sixteen weeks. Casting off 22 pounds like Beyoncé did is not only unhealthy, but it's also counterproductive in the long run since the elation of losing substantial weight is quickly replaced by despair when the old pounds come right back. Depressed dieters often cope by reverting back to deeply entrenched eating habits, which often leaves them weighing *more* than when they started the quick-loss diet in the first place.

Setting Sail

Perfect Weight Canada is about making a personal transformation in quantitative categories such as weight loss and reduction of disease risks, as well as qualitative improvements in mental acuity and physical vitality. Best of all, you will love the eating plan because you will consume an assortment of satisfying and delicious foods, as you will discover to your delight in chapter 3: "Eat for Your Perfect Weight."

In the following chapters, you'll learn how to:

1. Change your diet.

- Eat healthy so that you attain and maintain your "perfect weight."
- Eat for your individual nutritional type.
- Optimize your nutrient intake while cutting out unnecessary and unhealthy calories to ensure healthy weight loss.
- Learn about the nutritional supplements that can make a big difference in your health and vitality.
- Tap into the Perfect Weight Eating Plan, a sixteen-week, four-phase program that offers you approved foods while restricting others.

2. Change your life.

- Eliminate wastes and toxins as you undertake the Perfect Cleanse.
- Experience FIT, the exercise program that you can live with.
- Reduce toxins in your personal environment.
- Reduce stress and get more rest in order to unlock your health potential.
- Focus on mental, emotional, and spiritual balance for total body, mind, and spirit wellness.

3. Change your world.

- Learn simple steps you can take to live a "green lifestyle."
- Take weight off the planet, as well as off your body.
- Incorporate habits that promote sustainability for your health, the health of future generations, and the health of the planet.

I've spoken in a number of churches in my day, including several in Canada, and occasionally a heavyset member will ask me, tongue firmly planted in cheek, if he can still enjoy all of his favourite unhealthy foods and snacks and still get past the pearly gates. "Oh, sure, you'll get to heaven," I'll respond. "You'll just get there a lot sooner."

The line is always good for a chuckle, but those who've faced their mortality after a heart attack, debilitating stroke, or cancer diagnosis aren't laughing very loudly. They understand better than most that every minute they have on Earth is precious and should be valued.

If you're married with children, your family needs you and loves you. Don't you want to stay around for them? Every year you have more to offer, not less, because you have wisdom and experience on your side. Use that wisdom to establish a health legacy for yourself and for your future generations, and you won't live a life of regrets.

Living a long, healthy life matters more than you know. I lost both of my grandfathers way too early. My grandfather on my father's side was significantly overweight and died at the age of sixty-two from a heart attack. My grandfather on my mother's side was overweight as well, and he died of a heart attack at the age of fifty-five. Both of my grandfathers were gone before I turned ten years old. I wish I had known them longer, but I never got the chance.

You may be reading this, however, and thinking, "I've let myself go too far…I can tell when people are staring at me." Well, with *Perfect Weight Canada*, you will be empowered to do something about your health and excess weight from this day forward. The question now becomes: What are you going to do about it? Will you take the information and apply it to your life and perhaps those closest to you?

You don't have to die early, as my grandfathers did. You have a wonderful purpose in life—to be there for your loved ones. Chase your dreams, and live life to the fullest. When you change your diet, change your life, and change your world, you will become much more than you ever thought possible.

A Little Bit About Me

Before we go any further, now would be a good time to fully introduce myself. As the eldest of two children born to Herb and Phyllis Rubin, I grew up in South Florida. Dad was a naturopathic physician and a chiropractor. Mom was a home-maker who helped Dad with the office chores.

My parents were born after World War II and came of age in the 1960s. While they weren't exactly hippies, they were definitely countercultural. Not only did they adopt the back-to-nature lifestyle (as it was called back then), but my father also promoted it wholeheartedly during my early childhood, while he attended naturo-pathic medical school and chiropractic school, and later in his chiropractic practice, where he employed a more natural approach to treating patients who saw him for a variety of aches and pains. Unlike many of my parents' peers in the baby-boom generation, eating healthy was not a fad for them. Their motto was, "The more natural, the better," and they filled their cupboards with raw honey, wheat germ, and granola, and their refrigerator with farm-fresh organic fruits and vegetables.

Kids in my neighbourhood didn't exactly flock to our house after school because Mom banned potato chips, cookies, and candy bars. But if they wanted a wheat-grass smoothie or a Mason jar of homemade plain yogurt, they came to the right place. You could say that I was a granola kid growing up, but whenever I went to school or my friends' homes, I made a beeline for the junk food. Maybe it was the forbidden fruit syndrome at work. At any rate, I can remember trying to trade baby carrots for chips and cookies during school lunch. I never found many takers, though. Some of my classmates were willing to part with some of their chocolate-covered treats for a quarter, however, so I took them up on their generous offer.

Despite my occasional forays into junk food, I grew into a healthy, athletic teen-ager. I can't recall anything more serious than a cold or flu keeping me out of the classroom. After high school, I attended Florida State University and earned a spot on the cheerleading squad and a place on the Doak Campbell Stadium floor when-ever the 'Noles played at home.

Like someone passing through a buffet line for the first time, I put too much on my plate during my freshman year—literally and figuratively. We were expected to practice every weekday for the FSU cheerleading team; miss a day, and you were cut from the squad. I had a full slate of classes, several books to read each week, intramural football games, and various "functions" at my fraternity, Phi Kappa Alpha. I also was a member of a traveling music group for the college ministry.

I tried to eat healthy on campus, but that was pretty much impossible in those days. Breakfast was a softball-sized blueberry muffin or sugar-laden, fat-free yogurt. During my school day, I fell into a burger-and-fries-and-soft-serve-frozen-yogurt routine. On the plus side, I managed to stay away from the party scene because I didn't drink alcohol or do drugs.

After finishing a hectic first year of college, I went back home and picked up a few dollars by being a counsellor at a summer youth camp in the area. It was during that time that I started to experience terrible digestive upsets, painful mouth sores, and weakening fatigue.

I hung on as long as I could, but when I couldn't do my job—like helping kids do the ropes course—I knew it was time to see our family doctor. He poked and prodded, then ran a battery of tests. When they came back clean, he shrugged his shoulders and handed me a prescription for two antibiotics. He didn't see any reason why I couldn't return to Florida State in the fall.

If only my body cooperated. The fall quarter was hellacious: 104-degree fevers, listlessness and fatigue, and embarrassing digestive problems. Two months into the football season, I couldn't fool myself any longer. I was really sick.

I called home and described my plight to Mom, who had me fly home the next day. My health steadily worsened over the next six months, including a scary episode with a 105-degree fever that left me speaking gibberish. I was referred to gastroenterologists who felt that my symptoms—vomiting, fever, night sweats, loss of appetite, severe abdominal cramps, and bloody diarrhea—pointed toward a digestive disorder known as Crohn's disease. If I didn't get better soon, one specialist said, I would be a strong candidate for a colostomy, which was the surgical removal of the colon.

At age nineteen, a colostomy sounded like a fate worse than death. In an effort to avoid surgery at all costs, my parents and I embarked on an all-out odyssey to regain my health. Over time, I was seen by seventy doctors and medical practitioners, tried every dietary plan under the sun, and even traveled to Mexico and Germany to seek alternative treatments. My parents tapped into their home equity to cover the $150,000 in medical bills.

Nothing reversed the downward trajectory of my health. My diseases—doctors were also treating me for diabetes, arthritis, anemia, and chronic fatigue syndrome—exacted a heavy toll on my body. After six months, when my weight plummeted to under 110 pounds, I needed a wheelchair to get around the house. How humiliating! I looked like a skeleton after months of wasting away. My lowest point happened when I was hospitalized at Bethesda Memorial Hospital in Boynton Beach, Florida, where I barely survived a harrowing night. I heard a nurse crying in the hallway, choking back tears as she told another RN that I wasn't going to survive the night. I felt blank, perhaps lost, and wasn't sure if I would wake up in the morning. When my eyes flickered open, the morning nurse said she had some good news for me: I had gained 10 pounds in water weight since receiving the intravenous fluids. I was alive, barely, but I was still bedridden.

Jordan's experience and results were extraordinary.
Readers should not expect miraculous results.

Nearly two years into the battle for my life, my father happened to have an interesting phone conversation with William Keith, a San Diego nutrition expert. He believed he could help me overcome the chronic digestive diseases plaguing my body—the ones called "incurable" by my doctors.

Intrigued, and figuring I had nothing to lose, Mom and Dad agreed that I should fly out to California and meet with Mr. Keith. My parents purchased a well-used RV so I could get around and have a place to sleep near the ocean. As I detail in many of my previous books, my health rebounded after I began consuming healthy "live" foods that were rich in vitamins, minerals, enzymes, and friendly microorganisms called probiotics—foods that are part of the Perfect Weight Canada program. Over a forty-day period, I gained 29 healthy pounds and put myself on a path of recovery.

I left San Diego with a renewed sense of purpose and a burning desire to transform the health of North America one life at a time. I took a job at a health food store that introduced me to the natural health movement. Eager to increase my knowledge, I studied naturopathic medicine and was soon formulating my own nutritional supplements and functional foods. My entrepreneurial spirit prompted me to start a company called Garden of Life, Inc., in my early twenties, and I began formulating and marketing whole-food nutritional supplements, functional foods, and personal care products. In my personal life, I met a beautiful princess named Nicki, whom I married in 1999. After overcoming a two-and-a-half-year stint of infertility, we became the proud parents of Joshua Michael in May 2004.

Today, at the age of thirty-two, I know what my purpose and burning desire is in life: to share my message of health and hope as well as my improbable comeback story. It's a message that I've communicated in the *New York Times* best seller *The Maker's Diet*, as well as seventeen other books, which have prompted dozens of appearances on national TV and radio programs and features in major newspapers and magazines. I'm humbled that I've shared my heart before millions of viewers and tens of thousands at major conferences throughout the United States and Canada as well as in Australia, New Zealand, Malaysia, China, Indonesia, Singapore, South Africa, and the United Kingdom.

All along, my goal has been to impact the health of this world one life at a time, and today that message begins with you. If you are ready to change your diet, change your life, and change your world, now's the time to get started.

In our next chapter, we'll talk about how the expansion of American waistlines foreshadows all sorts of health challenges today and for the next generation. If you'll pardon my pun, there's a heavy demand among millions of Americans eager to reach their perfect weight, but before we get into the meat of *Perfect Weight Canada*, an introduction is in order.

Introducing Bernard Bulwer, MD

Note from Jordan Rubin: A couple of years ago, I received an e-mail from Dr. Bernard Bulwer, who said he watched several episodes of my half-hour health show on cable TV and liked what I had to say about eating healthy and my prescription for living a long and abundant life. Dr. Bulwer felt we were kindred spirits since he had written a book, *Your Doctor Can't Make You Healthy*, that contained his insights into protecting your health. Dr. Bulwer's book echoed many of the same points I was making.

I soon learned that Dr. Bulwer is a modest man because I practically had to drag out the information that he was an advanced clinical fellow in noninvasive cardiology (echocardiography) at one of the premier teaching hospitals at Harvard Medical School—the Brigham and Women's Hospital. We stayed in contact. After I traveled to Toledo to launch the Healthy Toledo initiative and began putting legs and feet to the Perfect Weight Canada campaign, I felt I needed a medical expert overlooking my shoulder. I wanted to make sure that this book, *Perfect Weight Canada*, was medically sound, which is why I asked Dr. Bulwer to review the manuscript and make pertinent observations throughout the book. I also want readers to get to know Dr. Bulwer, so I've asked him to share a little bit about his background.

I'm from Belize, Central America, a country half the size of Nova Scotia, with less than 300,000 inhabitants and English as its official language. My family was large, even by Belize's standards. My parents had twelve children—and no twins! Though my father and mother never went beyond a basic primary school education, they were exceedingly knowledgeable and intelligent, and they saw eight of their children through to foreign universities across the United States, Europe, Australia, and the Caribbean.

My parents were not "rich" by any stretch of the imagination, but the true wealth they invested in us were those precious things that money can't buy. They taught us the value of hard work, respect for others, and commitment to family. Mom ran a popular restaurant in the neighbourhood, and Dad loved farming, but he was best known for the elegant mahogany furniture he built. My father worked hard; two things he despised were laziness and idleness. "The devil finds work for idle hands" was one lesson I learned very early. Today I can say with certainty, and with much gratitude, that these and other lessons have served me well. Included among them is how much I know about food and farming.

Talk about exotic tropical fruits! We didn't have to be coaxed into eating five daily servings of fresh fruit in Belize. Those who've been fortunate enough to experience the tastes and the varieties of our mangoes would know exactly what I mean. If ever a Belize mango could, it would sue an "American mango" for defamation. The call to eat five mangoes in one sitting was normal behaviour—indeed too restrictive. So tempting—in both smell and taste—was the local fruit that for many neighbours, the most horrible thing about having fruits in season was that the neighbourhood children would not leave their fruit trees alone.

I graduated from high school at age fifteen and pursued premed in zoology, chemistry, and physics, before winning a scholarship to medical school at the regional University of the West Indies in Jamaica and Trinidad. I earned my MD at the age of twenty-four with distinctions in the anatomical and surgical sciences, but I had little desire to spend much of my medical life confined to an operating theatre.

Postgraduate studies took me to the University of London at King's College, where I completed a master's degree in nutrition. Specialty training fellowship in diabetes and metabolic medicine (preventive cardiology) in England followed. I had a passionate desire to impart what I learned, so I packed my bags and returned to Belize, where I started the local diabetes association. There, I began educating and empowering the public on how to look after their health. Having served as clinical director of an ambulatory care facility, including being the physician designate for the United States Embassy, I began writing my first book. My activities caught the attention of Dr. David Singer, a visiting physician from Harvard University in Boston, Massachusetts, and I was soon invited to pursue fellowship training in cardiovascular disease.

I finished my U.S. medical licensing exams within months and completed fellowship training in preventive cardiology and later noninvasive cardiology/echocardiography at the Brigham and Women's Hospital, a major teaching hospital of Harvard Medical School in Boston. During this period, I published my first book, *Your Doctor Can't Make You Healthy*—a reflection of my desire to inform readers that their health and health care are two very different things.

The explosion of lifestyle-inflicted diseases that now stalk North America will not be solved through magical "cures," our preoccupation with prescription drugs, or hospital-based care. Obesity does not respect any borders. Today, people in countries like Belize, and indeed throughout the world, have been seduced into forsaking their traditional organically grown produce in favour of "up market" processed foods. This development has not only upped their waistlines, but it has also upped their medical bills.

Though I am heavily involved in writing medical textbooks and multimedia teaching tools for medical students and doctors for upcoming cutting-edge technologies like ultrasound stethoscope, such cool tools are not the answer to the obesity and heart disease pandemic. The best answers will come when people take more responsibility and better care of their own health.

I made contact with Jordan because he was on the front lines *doing* something—even baring his life's experience and transforming his convictions into what I believe is a pivotal message. This affects people where they live—something that is not the priority at our academic ivory towers. Jordan is doing his part. I hope to do mine, and I sincerely hope you do, too. Your health is your biggest investment.

Chapter 1

Globesity

IN GREEK MYTHOLOGY, Atlas was commonly depicted with a great globe on his shoulders, like some overambitious shot-putter, holding up the world in an agonized asymmetrical position.

If Atlas were holding up the earth today, he'd better truss his loins to lift all of the overweight people inhabiting the planet. For what surely must be a first in the annals of recorded history, demographers have determined that there are more overweight people living among us than those who are undernourished. According to the World Health Organization, one billion adults are overweight (of which 300 million are obese), meaning they weigh at least 50 pounds more than their ideal body weight. At the other end of the spectrum, the number of rail-thin starving and undernourished individuals remains steady at 600 million.[1]

For thousands of years, our forebears eked out an existence that depended upon the sweat of their brows and whether or not nature provided bountiful crops at harvest time. Hunger was their constant companion; famine, their frequent worry. I can't imagine what went through the minds of desperate parents who held their starving, frightened children to their breasts and wondered what they could do to provide something to eat.

The miracle of modernization has taken care of much of that problem, although as someone who supports the relief efforts of Life Outreach and Compassion International, I'm aware that far too many fall asleep each night with gnawing hunger pangs in their growling stomachs. If the World Health Organization's figures are correct, at least one-sixth of the global population has a different dilemma—they're too big from engorging themselves with greasy, high-fat, low-nutrient, chemical-laced, mass-produced foods. The global growth of industry and technology has led to an abundance of cheap, high-caloric meals, unhealthy sugary snacks, and a steep decrease in physical activity, resulting in one of the most blatantly visible, yet most neglected, public health problems in the history of mankind.

The skyrocketing ascent of obesity in both developed and developing regions inspired the World Health Organization to coin a new phrase for this occurrence: *globesity*. A nutritional expert for the World Bank warned that if corrective measures aren't taken soon, globesity could become as devastating as malnutrition, especially to the economies of the poorest countries. In other words, the global obesity epidemic could become more harmful to the world community than starvation.[2]

What an astonishing turn of events! I can remember Mom reminding me to clean my plate because of the "starving children in China," but she would have to amend her example if she were raising me today. Ten percent of city-dwelling Chinese children suffer from obesity—a number that's increasing by a shocking 8 percent per year. In Japan, obesity in nine-year-olds has tripled. Twenty percent of Australian adolescents and children are overweight or obese.[3] "The prevalence of obesity in Europe has tripled in the past two decades; half of all adults and 20 percent of all children are overweight," according to an article by the Associated Press.[4]

That's just the tip of a massive iceberg that's threatening to sink the health of young and old from Anchorage, Alaska, to Zurich, Switzerland. The tentacles of globesity reach into every continent and grip every major city in the world. We're seeing hundreds and hundreds of millions consume Western-like convenience foods, shift away from physically demanding jobs in agriculture, and devote their growing leisure time to watching TV and surfing the Internet. They're adopting this new lifestyle rather rapidly, unaware that they are putting themselves at risk for chronic diseases that could shave years off of their lives. My colleague Dr. Bulwer says that fast food is everywhere in Belize, where eating "well" means eating like the Americans or the British—the greasy fried foods they see advertised on television.

Another telling example comes from the Japanese, who, after centuries of staying slim on a diet of fish, vegetables, seaweed, fermented soy, and rice, have developed a strong taste for American fast food. When the Japanese McDonald's introduced the Mega Mac—a four-patty burger—they sold 1.7 million in four days. The fascination with Yankee junk food is so widespread that the Japanese have coined a phrase—which translates to "in your face food"—to describe their apparent desire to escape the stresses of a pressure-packed society by satiating their stomachs with glazed doughnuts and quadruple-stacked hamburgers.[5]

The Japanese still have a long way to go before they catch up with Americans, though. Like an Olympic flag bearer, the American contingent is leading the globesity parade. Not only are we—speaking for my country—the fattest nation on Earth, but we're also ballooning to extremely obese proportions at an alarming rate. A staggering two-thirds of American adults aged twenty years and older are over weight (which is defined as having a body mass index or BMI of 25 or higher), while the number of those who are extremely obese—at least 100 pounds—overweight has *quadrupled* since the 1980s. Twenty years ago, one in two hundred adults were candidates to purchase two seats when booking a flight on Air Canada; today that number is one in fifty.[6]

The Canadian obesity statistics are better than what's coming out of America, but not by much. The disquieting trend is that the percentage of Canadians who are overweight or obese has risen dramatically in recent years. Just over 59 percent of adult Canadians are overweight, while nearly one-quarter (23.1 percent) of adults aged eighteen or over obese (compared to 33 percent in the United States), according to Statistics Canada's most recent Canadian Community Health Survey.[7]

South of the border, the alarm is being sounded. If people keep gaining weight at the current pace, U.S. researchers at Johns Hopkins University predict that 75 percent of U.S. adults will be overweight (and 41 percent obese) by 2015, which is just around the corner. "Obesity is a public health crisis," declared Dr. Youfa Wang, who led the study.[8]

Heavy Demand

I haven't met a heavyset person in the United States or Canada who wouldn't *want* to lose weight, but from my vantage point, many obese individuals harbour attitudes similar to the classic "five stages of grief," as articulated by Elisabeth Kübler-Ross in her seminal book *On Death and Dying*.[9] The five stages are:

1. Denial
2. Anger
3. Bargaining
4. Depression
5. Acceptance

I'm willing to wager that if you're battling your weight, you could place yourself among one of those five descriptions. You could be denying that you're *really* overweight, that all you have to do is set your mind one day to taking off those "extra" pounds on your waist and hips. You could be angry about your lacklustre physical condition and appearance, harbouring resentment that you've always been heavy or were born into a family that fed you crummy foods growing up. You could be at the bargaining stage where you'd do anything to lose weight—like undergo expensive gastric bypass surgery or take a pharmaceutical with dangerous and embarrassing side effects. You could be depressed and feel like you have no future and no hope of reaching your perfect weight. Or you could be at the final and most dangerous stage—acceptance, a feeling that you'll always be obese and there's nothing you can do about it.

I'm seeing more evidence that being overweight is a societal norm among the cultural elite. Weight and body image issues are squeezing into U.S. college course catalogues as "fat studies" emerge into a growing interdisciplinary field. At Harvard University, students can sign up for "Body Sculpting in America," which examines the social and political consequences of being overweight. The University of Wisconsin at Milwaukee offers a course called "The Social Construction of Obesity," which is taught by a human movement sciences professor who challenges the alarmist message about the obesity epidemic in America. I've yet to hear about "fat classes" in Canadian colleges, but I'm sure they're coming.

The big deal on U.S. campuses is groups that focus on promoting "fat acceptance." A San Diego State University graduate student cofounded Size Matters to fight the prevailing attitude that being fat is a moral failure rather than the result of complicated factors. The goal is to get members comfortable with saying, "I'm fat," with a sense of defiance and pride.[10]

I'm all for feeling good about yourself, but a sizable weight-loss industry has stepped into the vacuum on both sides of the border. Figures are hard to come by in Canada, but the U.S. weight-loss and diet control market was expected to swell to $58 billion in 2007, according to Marketdata Enterprises, with various options vying for attention:[11]

- Gastric bypass surgery, in which surgeons staple or bind the stomach with an adjustable band. Fewer than a dozen clinics do bariatric surgery in Canada, and most have long waiting lists for a complicated surgical procedure that creates a small pouch able to hold only a few ounces of food. The situation is different in the States, where gastric bypass surgery is becoming as common as a root canal. Celebrities like singer Carnie Wilson, reality show star Sharon Osbourne, and talk show host Star Jones Reynolds have sung the praises of this potentially dangerous surgery after shedding hundreds of pounds. *American Idol* judge Randy Jackson, who has advised less-than-svelte contestants that they might want to lose some weight, underwent gastric bypass surgery in 2003.[12]

- Commercial chains such as Weight Watchers, Jenny Craig, and Nutri-System, where dieters commit to "customized" diet plans. These structured programs often include "phone meetings" with a trained consultant as well as the consumption of diet meals purchased directly from the company.

- Over-the-counter diet pills such as Xenadrine EFA, CortiSlim, One-A-Day WeightSmart, and TrimSpa are easily available in Canada and are advertised on television and radio and in alluring ads in supermarket tabloids. They target the lose-weight-quick crowd with breathtaking copy describing how their "miracle ingredients" and "breakthrough formulas" are "clinically proven" and "guaranteed to work." Anna Nicole Smith, before her untimely death, was a TrimSpa endorser who claimed that she was "hotter than ever" after "just twelve weeks" of taking the diet pill.[13]

- Diet food home delivery, where affluent dieters pay as much as $1,200 a month (per person!) for healthy meals to be delivered daily to their doorstep. A handful of companies such as The Zone, Atkins, CarbControl, and Healthy Living have twenty-eight-day menu cycles available in Toronto, Vancouver, and Calgary.

- Weight-loss summer camps for heavy teens, which are a predictable outgrowth of the childhood obesity problem in this country. These types of camps didn't exist in my parents' time because the demand wasn't there. Today, teens seek to turn their lives around at places like Active Challenge, a weight-loss camp located at Bear Creek Outdoor Centre outside of Ottawa.

Adults don't have summer camps, although there are a number of discreet but expensive "fitness spas" that you can check yourself into if you have the time and the *dinero*. In the world of weight loss, anything is possible if you have the money and the opportunity.

Need a Cushy Seat for the Tush?

Talk about a growing market with room for expansion.

A host of entrepreneurial companies are marketing products promising to make life comfy and cushy for overweight people. WideBodies Furniture sells oversized sofas, love seats, and chairs. LiftChair .com has introduced recliner chairs that lift and tilt forward so that morbidly obese people weighing as much as 700 pounds can get in and out of them more easily. For those who need a different type of seating, the Big John toilet seat is a full 5 inches (12.5 centimetres) wider than the standard 14-inch-wide (35.5 centimetres) version—and more receptive to an oversized tush.

Consumer research has helped huge corporations like GM Canada and Ford of Canada, which have assembly plants in Ontario, tailor their products for the growing numbers of overweight people in North America. The automakers have quietly widened seats in their SUVs and light pickup trucks so that heavyset drivers will have "plenty of leg room." You can scroll through Sizewise.com to determine which cars provide the most interior room, but some obese drivers have to take their cars into auto upholstery shops to have seatbelt extenders installed. Those who can't squeeze in behind the wheel have smaller steering wheels mounted at body shops.

Businesses are feeling the weight of heavier customers and employees. Since wide-body jets are carrying a lot of wide bodies these days, the U.S. Federal Aviation Administration recently increased its "rule-of-thumb" advisory for calculating the weight of passengers. The airlines now expect male passengers to weigh 184 pounds (a 9-pound increase) and female passengers to weigh 163 pounds (a whopping 18-pound increase).[14] This means the airline industry must top off the tanks with an extra 350 million gallons of jet fuel annually to compensate for the increased "payload."[15] At a cost of $2 per gallon, that's a $700 million hit to passengers, who must pony up the extra cash to fly. This extra fuel usage not only hurts our economy but our environment as well.

Hospitals, no doubt seeing more obese patients since overweight people are hospitalized more often than the general population,[16] have installed patient hoists in certain rooms. They need the hoists on hand since orderlies cannot lift such large amounts of weight in and out of hospital beds without landing in the hospital themselves—with a hernia.

Before There Were Couch Potatoes

You could say that we haven't been at our perfect weight for a long time. If I had to pick a date, I would say things started going downhill after 1950. Television, which had been invented, wasn't commonplace, and the term "couch potato" wasn't part of the lexicon. Neither were *Hockey Night in Canada* and Don Cherry. Fast-forward more than a half-century, and televised sports has exploded, changing Canada and America from nations of doers to nations of *watchers*.

In my country, football is merely the top dog among a pack of televised sports barking for attention. The others are baseball, basketball, hockey, golf, auto racing, tennis, soccer, and even poker, which is considered a sport by some. Extreme sports like the X Games and Nathan's Famous Hot Dog Eating Contest also compete for eyeballs in a 500-station universe. Women have plenty of shows to keep them occupied as well: *Oprah*, *Rachael Ray*, and Lifetime movies, to name a few.

The U.S. government didn't start keeping records of how much Americans weighed until 1960, when the first National Health and Nutrition Examination Survey was completed. From that baseline, the National Center for Health Statistics says that adult men and women are roughly an inch taller than they were nearly fifty years ago but nearly 25 pounds heavier on average. The average BMI among adults has increased from 25 to 28.[17]

Meanwhile, the average weight for U.S. men aged twenty to seventy-four years rose dramatically from 166.3 pounds in 1960 to 191 pounds in 2002, while the average weight for women the same age increased from 140.2 pounds in 1960 to 164.3 pounds in 2002. Though the average weight for men aged twenty to thirty-nine years increased by nearly 20 pounds over the last four decades, the increase was greater among older men:[18]

- Men between the ages of forty and forty-nine were nearly 27 pounds heavier on average in 2002 compared with 1960.
- Men between the ages of fifty and fifty-nine were nearly 28 pounds heavier on average in 2002 compared with 1960.
- Men between the ages of sixty and seventy-four were almost 33 pounds heavier on average in 2002 compared with 1960.

For U.S. women, a similar trend occurred:[19]

- Women aged twenty to twenty-nine were nearly 29 pounds heavier on average in 2002 compared with 1960.
- Women aged forty to forty-nine were about 25.5 pounds heavier on average in 2002 compared with 1960.
- Women aged sixty to seventy-four were about 17.5 pounds heavier on average in 2002 compared with 1960.

Meanwhile, the report documented that average weights for children are also increasing:[20]

- The average weight for a ten-year-old boy in 1963 was 74 pounds; by 2002 the average weight was nearly 85 pounds.
- The average weight for a ten-year-old girl in 1963 was 77 pounds; by 2002 the average weight was nearly 88 pounds.
- A fifteen-year-old boy weighed 135.5 pounds on average in 1966; by 2002 the average weight of a boy that age increased to 150.3 pounds.
- A fifteen-year-old girl weighed 124.2 pounds on average in 1966; by 2002 the average weight for a girl that age was 134.4 pounds.

I know that was a ton of statistics to roll out, but the key point to remember is that overweight individuals, on the average, carry around 25 to 35 pounds of extra weight. The extra poundage taxes our health and portends all sorts of difficulties, some immediate, some long-ranging, and some permanent—like death.

"America's weight problem is rapidly overtaking cigarette smoking as the leading cause of preventable death," according to the U.S. Centers for Disease Control.[21] If you're 25 pounds too heavy, you're three times more likely to develop coronary heart disease, two to six times more likely to develop high blood pressure, and three times as likely to get type 2 diabetes. Heavier people are also at higher risk for developing arthritis, gout, gallbladder disease and the Big C—cancer. (See sidebar on the next page.)

The health risks associated with obesity are formidable. Let's take a closer look from descriptions provided by the Cleveland Clinic physicians behind WebMD .com.[22]

Heart disease and stroke

Heart disease and stroke are the leading causes of death and disability for people in the United States. (Cancer and heart disease are by far the leading causes of death in Canada, according to Statistics Canada.[23]) Overweight people are more likely to have high blood pressure, a major risk factor for heart disease and stroke, than people who are not overweight. High blood levels of LDL or "bad" cholesterol can also lead to heart disease and often are linked to being overweight. Being overweight also contributes to angina (chest pain caused by poor blood flow to the heart) and sudden death from heart attack or stroke without any prior warning signs or symptoms.

Diabetes

Type 2 diabetes reduces your body's ability to control blood sugar. It is a major cause of early death, heart disease, stroke, and blindness. Overweight people are twice as likely to develop type 2 diabetes compared to normal-weight people.

Cancer

Several types of cancer are associated with being overweight. In women, these include cancer of the uterus, gallbladder, cervix, ovary, breast, and colon. Overweight men are at higher risk for developing colorectal cancer and prostate cancer.

Gallbladder and liver disease

Gallbladder disease and gallstones are more common if you are overweight. Your risk of disease increases as your weight increases. Most gallstones are cholesterol-rich. When the cholesterol level in bile (stored in the gallbladder) increases, so does the risk of cholesterol stones. Increased production and excretion of cholesterol by the liver into the bile occurs in obesity.

Osteoarthritis

Osteoarthritis is a common joint condition that most often affects the knees, hips, and lower back. Carrying extra pounds places extra pressure on these joints and wears away the cartilage (or tissue that cushions the joints) that normally protects them.

Gout

Gout, a disease that affects the joints, is often triggered by high levels of a substance called uric acid in the blood. Obesity causes higher uric acid levels. Uric acid crystals can precipitate in the joints, causing severe joint pain, as well as in the kidney, causing kidney stones and chronic kidney disease.

Sleep apnea

Sleep apnea is a serious breathing condition associated with being overweight. Sleep apnea can cause a person to snore heavily and to stop breathing for short periods during sleep. Sleep apnea may cause daytime sleepiness and even heart failure.

Cancer and Being Overweight by Bernard Bulwer, MD

We all know that excess pounds raise the risk of heart disease, hypertension, diabetes, stroke, arthritis, and gallbladder disease, but few fixate on the relationship between obesity and cancer. According to the American Cancer Society, obesity is linked to cancer of the colon and rectum, esophagus, stomach, pancreas, liver, kidney, as well as multiple myeloma and non-Hodgkin's lymphoma.[24] These are mainly cancers of the gastrointestinal system, a reflection of what goes into our mouths. In women, obesity increases the risk of death from breast, uterus, cervical, and ovarian cancer. Obese men are at increased risk from prostate cancer. Note that obesity increases the risk of cancers that tend to target our reproductive organs.

Normally, our bodies repair themselves in an orderly fashion, with cell repair and replacement carefully monitored by in-built checks and balances. Excess body fat or adipose tissue, however, is more than just fat that sits idle; it is a major source of harm and mischief. Body fat is a major producer of the female hormone called estrogen. It also obstructs or interferes with the action of insulin—the major hormone regulator of how our bodies handle the food we eat. This spells double jeopardy because your body is suffering at least twice for the same offence. Higher levels of insulin and estrogen, which encourages cell proliferation, may be a time bomb. Unregulated cell growth is the cardinal feature of cancer, with abnormal precancerous or cancerous cells mushrooming into growth that we call tumours or cancer.

Cancer cells have two things in common: (1) they may grow uncontrollably, causing damage where they originate; and (2) worse still, they have the ability to metastasize, or spread to other parts of the body. For example, breast, bowel, or kidney cancer may more likely cause death from being spread to the brain rather than the original cancer itself.

Since cancer, by definition, occurs when damaged or abnormal cells assault the body, researchers have determined that some factors *inhibit* or *promote* the growth of cancer in the body. Examples of *inhibitors* would be nutrients found in fruits and vegetables, as well as properly raised meats and wild-caught fish. Drinking plenty of water allows the kidneys and liver to operate at full capacity and flush waste and toxins out of the body's digestive and urinary tracts, which is where cancer cells tend to congregate.

On the other hand, examples of *promoters* would be smoking cigarettes, eating highly refined high-sugar foods, feasting on fried foods rich in trans-fatty acids, or coming into contact with cancer-causing substances, also known as carcinogens. Tobacco smoke, pesticides, air pollution, and industrial chemicals (such as asbestos) can trigger the initiation of cancer, which can take years to develop into a mass and many more years to detect. This is all the more reason to adopt the principles of *Perfect Weight Canada*.

While environmental elements behind cancer are significant, at the end of the day, lifestyle factors are the main causes of cancer. While genetics and family history do play a role (between 5 and 10 percent of all cancers are clearly hereditary), the choices in the food we eat, the amount of time we exercise, the hygiene we practice, the stress we undergo, and the otherwise imbalanced lives we lead account for about 65 percent of cancer deaths in the United States, according to researchers at the Harvard School of Public Health.[25]

Since cancer is the leading cause of death in Canada, accounting for 27.2 percent of all deaths, lifestyle factors certainly count in your country as well.[26]

Whether it's one of the big three—cancer, cardiovascular disease, or diabetes—shuffling through life above your perfect weight *will* cut years off your life. A team of University of Illinois researchers recently stated that rising obesity rates could reverse life expectancy gains, which would be the first time this has happened since the U.S. government began keeping track of life expectancy in 1900. Obesity significantly increases the risk of premature death; among the severely obese, life expectancy is reduced by an estimated five to twenty years, according to one government study.[27]

Obesity is shrinking life expectancy expectations in Canada as well. More and more Canadian children are overweight—one in four are categorized as being overweight or obese. For the first time, the country's younger generations are expected to live shorter lives than their parents, according to a House of Commons committee report released in 2007.

Life expectancy in Canada recently surpassed eighty years for the first time, according to Statistics Canada, now standing at 80.2 years, ranking among the top half-dozen countries in the world.[28] That all could change in North America. Here in the United States, life expectancy is at a high of 77.6 years, but according to a study published in the *New England Journal of Medicine*, that could mean—and I have to emphasize the conditional here—that the generation of my preschool-aged son, Joshua, could live two to five years less.[29] Current trends indicate that the prevalence of obesity will continue to rise and affect ever-younger age groups.

The good news is that you can *extend* your life by reaching and maintaining your perfect weight. Using data from a large federally funded assessment of obesity rates, the researchers calculated how much longer life expectancy would be if everyone who were currently obese were to lose enough weight to obtain an optimal body mass index of 24. Under such a scenario, the authors "conservatively estimated" that the average U.S. life expectancy of 77.6 would be extended by four to eleven months longer for white men, four to ten months longer for white women, four to thirteen months longer for black men, and three to nine months longer for black women.[30] I am sure similar ratios would prevail in Canada.

Putting aside life extension for a moment, achieving your perfect weight can begin to reverse the ravages of obesity *now*. These benefits in quality of life—less arthritis pain, lower blood pressure, improved diabetes control, or even reversal, coupled with less dependency on prescription drugs—can occur while you're on the journey toward your perfect weight.

Seven Truths to Think About

According to obesity specialist Gus Prosch Jr., MD, a physician who practiced in Birmingham, Alabama, until his death in 2005, there are seven truths about obesity.[31] Think about each declaration for a moment before moving on to the next one:

1. If you're obese, you have a lifetime disease.
2. Your metabolic processes will always tend to be abnormal.
3. You cannot eat what others eat and stay thin.
4. Anyone can lose weight and stay slim provided the causes of weight gain are determined, addressed, and corrected.
5. Understanding insulin metabolism is the key to losing weight intelligently.
6. There is absolutely no physiological requirement for sugar or processed foods in your diet.
7. You must address all the contributing factors causing obesity.

You cannot lose weight and keep it off successfully by strictly and solely following any special diet, by taking a weight-loss pill, or by following an exercise program. In order to succeed in the fight against obesity, you must realize that losing weight must involve a major lifestyle change.

Taking Inventory

Most people don't have to guess whether they are at their perfect weight. A glance into a full-length mirror without clothes on usually provides enough evidence that they're not going through life at a healthy weight. At the same time, it's helpful to know your body mass index (BMI), the size of your body frame, and what percentage of body fat you're carrying so that you can soberly face the music.

Let's first examine the BMI, a fitness-scale method that has become the measurement of choice for physicians and researchers who study obesity, although the results have to be interpreted with some caution, as I'll explain shortly. The BMI uses a mathematical formula that takes into account a person's height and weight. As a strict formula, the body mass index equals a person's weight in kilograms divided by height in metres squared. For those of you keeping score at home, that's $BMI=kg/m^2$.

You may be saying to yourself, "I haven't done any equations since tenth grade trigonometry." Have no fear. On page 26 is a converted body mass index chart using inches and pounds. Just find your height in the left-hand column, and then swish your finger over to your weight. The column above your weight (a number between 19 and 40) is your BMI.

The BMI breakdown goes like this:

BODY MASS INDEX FOR ADULTS TABLE

	NORMAL						OVERWEIGHT					OBESE									
BMI	19	20	21	22	23	24	25	26	27	28	29	30	31	32	33	34	35	36	37	38	39
HEIGHT (INCHES)	BODY WEIGHT (POUNDS)																				
58	91	96	100	105	110	115	119	124	129	134	138	143	148	153	158	162	167	172	177	181	186
59	94	99	104	109	114	119	124	128	133	138	143	148	153	158	163	168	173	178	183	188	193
60	97	102	107	112	118	123	128	133	138	143	148	153	158	163	168	174	179	184	189	194	199
61	100	106	111	116	122	127	132	137	143	148	153	158	164	169	174	180	185	190	195	201	206
62	104	109	115	120	126	131	136	142	147	153	158	164	169	175	180	186	191	196	202	207	213
63	107	113	118	124	130	135	141	146	152	158	163	169	175	180	186	191	197	203	208	214	220
64	110	116	122	128	134	140	145	151	157	163	169	174	180	186	192	197	204	209	215	221	227
65	114	120	126	132	138	144	150	156	162	168	174	180	186	192	198	204	210	216	222	228	234
66	118	124	130	136	142	148	155	161	167	173	179	186	192	198	204	210	216	223	229	235	241
67	121	127	134	140	146	153	159	166	172	178	185	191	198	204	211	217	223	230	236	242	249
68	125	131	138	144	151	158	164	171	177	184	190	197	203	210	216	223	230	236	243	249	256
69	128	135	142	149	155	162	169	176	182	189	196	203	209	216	223	230	236	243	250	257	263
70	132	139	146	153	160	167	174	181	188	195	202	209	216	222	229	236	243	250	257	264	271
71	136	143	150	157	165	172	179	186	193	200	208	215	222	229	236	243	250	257	265	272	279
72	140	147	154	162	169	177	184	191	199	206	213	221	228	235	242	250	258	265	272	279	287
73	144	151	159	166	174	182	189	197	204	212	219	227	235	242	250	257	265	272	280	288	295
74	148	155	163	171	179	186	194	202	210	218	225	233	241	249	256	264	272	280	287	295	303
75	152	160	168	176	184	192	200	208	216	224	232	240	248	256	264	272	279	287	295	303	311
76	156	164	172	180	189	197	205	213	221	230	238	246	254	262	271	279	287	295	304	312	320

EXTREME OBESITY

BMI	40	41	42	43	44	45	46	47	48	49	50	51	52	53	54
HEIGHT (INCHES)	BODY WEIGHT (POUNDS)														
58	191	196	201	205	210	215	220	224	229	234	239	244	248	253	258
59	198	203	208	212	217	222	227	232	237	242	247	252	257	262	267
60	204	209	215	220	225	230	235	240	245	250	255	261	266	271	276
61	211	217	222	227	232	238	243	248	254	259	264	269	275	280	285
62	218	224	229	235	240	246	251	256	262	267	273	278	284	289	295
63	225	231	237	242	248	254	259	265	270	278	282	287	293	299	304
64	232	238	244	250	256	262	267	273	279	285	291	296	302	308	314
65	240	246	252	258	264	270	276	282	288	294	300	306	312	318	324
66	247	253	260	266	272	278	284	291	297	303	309	315	322	328	334
67	255	261	268	274	280	287	293	299	306	312	319	325	331	338	344
68	262	269	276	282	289	295	302	308	315	322	328	335	341	348	354
69	270	277	284	291	297	304	311	318	324	331	338	345	351	358	365
70	278	285	292	299	306	313	320	327	334	341	348	355	362	369	376
71	286	293	301	308	315	322	329	338	343	351	358	365	372	379	386
72	294	302	309	316	324	331	338	346	353	361	368	375	383	390	397
73	302	310	318	325	333	340	348	355	363	371	378	386	393	401	408
74	311	319	326	334	342	350	358	365	373	381	389	396	404	412	420
75	319	327	335	343	351	359	367	375	383	391	399	407	415	423	431
76	328	336	344	353	361	369	377	385	394	402	410	418	426	435	443

BMI Categories

- Underweight = < 18.5
- Normal weight = 18.5–24.9
- Overweight = 25–29.9
- Obesity = BMI of 30 or greater

Courtesy of National Heart, Lung, and Blood Institute, National Institutes of Health

- 18 or lower: underweight
- 19–24: normal
- 25–29: overweight
- 30–39: obese
- 40–54: extremely or morbidly obese

Nearly one-quarter of Canadian adults fall into the obese category. This number does not vary greatly by province. The obesity rate for men was higher in Newfoundland and Labrador, and Manitoba. The obesity rate for women surpassed the national average in Newfoundland and Labrador, Nova Scotia, and Saskatchewan.[32]

As I hinted at previously, the BMI is not a perfect measurement of where you stand with your weight. I offer myself as an example. I stand a little more than 72 inches tall (that's 6 feet) and weigh 184 pounds. My finger finds number 72 in the left-hand column, slides over to the 184 box, and that tells me I have a BMI of 25.

So am I a tad pudgy with a BMI of 25, which, according to the BMI scale, is borderline overweight? No, because I perform FIT—Functional Interval Training exercises. (You'll learn about this breakthrough exercise program in chapter 9, "Get FIT for Your Perfect Weight.")

I think you also have to weigh—pardon the pun—the BMI against your body frame size. Some folks are slight of stature; others are flat-out larger than others. Dr. Bulwer says this is the major fault of the BMI. You can have skinny legs and an obese abdomen and still have a normal BMI. On the other hand, a BMI of 25 or 26 ranks you as "overweight" just because you're pear-shaped. This, in itself, is not an unhealthy condition.

The simplest—but least accurate—method to calculate your frame size is to grab your wrist with the other hand and try to touch your thumb and index finger where the wrist meets the hand. If your fingers do not touch, you're a big-boned person with a large body frame. If your thumb and index finger just meet, you have a medium frame. If they overlap, you have a small frame.

What a Waist!

Did you know that the circumference of your waist, not your overall weight, is one of the leading indicators of mortality related to being overweight? For women, a generally recommended waist size is 32½ inches (about 83 centimetres)—with an increased risk of health consequences occurring when the waist size exceeds 35 inches (88 centimetres). For men, a generally recommended waist size is 35 inches—with dangerous health consequences increasing when 40 inches (102 centimetres) is reached and exceeded.

Canadians are short on waist-size knowledge: a recent poll found that fewer than 25 percent of Canadians could identify the danger zones for men, and fewer than 10 percent knew the cut-off point for women, according to the Canadian Obesity Network.[33]

Whether you have a large-, medium-, or small-sized frame, the fact of the matter is that you may have to lose less weight to reach your perfect weight, and that's a good thing. Or you may have to lose more than you thought, based on our next criteria—body fat.

Body Fat Distribution

It's helpful to know how much body fat your torso contains because new research is showing that your body fat—not just your body weight or BMI—is a better indicator of how healthy you are. This has generated new terms like apple- or pear-shaped obesity, or scientific terms like the metabolic syndrome or the insulin resistance syndrome. The different terms arose from different ways of measuring or describing mainly the same issue.

We all need some fat on our bodies since fat regulates body temperature, cushions and insulates our organs and tissues, and is the main form of the body's energy storage. However, there is a problem when there is extra fat stored in the body, which translates into extra weight and causes the heart to work harder.

Fat circulates in your blood, and if you were to take a vial of blood and let it sit in a corner, a fatty layer would rise to the top. The difference between what makes you fat or thin is not the amount of fat cells but the size of those cells. The fat globules within each cell increase as you store more fat. Muscles work the same way; you don't make more muscle cells—the muscle cells get larger when you exercise.

Much of the fat absorbed via the intestines gets stored in the *omentum*, which is a fatty apron or curtain that hangs from your stomach. The omentum stores fat that's quickly accessible to the liver but causes bad cholesterol and triglyceride levels to rise. It also takes insulin out of circulation, causing your blood sugar to rise. The more omentum fat present, the more abdominal obesity, high blood pressure, high cholesterol, and other risks associated with coronary artery disease.

Most fitness clubs have skinfold calipers that give a snapshot measurement of body fat by measuring a pinch of skin in several strategic areas of your body:

- Triceps (back of the upper arm)
- Chest (between the arm line and nipple)
- Subscapula (below the edge of the shoulder blade on the back)
- Waist (slight to the right of the navel)
- Suprailium (over the hip bone)
- Thigh (halfway between the hip and knee joints)

At least two measurements should be taken at each site to gain an accurate reading, and some measurements will vary depending upon your sex. If you don't belong to a fitness club, you can go online at find any number of body fat tests that you can take at home. You'll need a cloth tape measure to measure the circumference of your waist, hips, forearm, and wrist.

Once you have a number, compare it to the list below prepared by the American Council on Exercise, which has categorized ranges of body fat percentages as follows:

BODY FAT PERCENTAGE		
DESCRIPTION	WOMEN	MEN
Essential fat	12–15%	2–5%
Athletes	16–20%	6–13%
Fitness	21–24%	14–17%
Acceptable	25–31%	18–25%
Obese	32%+	25%+

Subcutaneous fat vs. visceral fat

If you're reading *Perfect Weight Canada* because you want to do something about the flabby tire around your midsection, then reaching your perfect weight means targeting the two kinds of fat in your body: subcutaneous fat and visceral fat.

Much of the fat we see in others and ourselves is subcutaneous fat—that jelly-like layer of fat found underneath the skin that gives people their pudgy look and men their famous beer bellies. Gender plays a major role in determining where your body stores subcutaneous fat: for most men, it's their bellies; for women, it's the hips and thighs.

Visceral fat, on the other hand, is found deep inside your body in the abdominal cavity, not just under your skin like subcutaneous fat. This type of fat may even infiltrate the internal organs, which contributes to a wide range of health complications. Visceral fat carries a reputation in the medical community as a "killer fat." The pesky cellulite padding your thighs won't lead to your demise; it's what lies beneath —the visceral fat, which is also known as white adipose tissue.

Golfer Phil Mickelson, who's flabby midsection stands out in contrast to flat bellies like Tiger Woods's and Mike Weir's, thinks he knows the difference between the two types of fat. "The one thing I wish was different about me was that I wish I had visceral fat instead of subcutaneous fat," he told one interviewer.[34]

Actually, Phil should be careful what he wishes for because this deeper, underlying fat, which clamps on vital organs like barnacles, is more likely to increase the risk for heart attacks than subcutaneous fat, according to researchers from Johns Hopkins Medical Institutions.[35] Visceral fat, or white adipose tissue, is also medically linked to various metabolic diseases like diabetes, and it may even present health risks for those who don't appear to have an ounce of fat on their bodies. Often invisible to the naked eye, visceral fat could be more dangerous than the "saddlebag" fat hanging on the frames of the overweight.

Dr. Jimmy Bell, a professor of molecular imaging at Imperial College in London, England, and his team scanned nearly eight hundred people with MRI machines to create "fat maps" showing where people store fat. The results were surprising: those who maintained their weight through diet rather than exercise were more likely to have major deposits of internal fat.[36]

Researchers at the Duke University Medical Center found that energetic exercise can significantly reduce your visceral fat. Lead author Dr. Cris Slentz said that the more people exercised, and the higher the intensity, the faster they lost their excess visceral fat.[37] Short, intense workouts, not low-impact walks through the neighbourhood or light steps on a treadmill, are foundational to my fitness plan described in chapter 9, "Get FIT for Your Perfect Weight." I've followed a program called Functional Interval Training (FIT), with a heavy emphasis on short spurts of intense exercise, followed by rest periods, that will burn both peripheral (subcutaneous) and visceral fat during and after your workout. As for those with the more noticeable subcutaneous fat, the Perfect Weight Canada dietary approach, with its emphasis on eating foods from organic sources and staying away from processed, high-sugar treats, will do something about the fat that everyone sees because of the reduction in caloric intake and the increase in fibre and nutrients.

Get on Board

The point of this discussion about the BMI, body frame size, and body fat is that no "perfect weight" can be applied across the board. God created everyone differently, and our bodies change shape as we grow older. While I don't think anyone can tell you what your perfect weight should be, the Pew Research Center reports that dieters say they are 29 pounds heavier than they would like to be.[38] If that number sounds like it's in your ballpark, then joining the Perfect Weight Canada campaign—and sticking to the program—will move you much closer to your perfect weight, help you feel much better about yourself, and even change the world around you.

I want to help you reach your perfect weight, but before embarking on any decision to get healthier and shed pounds, you should have a whole host of support around you. Begin with your health professional, especially if you have a family history of heart disease or other medical illnesses. Be sure to include your family as well as friends and co-workers who seek only the best for you. You do *not* need critics or negative people to be included in your network. They will only drag you down.

So how can we get to that perfect weight, Canada? In a nutshell, here are three guidelines for doing so—which are expanded on in the rest of this book:

1. Maximize food; minimize non-food

Losing weight is not necessarily eating less; it's about eating more intelligently—more of the "right" foods. Our bodies were designed with a biological instinct of how our bodies originally looked and functioned best. Knowledge and application of this knowledge is key to successful weight loss.

2. Maximize life; minimize life-drainers

Attaining and maintaining your perfect weight is individualized, even though it is important to include accountability and collaboration during this endeavour. You can't discuss weight issues without exploring the reasons why your individualized brain, hormones, and emotions may drive you to overeat. Take responsibility for your body—love it and then lose the weight—by yourself *or* with the help of others.

3. Maximize care; minimize carelessness

You need to understand how and why the body naturally stores fat—to protect itself in times when it needs to provide energy in the absence of food. The balance of nutrition and eating times and intervals, as well as types of foods, all figure into successful and sustained weight management.

Eating right (and frequently) with consistent functional integrative exercise is key to successful and sustained weight management. *Perfect Weight Canada* can work in ways that will teach your body to eat and work smart—resulting in "trimming the fat." Beginning in chapter 3, you will find out the foods you should be eating so that you can live a leaner and healthier life.

Attaining your perfect weight does not have to be a complicated, difficult, and starvation-like experience that becomes drudgery and causes you to lose hope instead of weight. You will learn that your diet and exercise program can be easily integrated into your life and be easily sustained. Your DNA is not necessarily your destiny in determining your weight and health. In fact, through diet and exercise, you can once and for all win the battle against chubbiness.

Before we get into specifics of the foods you should eat, the nutritional supplements you should take, and the sustainable lifestyle you should lead, we should talk about why many diets don't work, the often untold drawbacks of gastric bypass surgery, and how the media shapes our perceptions, which we'll do in our next chapter, "What Are You Failing For?"

Perfect Weight Recap: Globesity

- The percentage of Canadians who are overweight or obese has risen dramatically in recent years: 59 percent of adult Canadians are overweight, while nearly 23.1 percent of adults aged eighteen or over are obese.
- Many who have been overweight for years or decades exhibit attitudes mirroring the five stages of grief: denial, anger, bargaining, depression, and acceptance.
- Overweight individuals, on the average, carry around twenty-five to thirty-five pounds of extra weight. The extra poundage taxes our health and portends all sorts of difficulties, some immediate, some long-ranging, and some permanent—like death.
- Scientific researchers fear that rising obesity rates could mean that children born in this decade could see their expected life expectancy drop by two to five years.
- The body mass index (BMI) is the standard measurement for determining whether you're overweight or obese, but it's important to submit to other criteria such as body frame size and body fat.
- There are two types of fat in the body: subcutaneous fat and visceral fat. The fat you can't normally see—visceral fat—can actually be more dangerous to your health than the fat you can see around people's midsections—subcutaneous fat.

Chapter 2

What Are You Failing For?

STOP ME IF you've heard these clichés before.

- You have to eat a sensible diet and start exercising.
- Eat less and move more.
- Make healthy food choices and join a fitness club.

It's not difficult to decode most diet books. Many work on the principle of cutting 500 calories a day and burning another 500 on the treadmill. Keep that up for seven days, and the deficit of 7,000 calories results in the net loss of two pounds per week.

No one will argue with the admonition to get your buns moving, but simply cutting calories doesn't work for long. Continuous calorie restriction almost always backfires because your body thinks it's starving to death, so your brain sets off a chain of chemical processes, including the slowing down of the body's metabolic rate. A sluggish metabolism, however, allows the body to become *more* efficient at storing fat. When you stop eating rabbit food—or whatever the "special" diet calls for—and resume the consumption of your favourite edibles, your much slower and inefficient metabolism can't keep up. Bottom-line result: you gain the weight back even faster, even though you may be eating less than you were before you embarked on the diet.

"You can initially lose 5 to 10 percent of your weight on any number of diets, but then the weight comes back," said Traci Mann, a University of California at Los Angeles (UCLA) associate professor of psychology who analyzed thirty-one studies that followed people on diets for two to five years. In fact, said Ms. Mann, several studies found dieting was a consistent predictor of *future* weight gain. When asked what overweight people should do, Ms. Mann replied, "Eating in moderation is a good idea for everybody, and so is regular exercise."[1]

I disagree with this simplified, two-front approach, as you'll see in later chapters of *Perfect Weight Canada*. But since it is universally agreed that 95 percent of all diets fail,[2] which only keep overweight people in bondage and despair, what's the biggest reason why mainstream diets are so universally unsuccessful?

I think it's because dieters get too hungry.

The primal urge to open our mouths and receive sustenance is a survival instinct

32

that materializes from physiological and psychological needs. For example, when the clock says it's noon, many people salivate like Pavlov's dog and automatically become hungry. Hunger is also triggered by our senses, like the smell of frying potatoes or an alluring TV advertisement promoting a grilled chicken panini sandwich. Whatever the reason, the brain's thalamus in the limbic system—the seat of human motivation and emotions—converts the sensory information into a palatable craving. Depending on how hungry you become, that longing can range from "I think I'll snack on something" to "I'm hungry! I've got the munchies!" Very few can resist the siren call of food, glorious food, as Oliver Twist and his orphan colleagues sang.

No matter how hard you try to be "good," no matter how much you watch what you eat, satiating the appetite will overwhelm every instinct you have (except the will to live, of course). That's why simply slashing calories doesn't cut it and is doomed to failure. Physiologically speaking, hunger begins in the brain when the limbic system determines that the body is low in blood sugar, or glucose. Most of the food you eat is converted into glucose, much of which is converted by the liver into fat for later use. When glucose levels are low, the liver sends signals to the hypothalamus—the small but vital gland at the base of the brain below the thalamus—that blood sugar levels have dipped precipitously. The hypothalamus, in turn, triggers stomach contractions or hunger pangs, demanding a fill-up. When nothing happens, nasty growling noises ensue. The hunger cravings can drive you batty, making you feel light-heated and irritable. An oft-quoted proverb says it well: *The spirit is willing, but the flesh is weak.*

Scientists have known that the hypothalamus plays a key role in regulating food intake and body weight since the 1940s, but it's only been in recent years that they've discovered how a pair of "hunger hormones" secreted by the body—leptin and ghrelin—also reduce *or* spike hunger pangs. The hormone leptin, which is generated by fat cells, sends crucial signals to the brain's "satiety centre" to stop eating when the stomach is full, kind of like a yellow light at an intersection. The trouble is that many with weight problems have conditioned their bodies to ignore the internal cautionary reminder to stop grazing at the buffet table. With each additional bite, they speed past the intersection of appropriate satisfaction, which is the epicurean equivalent of running a red light—and just as foolhardy and dangerous.

As overweight people build up a resistance to the appetite-suppressing effects of leptin, levels of leptin continue to drop, which makes them even *hungrier*, says obesity expert Mary Dallman, PhD, from the University of California at San Francisco. This is another explanation for why many dieters eventually regain all the weight they lost.[3]

On the other hand, the hormone known as ghrelin *increases* appetite. Released primarily in the stomach, ghrelin level rises dramatically before you eat, then plays a leading role in determining how quickly hunger strikes back after noshing on a snack or meal. When your stomach feels empty, ghrelin levels spike again, which explains why you're ready to raid the refrigerator at midnight. Those who maintain a deprivation diet dial up the intensity of their hunger pangs, which prompts the body to secrete even *more* ghrelin. Any remaining willpower to "be good" melts in the face of such a hormonal onslaught.

All is not lost, however. Of the two hormones, leptin—the appetite suppressor—appears to be the bigger player in our bodies' energy balance. While one of leptin's duties is to inform the brain that the body has enough energy stores such as body fat, for some reason, many obese people don't respond to leptin's signals even though they have higher levels of leptin because they are desensitized or resistant to its effects. Those who need to lose the most weight are often the ones with the biggest appetites. Life becomes a vicious circle: as overeating causes weight gain, the body's ability to regulate its hunger hormones is reduced even more.

The most important thing you can do is recognize the body's yellow caution signals and take your foot off the gas when your stomach feels just right—satiated. Consciously ask yourself, "Am I full yet? Have I had enough to eat?" When you feel a sense of satisfaction, set the knife and fork on the plate and take a break. It will take time—as well as discipline—to become aware of the yellow caution lights. It may mean allowing yourself only one pass through the buffet table or saying no to seconds when offered at a dinner party. You must stop eating when you feel satisfied.

Word Play

Readers of the *Washington Post* newspaper are asked each year to participate in its annual "neologism" contest, where contestants are asked to supply alternate meanings for common words. Sample: *balderdash,* (n.) a rapidly receding hairline.

Here are two entries that relate to Perfect Weight Canada:

- flabbergasted (adj.), appalled over how much weight you have gained.
- abdicate (v.), to give up all hope of ever having a flat stomach.

Better Plan

People often follow the path of least resistance when hunger strikes by reaching for something convenient—a bag of salty potato chips or a bowl of candy—even though they know deep down that processed snacks and chocolate-coated treats will set them back. Reaching your perfect weight will involve *choosing something better* to eat rather than a quick fix to squelch hunger pangs.

The quick fix is the staple of today's 24/7 broadcast and print media—television, radio, and magazines, as well as the Internet. Not only is the mainstream media famous for having all the answers in a thirty-second sound bite or a "how to" article, but TV talk shows and women's magazines love promoting whatever's new in the weight-loss world—especially if a celebrity author is flacking a "new" diet.

Listen, I would appreciate any media attention for *Perfect Weight Canada*, although I'm not convinced that the media's short attention span will "get" what we're trying to accomplish here. They certainly haven't shown us why low-fat and low-carb diets—the two biggest dietary regimens of the last fifteen years—are ultimately destined to fail.

Back in the early 1990s, the conventional wisdom in the media was that foods containing *any* fats were to be avoided. If you were a teenager back then (as I was), you probably read influential articles in *MacLeans, Canadian Living,* or *Chatelaine* about how bad fat was for you. Your supermarket dairy case was public enemy No. 1: no butter, no eggs, no whole milk.

Media coverage at the time planted the notion that if you wanted to lose weight, then eating foods without fat would do the trick. Young girls took that advice to heart, believing they would be as thin as the supermodels taking flight down the runways of Milan and Paris if they eliminated fat from their diets. In a demonstration of the law of unintended circumstances, however, low-fat diets led to an unprecedented leap in anorexia and bulimia among weight-conscious teen girls.

One of the American media darlings behind the low-fat craze was an over-the-top woman with a platinum buzz cut named Susan Powter. Perhaps you saw her infomercial in Canada. Her mantra could be summed up in two sentences:

1. "Stop the insanity!"
2. "It's fat that's making you fat!"

Taking their cue from Ms. Powter, scores of magazine articles and newspaper features sang the praises of a low-fat, high-carbohydrate diet. Impressionable high school girls nodded their heads in agreement and gobbled up anything with the magic words *fat-free* or *reduced fat* printed on the packaging: cheese, crackers, cookies, yogurt, and ice cream. In high school, I can remember the cheerleaders studying the labels on packets of salad dressing to detect the presence of fat grams. Food manufacturers responded to this fascination with low-fat foods by flooding supermarket aisles with thousands of reduced-fat and nonfat products. Restaurants revamped their menus with low-fat entrees to suit the changing tastes of health-conscious consumers.

Did a low-fat diet make us any thinner? No, I'm afraid not. The problem with reduced-fat cookies and fat-free cream cheese was more than their low taste: these convenience foods had nearly the same amount of calories as the "full-fat" versions. People would eat more reduced-fat cookies because they thought they could, not knowing that food makers often replace the fat in snack foods with extra sugar, flour, and other waist-bulging ingredients.

After low-fat diets fizzled, the media was ready to pounce on the next get-thin-quick idea. They waited until the summer of 2002, when reporter Gary Taubes wrote a lengthy article in the *New York Times Magazine* about Robert Atkins, a Manhattan cardiologist who authored *The Atkins Diet Revolution* in 1972. The thrust of the *New York Times* article was that American doctors who recommended eating less fat and more carbohydrates—in other words, the essence of the low-fat diet—had it all wrong. Instead, it was low-carb diets that worked. Like a lone voice in the wilderness, "the unrepentant Atkins was right all along," Taubes declared.[4]

That was all that editors at the U.S.'s largest women's magazines—who live in the Big Apple and read the *New York Times* religiously—needed to jump on the Atkins bandwagon. Overnight, *Glamour, Redbook,* and *Cosmopolitan,* as well as NBC's *Dateline,* CBS's *48 Hours,* and ABC's *20/20,* cranked out features extolling the benefits of a low-carbohydrate, high-protein, high-fat diet. Readers and viewers learned that increasing their intake of protein from sources such as meat, fish, and dairy and reducing their intake of carbohydrates like bread, pasta, and rice would cause their bodies to burn excess body fat for fuel. Many dieters thought they had died and gone to heaven because they could gorge themselves with steaks, lobster, bacon, cream sauce, cheese, and eggs to their heart's content.

Overweight folks definitely lost weight following the Atkins diet, but they could never sustain a low-carbohydrate regimen. They got too hungry—the Achilles heel of many a diet—and when they fell off the Atkins bandwagon, they fell hard. Many binged on carb-heavy junks foods and gained all the weight right back—plus a few pounds more. That didn't stop the unquestioning media from changing its generally positive coverage of *Dr. Atkins' New Diet Revolution* as well as two other low-carb diets: *The South Beach Diet* by Miami cardiologist Arthur Agatson, MD, and *The Zone* by Barry Sears, PhD. It wasn't until Atkins Nutritionals, a company founded by the late Dr. Atkins that produced a line of low-carb convenience foods, snacks, and condiments, filed for U.S. bankruptcy protection in 2005 that the bloom fell off the low-carb rose. You can still find Atkins low-carb food at the Low-Carb Grocery in Toronto, however.

Unrealistic Expectations

Unwittingly or not, magazine feature stories and airbrushed advertisements set unrealistic expectations of what your perfect weight should be by highlighting celebrities and fashion models with tiny waists, large breasts, and great legs. Thin is in and has been for a long time. Wallis Simpson, the Duchess of Windsor and fashion icon from the 1930s, is famous for saying, "You can never be too rich or too thin."

With PhotoShop these days, digital photos are routinely manipulated to accentuate the positive, like the time a *GQ* cover shot of "healthy-sized" actress Kate Winslet was digitally altered to lengthen her legs and flatten her stomach. (The British film star was not pleased. "Like it or lump it, I'm not a twig and refuse to be one," she said.[5]) Another criticism levelled at today's advertising is the portrayal of unobtainable body images. We are so accustomed to seeing shirtless hunks with chiselled abs and bikinied women with knockout figures that we feel inadequate because we don't resemble them at all.

Consider these factoids:

- By the time a girl is seventeen, she has seen more than 250,000 messages about what she is supposed to look like.
- The average Canadian woman is a shade under 5 feet 4 inches tall and weighs approximately 153 pounds. The average American model is 5 feet, 11 inches tall and weighs 117 pounds.
- A survey of college-aged American women found that those who read magazines and watched television programs glamorizing thinness were more likely to have an eating disorder.
- Twenty-seven percent of American girls openly admit that the media pressure them to have a perfect body.
- Forty percent of newly identified cases of anorexia are in American girls aged fifteen to nineteen.
- Fashion models are 25 percent thinner today than models forty years ago.[6]

To achieve their ultra-skinny state, fashion models binge, purge, use laxatives, smoke, drink diet soda, and overexercise. These activities trigger a cascade of molecules in their blood to help them rebound from their severe diets, which causes them to overeat all over again. Thus they binge, purge, and diet even more rigorously. This turns into an ugly cycle that works in opposition to their body's natural chemical construction.[7]

Maybe Susan Powter's catchphrase—"Stop the insanity!"—needs to make a comeback. Fashion shows from Milan and Paris to London and Montreal are grappling with whether or not they should ban stick-thin models with BMIs less than 18.5 from the catwalk. Spanish officials in Madrid passed an ordinance doing just that after the eating-disorder deaths of two young models, Luisel Ramos, of Uruguay, and Ana Carolina Reston, of Brazil. Ms. Reston, who was 5 feet 8 inches tall and 88 pounds when she died, reportedly lived on a diet of apples and tomatoes in the weeks before her death.[8]

The point of these stories is that *no one* is satisfied with their weight when they focus on media-driven standards of appearance. Wherever you are on your journey to your perfect weight, it's more important to take control of your health than worry about what others think of how you look.

Advertising for Dollars

The media stay in business by selling advertising, and advertising works. Pizza delivery companies aren't stupid: on football weekends in the United States, they stack their cheesy ads in the first half and wait for the orders to pile in. Domino's typically sells more than one million pizzas on game days.[9]

Advertising foods to kids is like shooting fish in a barrel. Have you ever wondered why your kids pester you into buying something they want? In the United States, a Federal Communications Commission task force made up of FCC officials; members of the food, television, and advertising industries; and consumer health experts began studying the link between viewing habits and childhood obesity in 2007. It will be interesting to read the final report. Since Canadian children between the ages of two and eleven years watch more than fourteen hours of TV per week and view a barrage of advertisements for sugary cereal, candy, and fast food—I'm not sure what conclusion could be rendered except for the obvious: a barrage of junk food ads spurs sales of junk food.[10]

Soft drink makers, cereal makers, and candy makers target kids because they want them to become "brand loyal" consumers who will stay with the brand for their entire lifetimes. So billion-dollar titans square off like it's *Wrestlemania*: Pepsi vs. Coke or McDonald's vs. Burger King. Your kids are not the winners. Studies show that:

- American kids consume more than one-third of their daily calories from soft drinks, sweets, salty snacks, and fast food.
- Ads targeted to kids twelve and under lead them to request and consume high-calorie, low-nutrient products.
- A preschooler's risk of obesity jumps 6 percent for every hour of TV watched, 31 percent if the TV is in their bedroom.[11]

The reason junk food advertisers saturate the airwaves is because they're aware that children have "pester power," a unique ability to nag their parents into buying something they want. If your children are not at their perfect weight, you should limit their exposure to junk food advertising. Whether or not you're nodding your head in agreement, it's my contention that children aren't eating healthy because their *parents* aren't eating healthy.

Did I strike a nerve?

My Big Fat Greek Friend

Another topic receiving favourable media coverage is gastric bypass surgery, where you'll read nary a contrary word. To illustrate my concern with gastric bypass surgery, let me tell you about Nick Yphantides, MD, a San Diego family physician with whom I ate dinner one time and the author of *My Big Fat Greek Diet*. That evening he regaled me with a remarkable story of how he reached his perfect weight—and it wasn't by having his stomach stapled.

His story begins when Dr. Yphantides (a Greek name pronounced *ee-FAHN-tee-dees*) would treat indigent patients—mainly Hispanics—at a community health clinic in his hometown of Escondido. After a long day of office visits, he liked to reward himself by driving through his favourite fast-food joint, one that had a cult-like following in California—In-N-Out Burger. His order was always the same: a "4 x 4," large fries, and a Coke.

The "4 x 4"—four hamburgers and four slices of American cheese stacked in a hamburger bun with all the sauce and trimmings, plus the deep-fried fries and

16-ounce soft drink—contained 1,400 calories and 100 grams of fat, but that didn't bother Dr. Nick a bit. In his mind, the drive-through forays were just a snack, something to eat *before* dinner.

Dr. Nick had been gaining mounds of weight ever since medical school in the early 1990s, when he fortified his late-night study sessions with snack cakes and heaping bowls of rocky road ice cream. During interminable forty-hour shifts as an intern, he continually raided the hospital break room, where someone had set out a plate of sweets to be shared by the attending staff.

When Dr. Nick entered the public health arena as a family physician, he could be charitably described as "corpulent." He couldn't tell you how much he weighed, though, because he had stopped weighing himself. His expanding girth actually turned into an occupational blessing: his patients viewed Dr. Nick as a larger-than-life advocate for the poor, the big man with a big heart who cared for his community in a big way.

Overweight patients *loved* Dr. Nick because they knew they would receive tea and sympathy from someone who also shopped at the "big-and-tall" sections of department stores. From a doctor's perspective, he was always gracious with those who struggled with their weight. More than a few times, he looked a heavyset woman or large fellow in the eye and said with a smile, "Do as I say, not as I do."

Shortly after he turned thirty years of age, however, Dr. Nick began experiencing declining health and a host of unusual symptoms that led him to a doctor's examination room. A week later, he learned the bad news: he had testicular cancer. (Remember how I talked about the link between cancer and obesity in the previous chapter?)

The surgical excision of the right testes and aggressive radiation over twelve weeks saved his life—and caused some soul-searching. The way Nick saw it, he had dodged the cancer bullet, but there was another round in the chamber: his gargantuan weight had to be causing incredible amounts of stress on his organs—heart, lungs, and liver, as well as his skeletal frame. He wondered how much stress he was putting on his knees, which were bearing such a severe load.

One day, Nick planted his feet on two scales—one for each leg. Each needle came to rest on "233½." A fourth-grader could do the math: Dr. Nick Yphantides, the jolly doc with the Santa Claus–like image, weighed in at a hefty 467 pounds. Nick was scared. His cancer had forced him to face his mortality, and now he was sure that each bite of a burger brought him one swallow closer to the grave.

Something needed to be done. Nick was tired of dressing in XXXXL T-shirts. Tired of booking uncrowded red-eye flights so that he wouldn't have to buy a second seat. Tired of gawkers staring at his monstrous midsection in restaurants. Ahead of him was a future filled with high blood pressure, high cholesterol, and debilitating diabetes—unless he made a radical lifestyle change and lost a ton of weight. Well, maybe not a ton, but 200 pounds would be a good start toward his perfect weight, he figured.

In April 2000, Nick gave a one-year notice that he would be stepping down and leaving the Escondido Community Health Center. Then he began formulating a game plan. Since he wasn't going to work, he needed something to do—a diversion to keep his mind off being so hungry. That's it! Nick loved baseball, so he decided to drive around the country and visit all thirty major league ballparks—including Toronto's SkyDome and Olympic Stadium in Montreal before the Expos moved to Washington DC and became the Nationals. He calculated that he had been consuming 5,600 calories a day to maintain his weight. To lose weight slowly but surely, he would embark on a liquid diet—drinking a protein meal supplement offering just 800 calories a day, which is not exactly the eating plan recommended in *Perfect Weight Canada*.

On April 1, 2001, Nick sailed off in a used RV, a vehicle he christened the USS *Spirit of Reduction*, with the intention of becoming half the man he used to be. His father rode shotgun as an accountability partner. Going cold turkey from food gave Nick the shakes, just like any junkie coming down off a high. "I was so hungry at the ballpark that I would have eaten a cigarette butt dipped in mustard," he said.

At first, the pounds melted off Dr. Nick like a snowman standing in the Sahara Desert—17 pounds in the first week. After that initial surge of encouragement, his weight loss went from a gusher to a steady drip-drip as he continued to drink his protein shakes. He settled into an average of 1.1 pounds lost per day.

When Nick returned home in time for Thanksgiving, his mother was shocked by his appearance. Some of his nieces and nephews didn't even recognize him. Nick, now weighing 269 pounds, had shed nearly 200 pounds. He ate his first solid food in nearly eight months on Thanksgiving Day in America: some vegetables and a baked potato.

He continued to lose weight as he returned to solid food and his medical practice.

When I met Dr. Nick, he looked great. His weight had settled in at 220 pounds, and he had remained steady at that weight for five years. To this day, though, Nick said he still meets colleagues and acquaintances who casually ask him, "So, how did the surgery go?"

How did the surgery go?

They automatically assume that the only way Nick could have lost all that weight was by submitting to gastric bypass surgery, which is a radical form of "stomach reduction" or "bariatric" surgery. Such surgeries are aimed at either reducing the stomach size (by gastric banding or stapling) or bypassing the stomach altogether (gastric bypass).

In the last decade, hundreds of thousands of overweight people have barged down the doublewide doors of surgical centres in major U.S. cities and had their stomachs stapled. I realize that under socialized health care in Canada, gastric bypass surgery is performed at just a fraction of U.S. rates. The situation is far different in the States, where gastric bypass procedures have increased rapidly since 1998, when 14,000 were performed,[12] to a whopping 177,000 in 2006, according to the American Society for Bariatric Surgery.[13]

The reason for the explosive growth in the States has been the development of laparoscopic surgical techniques, which have made the invasive procedure less risky to the body. Gastric bypass surgeons staple the stomach—or bind it with an adjustable band—so that a small pouch is created to hold two or three ounces of food. This restricts food intake and interrupts the normal digestive process. People experience the sensation of being full after a few bites of food; if they eat any more, they often become nauseated.

A normal stomach can hold twenty-four ounces or seventy centilitres of food, which is a large plate of food. Gastric bypass surgery reduces the stomach to one-tenth of the size it used to be, so you'll lose weight because you can't eat any more. You don't have to be a brain surgeon to figure out that you're going to feel full very quickly.

The concept behind gastric bypass and gastric banding certainly sounds good: since most overweight people don't have the self-control they need to eat the way they should, let a team of doctors do some surgical rearranging of the stomach's gut to help them out. Several aspects to gastric bypass surgery, however, greatly concern me. I've met plenty of folks who've undergone the procedure, and I can see desperation written all over their faces. Their stories are almost universally the same: after losing a modest amount of weight, the pounds are coming back and they don't know what to do. They are like the baseball manager who's already used his last relief pitcher, but his team's getting shelled and there's no one left in the bullpen to call into the game. It's the same with gastric bypass: once you shrink-wrap your stomach, you're out of medical options.

The Next Step

Following the principles outlined in *Perfect Weight Canada* will give you a greater chance to reach your perfect weight than submitting to an uncertain medical procedure. Beginning with the next chapter, I'll get into specifics for:

- What you should eat
- What you should drink
- What you should snack on
- The importance of regular cleansing
- The key role of nutritional supplements, including the breakthrough new compound fucoxanthin
- Embarking on a FIT exercise program—Functional Interval Training
- The role of emotions and eating
- Ways to take weight off your world by adopting simple sustainability

A Closing Thought

Remember, the aim of Perfect Weight Canada is not to look like Kate Moss or even Kate Winslet. The goal is to reach a weight that makes you look and feel good about yourself and that will promote good health for the rest of your life—your perfect weight, to be exact.

I probably don't have to remind you that the way you view yourself—your self-image—has a profound effect on your weight. Your self-image is a combination of all the ideas you have formed about yourself over the years. Ever since childhood, you have developed a set of beliefs about who you are, what you look like, what you are worth, and what you deserve. These beliefs, over time, became part of your subconscious and help define who you are today.

The way you view yourself can be influenced by your self-talk and/or beliefs dictated by others, but only if you allow them to be. Thankfully, your self-image and the subconscious mind can be reprogrammed, as Dr. Nick told me. Over time, the subconscious mind will accept any thought you regularly think about yourself. Therefore, if you start to have positive thoughts, your self-esteem rises, and you feel better about who you are.

Next time you look in the mirror, don't zero in on the negative things you see. Find something you like and focus on that. As you begin to lose weight, say positive things to yourself like: "I can see the weight coming off, and I feel good about my results so far."

I've spoken with people who have reached their perfect weight but still had a negative view of their body and themselves. Self-worth is not equated with what the scales say; it is more about who you are. Your self-worth is measured in terms of the positive things you bring to people and events around you.[14] So find out what motivates *you* and be about it!

If there were an easier way to lose weight and change your life, someone would have found it by now. Losing weight should make you feel better about yourself, but don't forget the health benefits that come from a reduced risk of heart attack, diabetes, stroke, and cancer. Acting up the information contained in *Perfect Weight Canada* will likely improve your chances of living a longer, healthier, and, hopefully, a happier life.

Perfect Weight Recap: What Are You Failing For?

- The standard diet-book advice to cut calories and walk on a treadmill like a hamster rarely works over the long haul because dieters get too hungry. When they go back to their old comfort foods, the pounds—and then some—always seem to come back.
- Low-fat diets don't work because these foods often have the same amount of calories as their "regular" versions.
- Thanks to advances in laparoscopic surgical techniques and a growing population of overweight candidates, gastric bypass surgery—also known as "stomach stapling"—has become a viable option for the obese. The procedure has its risks, and some lose a modest amount of weight before the pounds start creeping back.

Section I
Change Your Diet

Chapter 3

Eat for Your Perfect Weight

TOLEDO'S FAVOURITE SON—AND biggest homegrown celebrity—is Jamie Farr, who played the comical role of cross-dressing Corporal Klinger on the hit TV show *MASH*. (I don't know how much the *MASH* sitcom was viewed in Canada, but I'm confident you've heard of the comedy program.) Often clothed in a spring dress with pumps and pearls, the otherwise dutiful orderly with the 4077th Mobile Army Surgical Hospital unit perpetually angled for a Section 8 discharge.

One of the inside jokes was that Corporal Klinger was a Lebanese-American from Toledo, Ohio, just like the real-life Jamie Farr. In several *MASH* episodes, Klinger rhapsodized about the chili-and-hot-pepper hot dogs found at Tony Packo's Café, located in the Hungarian/Polish neighbourhood of East Toledo. Another Toledo restaurant, though, had an even more special place in Jamie Farr's heart, as he described in the coffee-table book *Toledo: Treasures and Traditions*. Here's what the famous Hollywood actor wrote in the introduction:

> And who could forget one of the favourite meeting—and eating—places for the young and old, Chili Mac's. For a quarter, you could get the greasiest chili (or, some said, the chilliest grease) served on a mound of spaghetti and lined with the stalest soda crackers anywhere. You'd leave the joint with the worst heartburn—but with the best taste and best bargain in town. It always reminded me of one of Will Rogers' lines: about how chili was the world's most economical food because you eat it once and enjoy it for three days. Sadly, Chili Mac's is now but a memory.[1]

Although I haven't arrived at an age where I can appreciate nostalgia, I chuckled when I read Mr. Farr's reminiscences—and grimaced at the same time. His story demonstrates that dining out hasn't changed much in fifty years: you can serve the general public just about anything, and they'll eat it as long it tastes good going down and is easy on the wallet.

What *has* changed, though, is the restaurant scene. Beginning in the 1950s, greasy spoons like Chili Mac's closed down in droves after they couldn't compete with a new innovation—the fast-food restaurant and its assembly-line menu. When Ray Kroc opened the first McDonald's in 1955, he set the stage for a massive overhaul in the way Americans eat. "Great-tasting food at a reasonable price in a clean environment" became the mission statement of the fast-food industry. The success of McDonald's sired a stampede of imitators and matured into a colossal industry that collected $142 billion—that's *billion*—in 2006, according to the National Restaurant Association.[2]

I'm afraid that American-owned fast-food companies have invaded Canada like Visigoths of yore. In the last decade or so, fast-food restaurants have become as common as streetlights on every main boulevard and thoroughfare throughout Canada. From the crack of dawn to late-night runs, office workers, farmers, and families pass through drive-through lanes or line up at counters to order something quick and tasty.

It's safe to say that Americans and Canadians are hooked on greasy fried foods, captivated by sugar and sweets, and relatively clueless about what's healthy to eat. This obliviousness has exacted a heavy toll on our national health statistics: the scientific research on the link between obesity and fast food is unanimous on this, but a casual stroll through a crowded mall on a Sunday afternoon in December would confirm this. We're not even close to our perfect weight, in great part because of the lousy foods we eat—or what passes for inexpensive nutritional sustenance and familial enjoyment these days.

Frankly, we are an unhealthy people who haven't learned to discern. We traipse down supermarket aisles, pulling colourful and enticing boxes off the shelves and dropping them into the cart without a second thought—or a first thought regarding where the products came from, what the ingredients are, or how healthy they are to eat.

Brightly lit, gleaming supermarkets are the end product of the close and symbiotic relationship between big agriculture, mammoth food production companies, media advertising and tie-ins, and a sophisticated retail network that works together to grow, harvest, produce, market, and sell fresh, frozen, and processed foods to 33 million Canadians every day.

The good news is that we don't have a major hunger problem in North America, thanks to this interlocking economy. The bad news is what the food-industrial complex has wrought: homogenized, highly processed, and manufactured "products" of modern food science that are peddled to the masses for as cheaply as possible and to last on the shelves for as long as possible, thanks to chemical preservatives.

No wonder our taste buds have been manipulated by zillions of sweet and salty foods ready to be eaten or heated up in a microwave oven. Just about anything that comes in a box or a bottle is sweetened with sugar or high-fructose corn syrup or soaked in sodium. The strategy has worked: we're hooked on greasy foods high in calories, high in fat, high in sugar and salt, and—as a young Jamie Farr believed—high in taste. We're exiting convenience stores, supermarket check-out lines, ice cream stands, and fast-food restaurants with palate-pleasing foods pumped up with excess calories, and that's a root cause of our national health problems.

Making a Lifestyle U-Turn

I know what you may be saying: "But, Jordan, I don't want to go on a diet—diets don't work."

Here's the deal: if I followed you into a grocery store, shopping trip after shopping trip, week after week, month after month, I would see you purchasing the same thirty to fifty foods over and over again. The same milk. The same cereal. The same bread. The same meat. The same TV dinners. The same soft drinks. The same snacks. The same frozen vegetables, and the same occasional fruit and salad.

Each day you and your family eat the same things over and over again. In other words, you're already on a diet, and yours just stinks.

When it comes to a dietary strategy for winning the battle of the bulge, the most important step you can take is a lifestyle U-turn in what you choose to eat. You do that by following two fundamental principles for Perfect Weight Canada. They are:

1. Eat what God created for food.
2. Eat foods in a form healthy for the body.

Eating foods that God created means shopping for foods as close to the natural source as possible. I'm talking about:

- A wide array of organically grown fruits and vegetables
- Healthy dairy products like yogurt, cheese, and butter
- Healthy red meats like organic grass-fed beef, lamb, venison, and bison
- Cold-water fish caught in the wild
- Pastured or free-range chicken
- Whole grains like wheat and barley
- Nuts and seeds

These foods are part of the Perfect Weight Eating Plan, which I share in chapter 7. This sixteen-week plan has four phases and involves a comprehensive yet simple eating plan that will march you toward your perfect weight. This information, combined with a personal hydration program, proactive snacking, cutting-edge nutritional supplements, and a breakthrough exercise program comprise the total Perfect Weight Canada program.

As you can probably guess, I'm a proponent of natural foods grown organically and sustainably. Organic means the fruit or vegetable was grown without the use of most synthetic and petroleum-derived pesticides and fertilizers, antibiotics, genetic engineering, irradiation, and sewer sludge for three consecutive years. Organic meats must come from animals that eat 100 percent organic feed without any animal by-products; for dairy cows, the whole herd must have eaten organic feed for the previous twelve months. As for the term *sustainably*, this refers to a system of farming that maintains and replenishes soil fertility without the use of toxic and persistent pesticides and fertilizers. Livestock are pasture raised and grass fed, and fish are not pulled from the ocean faster than they can reproduce or caught in ways that destroy other sea life or undersea habitat.

"Organic" claim regulations are similar in the United States and Canada, but certification procedures are quite different in Canada. Currently, multiple organic standards are used to certify products as organic in Canada. As a result of the desire for a single national standard, the Canadian organic industry has requested federal regulators to establish organic guidelines. A new federally managed organic office should open soon. In the meantime, organic certification is provided by private sector organizations like the Bio-Dynamic Agriculture Association of British Columbia or the Nova Scotia Organic Growers Association in Canning, Nova Scotia.

The quest for a national organic standard needs to happen soon because organics is the fastest-growing sector in Canadian agriculture, with sales increasing at a steady 20 percent clip per year. In 2005, the most recent year for statistics, Canada had 3,618 certified organic farmers. Another 241 farmers were making the transition from conventional to organic farming.[3]

Most organic farms are found on the prairies, where grains and pulses are grown. Wheat is Canada's largest organic crop with over 187,000 acres in production. Most certified organic tree fruit is grown in central British Columbia, and organic dairy producers are found primarily in Ontario and Quebec. Organic livestock production has increased dramatically in recent years, with year-to-year gains of 20 percent.[4]

Beware of Frankenfood

If you pull a box of breakfast cereal off the supermarket shelf, there's a strong chance that the grains came from genetically modified (GMO) crops, which are created in the laboratory by taking genes from one organism and inserting them into another to make them grow higher, larger, denser, and more resistant to insect infestation. While this is a laudable goal, the problem is that scientists are adding a gene to a food that wasn't originally part of that food, which is unnatural and changes the DNA character of the crop. "You just can't get an elephant to mate with a corn plant," said Margaret Mellon of the Union of Concerned Scientists. "Scientists are making combinations of genes that are not found in nature."[5] My friend Jeffrey Smith, author of the groundbreaking book *Genetic Roulette*—which I highly recommend—quipped that GMO should stand for "God, Move Over."

While the science behind this technology is breathtaking, it's also stunning how quickly GMO crops have made it into the food chain. U.S. acreage has grown substantially in the last decade: today, 89 percent of soybeans, 83 percent of cotton, and 61 percent of corn is genetically engineered to resist weed-killing chemicals or help the plants make their own insecticides.[6]

How common are genetically modified crops in Canada? Doug Powell, assistant professor at the University of Guelph's Department of Plant Agriculture, says they are extremely common. "I can say with pretty good confidence that in Ontario, 35 per cent of the feed corn is genetically engineered Bt-corn," Powell declared. "I can say with reasonable confidence that slightly over 50 per cent of the canola in Canada is genetically engineered."[7]

While you won't find many GMO whole fruits or vegetables in your local supermarket—watch out for seedless watermelon and seedless grapes, however—it's estimated that 75 percent of the processed foods in this country (breakfast cereals, baked goods, vegetable oils, and so on) contain a potpourri of genetically modified ingredients.[8] I find this to be an amazing development because GMO crops such as corn, soybeans, and potatoes have only been around since the mid-1990s. I wouldn't be surprised if 100 percent of processed foods are made with GMO elements a decade from now.

As an aside, you can determine if your produce is GMO by looking at the sticker plastered on the fruit or vegetable. These little stickers contain different PLU codes that tell you whether the fruit was conventionally grown, organically grown, or genetically engineered. (PLU stands for Price Look Up and is a standard number in the United States, Canada, Europe, Australia, and South Africa.) The PLU code for conventionally grown fruit consists of four numbers, organically grown fruit is five numbers prefaced by the number 9, and GMO fruit is five numbers but prefaced by the number 8.

For example:

- A conventionally grown PLU would be 4446
- An organically grown PLU would be 94446
- And a genetically modified PLU would be 84446

Proponents of GMO foods believe they are riding the wave of the future, but I'm worried that we may be unleashing a form of "agricultural asbestos" on the American public. Genuine concerns about GMO foods have been raised worldwide, particularly in Europe, where they refuse American GMO imports.

I will not purchase, or knowingly eat, foods produced from genetically modified ingredients until we have a solid body of research regarding the short-term and long-term effects of eating GMO foods—and that doesn't look like it's happening any time soon. Until then, my family and I will sit on the sidelines and continue to shop for organic fruit, vegetables, grains, and meats. Besides, just on taste alone, organic foods have genetically modified crops beat by a country mile.

Organic is the popular buzzword these days as word gets around that there's a much healthier option to eating processed foods and meals-on-the-go. Sales of organic groceries in Canadian supermarkets skyrocketed by 28 percent from 2005 to 2006, according to the Nielsen Company, totalling $412 million in sales of certified organic food products in 2006.[9] Industry experts are forecasting continued rapid growth in the next decade. Progressive markets like Planet Organic, Capers, Choices, and Whole Foods (the biggest natural foods grocery chain in United States) have sprouted up like spring mushrooms to meet the surging demand for organic foods. Traditional grocers are not sitting idly by: Loblaw, Canada's biggest supermarket chain, created a private label, President's Choice Organics, to sell organic products to customers, and other major grocery chains—Sobeys, A&P, and Safeway—have been stocking up on a widening assortment of organic foods. Even the cavernous Costco warehouse clubs offer dozens of organic products to customers.

I like the direction Canada is heading.

Nicki and I do the bulk of our food shopping at two places: Nutrition S'Mart, a small chain of Florida health food stores, and Whole Foods, a luminous 39,000-square-foot natural foods market that's packed with organic fruits, vegetables, dairy products, breads, cereals, canned soups, frozen pizza, ice cream, tortillas, chips, and dip—everything a regular supermarket would stock. The notable difference between a Whole Foods and a regular store is that the former only sells products, for the most part, that are either natural or organic.

Americans are increasing their consumption of organic foods for a variety of reasons similar to why the Canadian public is purchasing more and more organic food. Health-minded individuals on both sides of the border believe organic foods are better for the environment (58 percent) and better for their health (54 percent). Almost one in three Americans (32 percent) believes organic products taste better, and 42 percent believe organic foods are better quality.[10] Americans also cite health as a key motivation in food purchases, declaring that they are eating healthy food to avoid illness later in life.

Food Additives and the Chinese Connection

China exports a lot more than cheap toys and plush animals to Canada. In the last decade, China has become the world's leading supplier of food flavourings and preservatives. China exported $2.5 billion of food ingredients to Canada and the rest of the world in 2006, a staggering 150 percent increase from just two years earlier.[11] The reason? Because they're cheaper, which fattens the bottom line of food conglomerates.

Here's a look at three of the most common food additives imported from China:

- Citric acid, used to give foods a tart taste and enhance fruit flavours, is used in soda, fruit-flavoured beverages, candy, and flavoured syrups.
- Sorbic acid, a preservative that inhibits the growth of mould and yeasts, is used in cheese, baked goods, and wine.
- Vanillin, an ingredient often made from wood pulp, is used in chocolates and cookies as an artificial vanilla flavour.

Good and Healthy vs. Bad and Unhealthy

Eating healthy, organic whole foods will give you the most nutritious, healthy fuel you need to attack the day *and* reach your perfect weight.

Consider these points:

- Good, healthy foods satiate you, are nutrient-dense, make you feel and look younger, decrease inflammation in your body, and help put an end to yo-yo dieting.
- Bad, unhealthy foods make you hungrier, are nutrient-deficient, prematurely age you, increase your body's inflammation levels, and perpetuate the yo-yo dieting pattern.
- Good, healthy foods are nutritional gold mines and contain no refined or processed carbohydrates and no artificial sweeteners.
- Bad, unhealthy foods are nutritional wastelands and contain genetically modified ingredients, unnatural additives, and potentially dangerous preservatives.

- Good, healthy foods come from natural and organic sources and are raised humanely and sustainably.
- Bad, unhealthy foods are produced by assembly-line workers in white lab coats or teens in hairnets manning fast-food kitchens.
- Good, healthy food takes time to prepare.
- Bad, unhealthy food is prepared in a hurry and often subjected to ionizing radiation.

Eat Less and Live Longer?

These days, I'm intrigued by a concept called "calorie restriction with optimal nutrition," or CRON. The idea is that reducing the intake of calories by 20 percent to 40 percent will improve health and extend your lifespan.

It's a concept that's been studied since the 1930s in laboratory settings. One of the researchers, Dr. Roy Walford of the UCLA pathology department, conducted experiments in which laboratory mice were given less and less to eat—but always enough to live on. Surprisingly to Dr. Walford, the deprived mice lived longer than their well-fed counterparts.

Dr. Walford then wondered if the same theory held true for humans. Offering himself as a human lab experiment, the research scientist voluntarily chose to eat very little for more than twenty years. His search for the fountain of youth led to a dietary regimen that consisted of small servings of low-fat milk shakes, vegetable salads, fish, and baked sweet potatoes. His daily calorie count of 1,600 was about half the 3,000 calories per day consumed by most Americans and Canadians.

Dr. Walford, who was widely featured in the U.S. media—*New York Times* and *Newsweek*, and on newsmagazine shows like *Dateline* and *Nightline*—was the author of *Beyond the 120-Year Diet: How to Double Your Vital Years*. Unfortunately, he didn't make it to 120 years of age. Dr. Walford died in 2004 at the age of 79 following a battle with amyotrophic lateral sclerosis, commonly known as ALS or Lou Gehrig's disease.

Scientific research has yet to support or refute whether a CRON diet extends life for humans. Julian Dibbell, writing in *New York* magazine, said that following the CRON diet meant living "as close to the brink of starvation as your body can stand."[12] I don't think God, who gave us wonderful foods to eat from His creation, wants us to go through life hungry. Neither does He want us to abuse our bodies by stuffing our mouths with junk food.

A happy medium must be found, but the idea of trimming the caloric sails a bit could make for a longer passage through life. It is my hope that by following the eating principles behind Perfect Weight Canada, you will not only live longer, but you will also live better.

Eating foods that God created and in a form healthy for the body contain far fewer calories, and calorie restriction with optimal nutrition is an important component of the Perfect Weight Eating Plan in chapter 7. As a way of example, you consume only 60 calories when you eat one of these foods as a snack, according to the Mayo Clinic in Minnesota:[13]

- One small apple
- One-half cup of grapes

- Two plums
- Two tablespoons of raisins
- One and one-half cups of strawberries
- Two cups of shredded lettuces
- One-half cup of diced tomatoes
- Two cups of spinach
- Three-fourths cup of green beans

On the other hand, a Cold Stone Creamery treat—a medium-sized mocha ice cream with Reese's Pieces and Oreo cookies mixed in and topped with pistachio nuts—comes out to a whopping 1,150 calories, or *twice* the amount of calories contained in *all* the fruits and vegetables I just listed!

"But, Jordan," you may be saying, "if you're telling me to just eat more fruits and vegetables to reach my perfect weight, it can't be this simple." Well, just so you know, I'm not advocating a diet of strictly low-cal fruits and vegetables, which doesn't provide the body with the full slate of nutrients that it needs. What I'm saying is that too many of us—when given the choice—will choose a Cold Stone ice cream for dessert rather than a bowl of fresh strawberries. I guess it's true what Irish dramatist and novelist Oscar Wilde said years ago: "I can resist anything but temptation

I want to help you discover—or rediscover—foods found in nature, as well as to retrain your taste buds. Do you have to think hard to remember the last time you bit into fresh raspberries, scooped up a handful of raisins, or supped on lentil soup? These listed foods are nutritional gold mines and contain no refined or processed carbohydrates and no artificial sweeteners. A diet based on consuming whole and natural foods fits within the bull's-eye of eating foods in a form healthy for the body. The basic components of a healthy diet include the right amount of:

- Protein, which is found in fish, meat, poultry, dairy products, eggs, and beans
- Fat, which is found in animal and dairy products as well as nuts and oils
- Carbohydrates, which are found in fruits, vegetables, whole grains, beans, and other legumes
- Vitamins such as vitamins A, B, C, D, E, and K
- Minerals such as calcium, potassium, and iron[14]

You'll see how all these nutrients come together in the Perfect Weight Eating Plan, but the Cliffs Notes version on reaching your perfect weight means that you will:

1. Eat foods low in sugar and refined carbohydrates, which will lower your daily glycemic load.

2. Add more omega-3 fats from wild-caught fish, grass-fed beef and game, and wild plants.
3. Try to balance your consumption of protein, fat, and slowly absorbed carbohydrates during your main meals.
4. Consume an abundance of vitamins and minerals from foods and whole-food nutritional supplements.
5. Eat foods high in alkalizing minerals, such as vegetables, which will prevent your blood from becoming too acidic.
6. Lower your intake of sodium.
7. Consume a high amount of antioxidants from foods, snacks, and whole-food nutritional supplements.
8. Eat foods with a high fibre content.

This last point needs to be circled in red because fibre is a natural appetite suppressant that curbs the appetite and keeps your cholesterol and blood sugar at optimal levels and your bowels functioning smoothly. High-fibre foods give you the biggest bang for your caloric buck because they pack a high volume of content into a low-calorie package. The reason you feel satiated when you eat fibre-rich foods is because fibre interacts with a gastrointestinal hormone called cholecystokinin—or CCK for short—that is secreted by the small intestine to signal the body, "Hey, we're getting full down here!" High-fibre foods promote and prolong the elevation of CCK in the blood, which in turn allows you to feel full for longer periods of time.[15]

Increasing your levels of CCK throughout the day will make it easier to decrease your caloric intake and still feel satisfied. Fibre also has a "flushing" effect on the bowels, which is why I recommend eating high-fibre foods during quarterly, ten-day detoxifying cleanses described in chapter 8, "Cleanse for Your Perfect Weight." Not only do the water and fibre in food flush toxins out of the body, but fibre also reduces the absorption of calories from food that you've already consumed.

How does this happen? People who eat diets high in fibre excrete more calories in their stool for the simple fact that fibre is not digestible. (A random thought, but how would you like to be lab tech given the chore of determining the amount of calories in a stool sample?) The "flush effect" means that when you go to the bathroom, you are eliminating 7 calories per gram of fibre that exit the body, unused.

You will have to up your intake of fibre-rich foods to get there. Here's a list that you can draw from, but keep in mind that scientists haven't been able to ascertain the exact total content of fibre in foods, especially fruits and vegetables, because of their complexity.[16] I found it interesting that many of the vegetables, when cooked, had twice the fibre than when eaten raw:

FRUITS	SERVING DESCRIPTION	FIBRE
Apples	One medium	4.0 grams
Blackberries	Half-cup	4.4 grams
Figs	Three	10.5 grams
Oranges	One large	2.4 grams
Peaches	One medium	2.3 grams
Pears	One medium	4.0 grams
Red raspberries	Half-cup	4.6 grams
Strawberries	One cup	3.0 grams

VEGETABLES	SERVING DESCRIPTION	FIBRE
Broccoli	¾ cup, fresh and cooked	7.0 grams
Carrots	Half-cup	3.4 grams
Corn	One medium ear	5.0 grams
Green peas	Half-cup, fresh	9.1 grams
Spinach	Half-cup, cooked	7.0 grams
Yams	One medium, cooked	6.8 grams

MISCELLANEOUS FOODS	SERVING DESCRIPTION	FIBRE
Black beans	One cup, cooked	19.4 grams
Lentils	⅔ cup, cooked	5.5 grams
Pinto beans	One cup, cooked	18.8 grams

Other high-fibre sources include:

- Most berries
- jBarley
- Cauliflower
- Celery
- Sprouted nuts and seeds
- Oat bran
- Oatmeal
- Brown whole-grain rice
- Vegetables with edible skins

Besides its "flushing" effect, fibre performs many important functions in the body. Fibre protects the health of the intestinal tract by increasing stool bulk and decreasing transit time, which minimizes the contact of carcinogenic and harmful elements with the intestinal lumen. Be aware that there are two kinds of fibre, soluble and insoluble. Water-soluble fibres are the slippery type found in grains such as oats, seeds, legumes, and pectins that make up part of the edible portions of seeds, vegetables, and fruits. Insoluble fibres are cellulose and lignin, found in the bran of wheat and other whole grains, and hemicellulose, found in whole grains, nuts, seeds, fruits, and vegetables.[17] This is the type of fibre Grandma calls "roughage."

Fibre helps with weight loss by satisfying your hunger so that you're not tempted to fill up on fatty and sugary foods. Good sources of fibre are nuts; seeds; beans; whole-grain sprouted breads; whole grains such as quinoa, amaranth, buckwheat, millet, and brown rice; green peas; carrots; cucumbers; zucchini; tomatoes; and baked or boiled unpeeled potatoes. Green leafy vegetables like spinach and fresh fruit are also fibre rich.

You will see that I include generous amounts of fibre-rich foods in the Perfect Weight Eating Plan in chapter 7. In practical terms, this means upping your consumption of vegetables with your meals and eating fruits for dessert. Fibre is like a sponge that soaks up fat and sugar in your gut and both slows and prevents some of their absorption, which helps you lose weight.[18] The addition of fibre to your diet is a miracle ingredient when it comes to losing weight.

What Ottawa and Washington Are Saying

Canada's Minister of Health released its latest *Canada's Food Guide* in the fall of 2007, complete with governmental recommendations for the number of servings per day of vegetables and fruit, grains and dairy products, and meat and vegetarian recommendations.

I took a look at Canada's Food Guide, which is remarkably similar to the food pyramid produced by the United States Department of Agriculture, which has become the basis of school lunch programs, hospital and nursing home menus, and all federally funded institutions that serve food in my country. After the government-sponsored food pyramid was introduced in 1992, my country reduced its intake of fat; increased its consumption of bread, rice, pasta, and cereals; and doubled its rates of obesity.[19] Not coincidentally, I might add. I'm not sure what the story is in Canada, but what has happened in the States can be instructive to Canadians.

The primary purpose of the USDA is not *your* health. It is to promote American agriculture—meaning big food. Experts on this subject, like Walter Willett, MD, and chairman of the Department of Nutrition at the Harvard School of Public Health, and professor Marion Nestle, PhD, have indicated in their books and writings that no food advice ever gets told to the American public that directly challenges the bottom line of the American food industry. Nutritional advice always gets yanked or watered-down by special interests. The end result: we all lose. Marion Nestle, in particular, has been a recipient of a number of letters and threats of lawsuits clearly designed to silence her or wear her down. Who writes these letters? They come from the food-industrial complex, of course—like Big Sugar.

Case in point: the original USDA food pyramid, which was terribly misleading as well as fundamentally flawed, according to Dr. Willett, who says that we're still trying to recover from the damage done by the media. The following axioms have been trumpeted in the mainstream media since the food pyramid's introduction more than fifteen years ago:

- All fats are bad.
- All complex carbohydrates are good.
- Protein is protein.
- Dairy products are essential for calcium intake.
- Potatoes are good for you.

In addition, the food pyramid made no recommendations regarding exercise or taking vitamins. After Dr. Willett and his team thoroughly researched those declarations, the Harvard professor shot them down like so many clay pigeons. His findings:

1. All fats are bad.
Not true, said Dr. Willett. While trans fats are bad for your health, monosaturated and polyunsaturated fats, as well as fats from fish, nuts, olive oil, and grains, are good for you.

2. All complex carbohydrates are good.
Not true, again. Besides, the food pyramid's recommendation to eat six to eleven servings of carbohydrates daily was way too much, Dr. Willett declared. The original food pyramid did not differentiate between refined carbohydrates (such as commercial pasta) and healthy carbohydrate foods (fruits, vegetables, whole grains, and whole-grain bread).

3. Protein is protein.
Again, the Harvard doctor disagreed. Some sources of protein are better for you than others. For example, red meat is a high-quality protein that's high in saturated fats, and wild-caught salmon is rich in heart-healthy omega-3 fatty acids.

4. Dairy products are essential for calcium intake.
According to Dr. Willett, this is also not true. He insists that there is not a calcium crisis in the United States. "In reality," he said, "there are studies that suggest that too much calcium can increase a man's chances of getting prostate cancer or a woman getting ovarian cancer."

5. Potatoes are good for you.
This claim didn't make any sense to Dr. Willett, who pointed out studies showing that eating a baked potato increases blood sugar levels and insulin faster and higher than an equal amount of calories from pure table sugar.

Finally, according to the Harvard professor, a healthy diet without exercise is counterproductive and adding vitamins and minerals to your diet is important.[20]

The USDA issued a revised set of food guidelines in 2005, but the new food pyramid was only a mild improvement, remarked Mark Hyman, MD, author of *Ultrametabolism: The Simple Plan for Automatic Weight Loss*. "Rather than educating about the dangers of refined carbohydrates and sugars, they [the USDA] meekly advised us to 'choose carbohydrates wisely,'" stated Dr. Hyman.[21]

What Nutritional Type Are You?

While boosting the amount of fibre in your diet is an important first step to reaching your perfect weight, you need to understand that the nutrients in our food—proteins, fats, and carbohydrates—are like putting fuel in your car's gas tank. When you eat the right foods, you should notice an improvement in your energy level, an uptick in your mental agility, a stabilization of your emotional well-being, and an overall feeling of well satisfaction. But if you finish a meal and notice your energy level dropping, or you're as grumpy as an airport security screener, then you have eaten an improper combination of proteins, carbohydrates, and fats.

Since we're born with different metabolisms, it stands to reason that certain foods can affect you in different ways, which, in turn, can positively or negatively influence your digestion, your mood, and, ultimately, your perfect weight. The idea of eating for your unique metabolism is a concept called "metabolic typing," which was introduced by William Kelley, DDS, in the 1960s and today is championed by several health experts, including Dr. Joseph Mercola, author of *Take Control of Your Health*, and researcher William L. Wolcott, author of *The Metabolic Typing Diet*.

Wolcott believes you can determine how well your body processes macronutrients—the proteins, the fats, and the carbohydrates—and use that information to make specific dietary recommendations.[22] He says people fall into three general metabolic types:

1. Protein types burn, or oxidize, carbohydrates quickly and must eat protein and fat to slow down this process. Protein types tend to be frequently hungry and often feel edgy and anxious.
2. Carb types have generally weak appetites, love sweets, have problems keeping weight off, and are often hooked on caffeine.
3. Mixed types generally have average appetites, no huge cravings for sweet and starchy foods, keep their weight under control, but tend to feel fatigued, anxious, and nervous about life.

Shortly, I'll present a simple test—although it's not foolproof—to determine what metabolic type, or what I prefer to call "nutritional type," you are. Before we get there, however, let me give you some more background information on protein and carbohydrates and how these nutrients impact your body.

The Power of Protein

Proteins, one of the basic components of foods, help you feel fuller than do carbohydrates or fats, so along with eating more fibre, you will need to eat adequate amounts of lean protein to control your hunger and food intake.

Proteins are the worker bees: they provide for the transport of nutrients, oxygen, and waste throughout the body and are required for the structure, function, and regulation of cells, tissues, and organs. Consuming meals rich in high-quality protein—chicken, beef, lamb, dairy, eggs, and so on—will leave you feeling full and satisfied, which supports weight loss.

The best and healthiest sources of protein are organically raised cattle, sheep, goats, buffalo, and venison. Grass-fed beef is leaner and lower in calories than grain-fed beef. Organic beef is higher in heart-friendly omega-3 fatty acids and important vitamins like vitamins B_{12} and E, and way healthier for you than meat from hormone-injected cattle eating pesticide-sprayed feed laced with antibiotics.

Even better, as it relates to weight loss, is that grass-fed beef is high in conjugated linoleic acid (CLA), a fatty acid that appears to modestly reduce body fat while preserving muscle tissue, according to researchers at the University of Wisconsin School of Medicine. Those participating in the study who took 3.2 grams of CLA each day had a drop in fat mass of about 0.2 pound per week, or around a pound a month, compared to those given a placebo.[23] Grass-fed animals have three to five times more CLA than grain-fed animals.

Fish with scales and fins caught from oceans and rivers are also lean sources of protein and provide essential amino acids. Canada, by virtue of its great fisheries, produces some of the world's healthiest-to-eat—as well as best-tasting—fish: wild salmon, walleye, Northern pike, smallmouth bass, and lake trout, just to name a few. Consuming fatty fish—wild salmon, mackerel, and sardines—comes with additional benefits. They provide the healthy omega-3 fats described earlier.

Protein is important when trying to reach your perfect weight for these reasons:

- Chicken, beef, fish, beans, and other high-protein foods slow the movement of food from the stomach to the intestine.
- A stomach that slowly empties means you feel fuller longer and get hungrier later.
- Protein's gentle, steady effect on blood sugar avoids the quick, steep rise in glucose levels that occurs after eating a rapidly digestible carbohydrate like white bread or baked potato.[24]

So If You're a Vegetarian . . .

That complicates things, especially if your nutritional type is skewed toward protein. Lacto-ovo vegetarians can get along fine if they consume lots of high-quality protein sources such as organic eggs and cultured dairy, but strict vegetarians will have a more difficult time meeting their protein needs on the Perfect Weight Eating Plan. You will need to substitute other foods for your protein needs, such as nuts, seeds, legumes, and cereal grains. Since these foods are only decent protein sources, however, you should seek the advice of a nutritionist who can offer nutritional guidance.

Many vegetarians, due to the nature of vegetarianism, eat an excess of carbohydrates and not enough proteins and fats. This is why you can be overweight while being a "perfect" vegetarian. A vegetarian diet of cereals, pastas, breads, and sweets is not helpful—for reasons aforementioned.

A good vegetarian diet should emphasize coconut, chia, avocado, tempeh (fermented soybean loaf), seeds, legumes, nuts, and whole grains such as amaranth, buckwheat, millet, and quinoa to get all the protein you need. A good vegetarian diet also provides healthy fats from extra-virgin coconut, olive, and flaxseed oils. You will find it necessary to mix and combine foods to get the needed nutritional balance at every meal. While being a vegetarian demands more planning and work to pull off, reaching your perfect weight can still be done.

Killing Those Carbs Softly

If protein and fats don't cause people to get fat, what's left?

You're right—carbohydrates. Too many carbohydrates, especially those from refined sources, are the culprits. Pigging out on refined carbs forces the body to convert any excess carbohydrates into body fat, which keeps pounds resting on the midsection.

You won't lose weight and keep it off when your diet is heavy in refined carbohydrates. Refined foods, a process in which fruits, vegetables, and grains are stripped of their vital fibre, vitamins, and mineral components, will never match up to the nutritional power of fresh produce and grains.

At the same time, carbohydrates are the body's chief source of energy. Carbohydrates are necessary for the digestion and assimilation of other foods, and they help regulate protein and fat metabolism. Fats require carbohydrates to be metabolized in the liver. We need carbohydrates. We just don't need the carbs from refined foods.

In response to the intake of too many carbs, your body is forced to produce extra insulin in order to prevent large spikes in blood sugar. Dr. Bulwer says this spike in insulin levels can overcorrect and cause blood sugar to transiently go too low in the short term—a state called hypoglycemia. This typically causes hunger pangs and a headache and leads to craving for more sweets. "Clearly, this leads to weight gain," he said. "A state of habitual high carb intake and progressive obesity leads to a state of hyperinsulinemia, where circulating insulin levels may increase two- or threefold."

If there's too much insulin in the bloodstream, which often happens when you eat highly refined, high-carb foods like rolls, pastas, and sweets, the body stores the extra sugar as fat. Cutting way back on refined carbs, however, will reduce the insulin and blood sugar roller coaster and cut down on fat production.

Apart from dietary fibre and sugar sweeteners, the other main carbohydrate form is starch, which is found in plant-based foods such as rice, potatoes, corn, and grains. When starchy foods are eaten, the digestive tract breaks down these long-chained starches into simpler sugars and finally into glucose (blood sugar), which is a source of immediate energy. If these calories are not expended, however, the body stores them as fat, which becomes a weighty problem—and is why high-starch foods should be eaten judiciously.

How fast the body turns these starches into blood glucose is a measure of the glycemic index, known as GI. The glycemic index is a ranking of foods based on their immediate effect on blood sugar levels as well as a measurement of how quickly the carbohydrates in food are digested. Carbohydrate foods with a high glycemic index, such as white breads, starchy potatoes, and sugary desserts, raise your blood sugar levels dramatically.

Carbohydrate foods with a low glycemic index, such as certain fruits, vegetables, salads, and organic whole-grain products, take your blood sugar to levels right where they should be. "Entry of glucose into the bloodstream occurs more slowly and smoothly," said Dr. Bulwer. "One thing that should not be forgotten is that the *quantity* of carbohydrates you eat is perhaps even more important than *what* you eat in terms of the degree of spike in blood sugar. This has given rise to the term that some prefer: glycemic load."

As I mentioned in chapter 2, diets that generally strike carbohydrates from your eating plan are doomed to failure. The human body, especially the brain, needs a constant supply of glucose because glucose levels that drop too low can result in weakness and fatigue. It's better to eat small, frequent meals that focus on fresh fruits and vegetables, whole grains, seeds, nuts, legumes, and healthy dairy foods. These foods that God created will help stabilize insulin and blood sugar levels. This doesn't mean that you should be nibbling all day long, however. Even too much of a good thing isn't good for you.

You will have to be careful about the type of carbs you eat. It's always best to consume proteins, fats, and foods lower in carbohydrates, like fresh vegetables, before eating any high-starch carbohydrates like potatoes, rice, grains, and bread. I know when you go out to a neighbourhood trattoria it's tempting to fill up on the delicious Italian panini and butter before the chicken cacciatore arrives. That's the absolute wrong way to eat, however. Leave the bread and rice or potatoes until the end of the meal, or, better yet, leave them out altogether if you're feeling satisfied.

The Skinny on Fats

Fat—along with protein and carbohydrates—is the third major nutrient found in food. If you recall from our last chapter, it's not fat that's making you fat, so there's no need to remove fat from your diet. Actually, we need to eat *some* fat: fats are a concentrated source of energy and source material for cell membranes and various hormones, have a protective effect against heart disease, play a vital role in the health of your bones, protect the liver from alcohol and other toxins, and guard against harmful microorganisms in the digestive tract. All fat-soluble vitamins—A, D, E, and K—need fat in the diet for their absorption and utilization.

Misconceptions are hard to overturn, however. For decades, the media have reported on studies that vilified fats, especially saturated fats, for those experiencing cardiovascular disease. The researchers conducting these trials, however, totally ignored the evidence that their subjects were carbo-loading on pasta, bread, cereal, muffins, doughnuts, Danishes, and desserts while failing to exercise; they were also drinking too much alcohol, which prolonged high insulin levels. Because insulin influences the biochemical processes that lead to atherosclerotic plaque formation in arteries, these subjects had higher rates of heart disease.

The Holy Grail of the "diet-heart" connection is the Framingham Heart Study, which began in 1948 when researchers recruited 5,209 men and women between the ages of thirty and sixty-two from the town of Framingham, Massachusetts. The study conducted extensive physical examinations and lifestyle interviews with participants in a search for common patterns relating to cardiovascular disease development; it has been used as the benchmark for cardiovascular health in Canada as well.[25]

In the Framingham study, researchers found that those who consumed more saturated fat and cholesterol in their diet actually weighed *less* and had a *lower* risk for heart disease, yet the Framingham study is often cited by the media as proof that fat and cholesterol are harmful. Now, other voices are being heard. One of them is the physician who was the associate director of the Framingham study for three years, George Mann, MD, who edited a book called *Coronary Heart Disease: The Dietary Sense and Nonsense*. In that volume, Dr. Mann provided powerful evidence that saturated fat is *not* the cause of heart disease.[26]

Another author, Diana Schwarzbein, MD, who wrote *The Schwarzbein Principle: The Truth About Losing Weight, Being Healthy, and Feeling Younger*, states that eating the right fats causes you to lose body fat and reach your ideal body composition.[27] The "right fats" are healthy saturated fats, omega-3 polyunsaturated fats, and monounsaturated (omega-9) fatty acids. You can find these fats in a wide range of foods, including salmon, lamb, goat's and sheep's milk and cheese, coconut, walnuts, olives, almonds, and avocados.

"My clinical experience with thousands of people has shown that eating saturated fats is not the culprit!" Dr. Schwarzbein exclaimed. "On the contrary, the patients I have followed, who have increased their consumption of saturated fats (as well as all other good fats), have improved their cholesterol profiles, decreased blood pressure, and lost body fat, thereby reducing their risk for heart disease. Eating saturated fats should be part of your balanced diet while, at the same time, your focus should be on reducing all the factors that increase insulin levels."[28]

The more healthy fats you eat, the healthier you'll become. The Inuits, who inhabit the Arctic region in the Northwest Territories, are well known for their high consumption of fats—mainly omega-3 and saturated fats from fish, seals, reindeer (caribou), and whales, including their fatty blubber. They have traditionally enjoyed very low rates of heart disease.

Below is a list of saturated, monounsaturated, and polyunsaturated fats that are good for you, along with some of the foods and where they are found. Within this list, be sure to shop for "pure cold-pressed" oils. The cold-pressing process, used to extract oil from natural sources, does not damage the fat. When heat processes are used to extract sunflower oil from sunflower seeds, for example, that damages the fat. This is an important point because your body cannot easily metabolize damaged fat.

Saturated fats (saturated fat oils are best for cooking)

- Butter
- Cheese
- Coconut and palm oils (look for extra virgin, as they are healthier than refined)
- Cream, dairy only
- Beef, venison, buffalo, and lamb fat (when found within the meat and raised organically)
- Eggs
- Ghee (clarified butter)
- Sour cream
- Chicken, duck, and turkey fat (when found within the meat and raised organically)

Monounsaturated fats (these oils can also be used for cooking but are less preferable to saturated oils)

- Avocados (they contain almost as much healthy monosaturated oleic fats per gram as olive oil—a whopping 70 to 75 percent)
- Almond oil
- Grapeseed oil
- Peanut oil
- Extra-virgin olive oil (best used on salads; should *not* be heated)

Keep in mind that not all olive oils are the same: olive-pomace oils, from the last dregs after pressing, are highly refined, chemically treated, and not recommended.

Polyunsaturated fats (for polyunsaturated fat oils, use only those that are cold pressed; they are not to be used for cooking purposes since heat damages these fats)

- Flaxseed oil
- Chia seed oil
- Hemp seed oil
- Sunflower oil
- Safflower oil
- Cod liver oil
- Herring oil
- Menhaden (fish) oil
- Salmon oil
- Sardine oil
- Sesame seed oil
- Wheat germ oil[29]

In addition, your diet should be rich in healthy fats from the following sources:

- Omega-3, free-range eggs
- Grass-fed red meat
- Free-range chicken
- Wild fish
- Nuts and seeds

Polyunsaturated fats are made up of high levels of omega-3 fats and omega-6 fats, known as essential fatty acids (EFAs). Omega-3 fats can improve cardiovascular health and help balance insulin and inflammation levels. Wild-caught fish, free-range eggs, walnuts, and flaxseeds are excellent sources of these important omega-3 fatty acids.

The types of fats you *really* want to run away from are trans fats, which have been vilified in the mainstream media for the last few years—and rightfully so. These horrible, artery-clogging fats are produced by heating liquid vegetable oils in the presence of hydrogen to make them solid at room temperature—a process known as hydrogenation. Food conglomerates routinely utilize hydrogenated oil inside their manufacturing plants, which means that trans fats are found in nearly all of our processed foods. The reason food producers employ so much chemistry in the hydrogenation process is because it allows them to produce a more competitively priced product with a longer shelf life.

The list of foods containing trans fats is endless: vegetable shortening, frozen pizza, ice cream, processed cheese, potato chips, cookie dough, white bread, dinner rolls, snack foods, doughnuts, candy, and salad dressing. The worst offender is margarine, even those touted in "heart healthy" tubs. Commercially prepared fried foods, like french fries and onion rings fried in polyunsaturated vegetable oils, also contain gobs of trans fat. Anything deep-fried in polyunsaturated oils—chicken, steak, or fries—contains higher-than-average trans fat levels. Canadians have a particularly high level of trans fats in their diet because of amount of canola oil they consume.

Mark my words: trans fats are horrible for your health, and that's the reason why they are in the crosshairs of politicians these days. Calgary may be known as the "Fat Cat City" for its booming economy, but Calgary is poised to become the first Canadian municipality to trim artery-clogging trans fats off menus, as well as packaged baking. A ban on trans fat in all foods could come into affect as early as October 1, 2008. The Calgary Health Region, which includes rural areas such as Banff and Lake Louise, decided to take action after Ottawa decided to allow businesses another two years to make voluntary changes in eliminating trans fats.[30]

Although Toronto is considering a similar ban, Canadian cities are playing a bit of catch-up to what's happening in the States. City officials in Tiburon, California, an exclusive enclave on the San Francisco Bay, successfully coaxed the city's eighteen restaurants to voluntarily stop using trans fats in their cooking oils in 2004. News of Tiburon's voluntary trans fat prohibition prompted cities like Philadelphia and New York City to pass laws banning restaurants from serving foods cooked or fried with oils that contain or produce trans fats. Eateries in both major cities have until the summer of 2008 to be in compliance. Metropolises such as Boston, Chicago, and Los Angeles may soon join them, and at least thirteen states are considering a trans fat ban, including a bellwether state, California. This will be interesting to watch unfold.

In Europe, the Danes are way ahead of North Americans. Denmark passed laws effective in 2004 restricting the use of industrial trans fats to a maximum of 2 percent of the fat in any food product. American multinationals like McDonald's and KFC had to comply with new oils in their fryers, so it *is* possible.

Beware of the Trans-Fat Gimmick! by Dr. Bernard Bulwer

Question: Can you explain how it's possible—since food packaging on both sides of the border require the amount of trans fats to be listed on food labels—that products with hydrogenated or partially hydrogenated fats (the source of bad trans fats) can still splash their packages with phrases like "Trans Fat Free" or "Zero Trans Fat"?

Answer: Because of the verbal gymnastics allowed by government loopholes. Even though the packaging says the food is trans fats free or has zero trans fats, manufacturers can still put dangerous trans fats in your food—as long as they ensure there's less than 500 milligrams of trans fat per serving.

The problem is that when you multiply 500 milligrams by the amount of servings you consume, then eat many different foods that play the same tricks with their labels, you're consuming trans fats when you thought you were being "good" and staying away from these menacing compounds.

Now you understand the deception, and it's all legal. Read your ingredient labels, and if you see the words *hydrogenated* or *partially hydrogenated* listed, figure that you'll be ingesting some amount of trans fat, no matter what the colourful label promises.

What's Your Nutritional Type?

Now that you have a better understanding of protein, carbohydrates, and fats, what nutritional type are you? Instead of categorizing people as protein, carb, or mixed types, I've simplified things by coming up with two categories:

1. Meat types, for their need to eat a higher-protein diet
2. Potato types, for their need to eat a diet higher in carbohydrates

You can determine, generally speaking, your nutritional type by answering the following questions adapted from Dr. Mercola's book *Total Health Program*, which will give you a broad idea of whether you are a meat type or a potato type:

1. When you eat or snack on high-carb foods like bread, cereals, fruits, grains, or vegetables, are you satisfied, or do you want to eat more?

   a. I'm generally satisfied after eating these high-carbohydrate foods.
   b. I'm in the middle—not satisfied but not hungry for more.
   c. I'm still hungry.

2. When you eat red meat regularly, do you lose or gain body weight? Do you feel slimmer?

   a. The bathroom scale confirms that I've gained weight.
   b. Eating red meat doesn't affect my weight either way.
   c. I actually lose weight when I eat red meat.

3. Do you think about food all the time? Are you one of those persons who live to eat?

   a. No, I'm not hung up on food.
   b. I'm in the middle: not hung up on food or crazy about it.
   c. I can't wait to chow down again.

4. What is your appetite like at breakfast?

   a. I'm not hungry at all.
   b. I can eat, but I'm not super hungry.
   c. I'm definitely hungry.

5. What is your appetite like at lunchtime?

   a. I'm not hungry at all.
   b. I can eat, but I'm not super hungry.
   c. I'm definitely hungry.

6. What is your appetite like at dinnertime?

   a. I'm not hungry at all.
   b. I can eat, but I'm not super hungry.
   c. I'm definitely hungry.

7. Does eating something higher in fat and/or protein (macadamia nuts, yogurt, whole milk, cheese, and guacamole) within an hour or two of bedtime help you sleep better?

a. No, not at all.

b. Eating those foods just before bedtime doesn't affect one way or another.

c. I sleep like a log when I snack on those foods.

8. Do you need to eat frequently, or can you eat three square meals and not feel the need to snack in between?

   a. I only need to eat one or two times a day, including snacks.

   b. Three square meals is all I need.

   c. I have to snack in between meals; otherwise I won't make it.

9. How much do you enjoy eating fermented foods like pickles, sauerkraut, or beets?

   a. I love them.

   b. They're OK, but I'm not a huge fan of fermented foods.

   c. I can't stand them.

10. When the Thanksgiving turkey is being carved, are you a white meat or dark meat type of person?

    a. I always eat the breast—white meat.

    b. I like both kinds of meat.

    c. I always go for the dark meat.

Add up your score of a, b, and c answers. If most of your answers were in the "b" and "c" categories, you're a meat type, someone who should be eating more protein foods. If most of your answers were in the "a" category, you're a potato type, someone who should consume a diet higher in carbs.

Meat types, as you would expect, do better eating higher protein and lower carbohydrate foods that include plenty of the "good" fats. Meat types burn fuel quickly, which is why they are known as "fast oxidizers." My experience has been that meat types like sweets but perform better on healthy protein foods. They have big appetites and also tend to crave salty and fatty foods, burning carbohydrates quickly. Eating more protein and more fat will slow this process.

Potato types feel bullish about the world when they're eating lots of carbohydrates, which ain't gonna happen on the Perfect Weight Canada program. They feel best when their plates are filled with carbohydrate foods like breads, grains, and vegetables. The danger is that this type of diet can increase fat storage. Pigging out on too many carbohydrates, especially those from refined sources, forces the body to convert any excess carbohydrates into body fat, which keeps pounds resting on the midsection. Potato types are also "slower oxidizers," meaning their bodies don't burn proteins and fats as efficiently. This explains why potato types tend to struggle when they go on a low-carb Atkins-type program—their bodies demand more carbs.

You should start by paying attention to the amount of proteins, carbs, and fats in your diet, and then adjust the proportions according to your taste and appetite. See how you feel as you go about your day. If you do not react optimally to your meal, you can change the ratios the next time around and analyze your reactions, fine-tuning each meal to the ratios of proteins, carbs, and fats that are just right for you.

Let's say you have a bland chicken breast with salad for lunch. If within an hour or two you feel absolutely famished, you probably need more fat in your salad. Next time, add an extra tablespoon of healthy salad dressing, extra-virgin olive oil, cheese, avocado, or almonds, and see if your mid-afternoon cravings disappear. Generally speaking, you should feel terrific for at least one hour after you eat. If you are still having food cravings or a noticeable dip in energy level, these are clues that you're probably not eating appropriately for your nutritional type.

I've designed eating plans for meat and potato types that can be found in chapter 15, "The Perfect Weight Daily Health Plan." If you want to receive a personalized daily eating program, go to www.PerfectWeightCanada.com.

The Concept of Food Combining

There's another aspect to eating that I want you to be aware of: the concept of "food combining," which encourages separating specific foods and eating certain ones together. A New York physician, William Howard Hay, MD, introduced the food combining concept nearly a century ago when he suggested that certain foods, when broken down, leave an acid pH, and other foods leave an alkaline pH. Translated into plain English, Dr. Hay believed food combining means not eating carbohydrates and protein at the same meal.[31]

Medical research has not been able to support Dr. Hay's food-combining theories, and no scientific proof asserts that foods digest better when carbohydrates and protein are eaten separately. I believe digestive systems were created to handle a variety of nutrients coming down the pike at the same time. If you happen to eat carbohydrates like grains, breads, pasta, cereal, fruits, and veggies with certain proteins like meat, fish, poultry, beans, and nuts, but don't appreciate the way your stomach feels afterward, feel free to experiment. You may find that nonstarchy green vegetables like broccoli, mushrooms, and zucchini work better with lean meats, eggs, and cheeses.

Some people say that combining fruit with any other food delays digestion and causes gas and bloating to occur. We know physiologically that fruits stay in the stomach for only a short time—twenty to forty-five minutes. For myself, I've found that I need to be careful about the fruits I eat and when I eat them. I've always remembered an old expression about melon that Dad used to say when I was growing up: "Eat it alone, or leave it alone." Since melons are comprised of 90 percent water, he said, they leave the stomach faster than other foods, including other fruits. That's why I eat melon alone as a snack. You may find that sweet fruits like bananas, dates, and figs aren't compatible in your stomach when consumed with acidic fruits like grapefruit, pineapple, or oranges. While I'm not totally onboard with the principles of food combining, it never hurts to listen to your body.

Along these lines, I recommend consuming fibre and fat with every meal and not eating your carbohydrates naked. Fibre and fat slows the absorption of sugar into the bloodstream, which keeps insulin levels in check.

Eat Your Colours

Have you noticed the lack of colour in a McDonald's value meal? Once you get your sandwich out of the wrapper, a Quarter Pounder and medium french fries is monochromatic beige. Same thing over at the Colonel's, where a plastic plate of KFC extra-crispy chicken, mashed potatoes, gravy, and corn are mainly lighter and darker hues of brown with a dash of pale yellow.

You usually don't find many colourful foods in fast-food restaurants, unless you order a salad. Contrast this with a visit to the produce department at an upscale health food store, where fruits and veggies with vibrant reds, greens, oranges, purples, and yellows are on display. Whether you're cooking at home or ordering out in a restaurant, you'll never go wrong eating foods exhibiting the pulsating, radiant colours of the rainbow. At one of my favourite restaurants, P. F. Chang's China Bistro, I'm partial to the Oolong Marinated Sea Bass entrée that's broiled and served with sweet ginger soy, baby corn, and spinach. Since we eat with our eyes first, this type of meal just *looks* better and healthier.

Many of the vivid colours in fruits and vegetables come from phytochemicals like anthocyanins, phenolics, lutein, indoles, flavonoids, and carotenoids like lycopene. These nutrients help the body maintain memory function, cardiovascular health, and a healthy weight. Pigments with health-promoting properties colour every fruit and vegetable, and their benefits are unique to each colour. For instance, blueberries—my favourite berry—are coloured by the phytochemical anthocyanin. Green vegetables owe their pigment to chlorophyll. Another phytochemical known as lycopene is the reason why tomatoes and watermelon are red. The nutrient fucoxanthin is a pigment that makes brown seaweed brown. All these phytochemical pigments offer antioxidant protection as well as other health benefits.

Being mindful of adding colour to your plate at a place like a Chili's-type restaurant means ordering a spring salad instead of french fries to go with your sandwich. When you're making a sandwich for work, add a leaf of lettuce and a thick slice of tomato to your turkey, tuna, or chicken. Shredded carrots bolster the look of tuna salad, and fruit salad with green grapes, red raspberries, and white banana add a pleasant ending to any meal.

What colour has your diet been? For some of you, it's been beiges and browns, the colours of restaurant food and frozen dinners. Perfect Weight Canada illuminates your diet with the following colours:

- Red: tomatoes and tomato sauces, raspberries, apples, strawberries, pomegranates, cherries, peppers, radishes, and watermelon
- Purple-blue: plums, grapes, prunes, blueberries, blackberries, red cabbage, beets, and eggplant
- Orange: oranges, sweet potatoes, cantaloupe, carrots, winter squash, apricots, peppers, and mangoes
- Orange-yellow: tangerines, oranges, peaches, papayas, pineapples, peppers, and nectarines
- Yellow: corn, lemons, peppers, and yellow squash
- Green: salad greens, kiwi, broccoli, avocados, brussels sprouts, chives, green onions, parsley, cilantro, green beans, spinach, peppers, Swiss chard, and kale
- White-green: celery, asparagus, honeydew, and pears
- White: mushrooms, onions, cauliflower, garlic, leeks, shallots, bananas, artichokes, and bamboo shoots

That's just a partial listing of all the colourful foods in God's creation, but the next time you sit down for a meal, regard what's on your plate or in your hand, and you'll find your dietary true colours.

The Five Tastes

The ten thousand taste buds on your tongue can detect five tastes: sweet, sour, salty, bitter, and umami. The latter one, umami (pronounced *oo-MAH-mee*) is a meaty, savoury taste that's responsive to free glutamates—like monosodium glutamate (MSG)—as well as the savoury tastes of Parmesan and Roquefort cheese. Since we were created with five distinct tastes, it's important to consume foods and beverages that supply *all* these tastes, not just the sweet and salty foods that define much of the Canadian diet. Exposing yourself to all five food tastes will open your palate to a wider variety of foods and the beneficial properties they impart to the body.

Given a little time, you could have a hankering for venison, goat's cheese, and kefir—three of my personal favourites!

Eating With the Seasons

My grandmother Rose, the youngest of seven children, grew up on a Polish farm the first thirteen years of her life. Her father owned a mill where they pressed poppy seeds and flaxseeds into oil during the fall harvest. She and her brothers and sisters loved gathering the pressed seeds and patting them into hard cakes, which were dipped into *schmaltz,* the rendered fat from chicken soup.

When autumn gave away to the inevitably harsh winter, the Catz family consumed only cooked foods, save for the barrel of sauerkraut they kept in the cellar as a source of veggies. They ate what was in season because they had no other choice.

Today, thanks to hulking container ships the size of football fields and fleets of interstate truckers, we can shop for fresh fruits and vegetables year-round: table grapes from Chile, ruby red strawberries from New Zealand, Haas avocados from Mexico, and pineapple and papaya from Costa Rica. Even though we can shop for great-tasting produce any day of year, should we?

Not necessarily. Traditionally throughout history, people have eaten the foods that were available in season, just as Grandma Rose did when she was a young girl. While it's not the end of the world if you snack on a bowl of Chilean grapes while watching the snow pile up outside your living room window, it makes more sense to eat warm foods when there's a blizzard outside—just as it's common sense to consume mouth-watering fruits during a heat wave. I know that Nicki instinctively craves homemade chicken soup when Florida winter nights turn cool, and I could eat watermelon all day long when our summer heat feels like an inferno. In traditional Chinese medicine, it is believed that cooked foods impart warming properties to the body and raw foods impart cooling properties.

Many Canadians who suffer from metabolic or thyroid issues have a low basal body temperature, so consuming cold, raw foods during the middle of winter makes things worse. That's why someone living in Medicine Hat, Alberta, in the month of January should consume mostly cooked vegetables, plenty of nourishing soups, cooked healthy meats, and whole grains cooked with healthy oils. Those living in West Palm Beach in the month of July should consume lots of raw fruits, salads, and juices.

If you've never given the concept of "eating with the seasons" a thought, then begin paying attention to what you eat based on the time of year and the temperature outside. Speaking in general terms, here's how I see the ratios breaking down:

- In winter, try to eat 75 percent cooked foods and 25 percent raw foods. Eat warming foods like fish, chicken, beef, lamb, and venison. Potatoes, onions, and garlic fit well, as do eggs.
- In spring, try to eat 50 percent cooked foods and 50 percent raw foods. This time of year, tender, leafy vegetables are popping up in stores: Swiss chard, spinach, romaine lettuce, fresh parsley, and basil.
- In summer, try to eat 25 percent cooked foods and 75 percent raw foods. Peaches, cherries, watermelon, strawberries, pears, and plums are in their seasonal glory.
- In fall, try to eat 50 percent cooked foods and 50 percent raw foods. Look for more warming foods like root vegetables, sweet potatoes, onions, and garlic.

Here's a guide to when certain fruits and vegetables are at their peak:

- **Spring:** asparagus, blackberries, green onions, leeks, lettuces, new potatoes, peas, red radishes, rhubarb, spinach, strawberries, and watercress.
- **Summer:** apricots, blueberries, cherries, eggplant, fresh herbs, green beans, hot peppers, melon, okra, peaches, plums, sweet corn, sweet peppers, tomatoes, and zucchini.

- **Fall:** apples, broccoli, brussels sprouts, cauliflower, collards, grapes, kale, pears, persimmons, pumpkins, winter squash, and yams.
- **Winter:** beets, cabbage, carrots, citrus fruits, daikon radishes, onions, rutabagas, turnips, and winter squash.

Eating with the seasons is a concept that's been forgotten in this country, thanks to modern-day shipping, but the seasons form a natural backdrop for eating and a source for diversity. When you buy foods produced from distant areas, this weakens the market for locally grown food and dampens regional economic viability. This is a truly green concept since when you shop locally for local produce, you reduce fuel consumption by shipping and trucking, and hence greenhouse gases, while supporting local enterprises.

The Dirty Dozen

No matter what time of year, you will be stealing from your future *and* robbing your health if you eat any of these foods that I call the "Dirty Dozen."

I wouldn't be surprised if some of these are among your favourite foods to eat. Nor would I be surprised if you find my list of "Dirty Dozen" foods to be controversial. When you eliminate these foods from your shopping list and/or toss out what's left in your cupboards and refrigerator, however, you will take a major step toward excellent health and reaching your perfect weight.

The following "Dirty Dozen" items should never find a way onto your plate or into your hands:

1. All pork products

Did you just sit up in your chair? I'm sure I got your attention because Canadians and Americans *love* pork. Fast-food establishments have watched their earnings sizzle by topping every hamburger and chicken sandwich in sight with strips of salty bacon; they go by names like Bacon Mushroom Melt, Big Bacon Classic, Cravin' Bacon Cheeseburger, Mesquite Bacon Cheeseburger, and Arch Deluxe with Bacon. I would imagine that Canada's favourite pizza toppings are pepperoni (a pork product) and Hawaiian (pineapple and ham). Only the Chinese, who have four times the population of the United States and Canada, consume more pork meat than us.

I've met people who have told me they have an emotional attachment to bacon for breakfast and pork chops with mashed potatoes and gravy for dinner. That was how they were raised, and maybe you feel the same way. Marketed brilliantly as "the other white meat," pork chops and pork ribs are usually the most inexpensive meats on display at the supermarket. Many folks eat pork three times a day: ham and eggs in the morning; a "BLT" sandwich—bacon, lettuce, and tomato—or a bacon-topped burger for lunch; and pork "barbecue" or pork tenderloin for a hearty supper. Others love snacking on pork rinds—the cooked skin of pigs. (I think I'm going to lose my lunch.)

So what's my beef with pork? My aversion to sowbelly is partly based on a pig's physiology. A pig's fast-acting physiological makeup and instinct allow them to eat any swill thrown at their muddy feet. Well, maybe swill isn't the right word. Actually, I'm thinking about the old saying: *Happy as a pig in slop.*

Yes, pigs will chomp on pails of you-know-what and not be bothered in the least. They will derive nutrition from human excrement dredged from a latrine pit, eliminating a sanitary problem for their rural masters. Even their own waste tastes fine to them. Although it's anecdotal, I heard the story about the pig farmer who stacked ten pigs in individual wire cages, one on top of another. All the farmer had to do was feed the pig in the penthouse cage and let trickle-down economics prove itself. As I'm fond of saying in my seminars, "Remember, if you eat the meat of animals, you are not just what you eat; you are what they ate!"

As for their physiology, pigs have a simple stomach arrangement. Whatever a pig eats goes straight into a simple stomach, where's it's rudimentarily digested and pushed out the back end. Total transit time: four hours.

Now compare the pig's digestive tract to animals that are OK to eat, such as cows, goats, sheep, oxen, deer, buffalo, and so forth. These animals put their vegetarian diet—they usually chomp on grasses, alfalfa, and hay—through a "wash and rinse cycle," thanks to a stomach and a secondary cud receptacle available for the task. Instead of a speedy four hours to digest and eliminate their waste, these animals take a more leisurely twenty-four hours.

Another reason I don't eat pork is my Jewish background. In Leviticus and Deuteronomy, two of the first five books of the Torah (if you're Jewish) or the Bible's Old Testament (if you're Christian), God forbade the Hebrew people to eat swine:

> You shall not eat any detestable thing. These are the animals which you may eat: the ox, the sheep, the goat, the deer, the gazelle, the roe deer, the wild goat, the mountain goat, the antelope, and the mountain sheep. And you may eat every animal with cloven hooves, having the hoof split into two parts, and that chews the cud, among the animals. Nevertheless, of those that chew the cud or have cloven hooves, you shall not eat, such as these: the camel, the hare, and the rock hyrax; for they chew the cud but do not have cloven hooves; they are unclean for you. Also the swine is unclean for you, because it has cloven hooves, yet does not chew the cud; you shall not eat their flesh or touch their dead carcasses.
>
> —Deuteronomy 14:3–8

The Scriptures used Hebrew words that can be translated as "foul," "polluted," and "putrid" to describe these "unclean meats" that were to be banished from their diets. What were God's reasons for doing so?

It wasn't because the Israelites didn't have refrigerated trucks following them from Egypt to the Promised Land to keep ham, bacon, or baby back ribs in a cool environment "safe" for consumption. No, God scratched pork from their meal plan because He knew all about their physiology, and He created them to be nature's garbage cleaners.

If you decide to strike pork from your diet, I'm predicting that you won't miss sausage, bologna, salami, bacon, and butchered cuts from the hog at all. I promise you there are great alternatives.

Some of you will feel that swearing off pork completely is too drastic—too radical given your attachment to Easter ham and Canadian bacon on your pizza. If that's the case, remember that every time you choose beef, chicken, or fish—especially from organic sources—you are taking a fantastic leap forward in your health, but each time you take a bite of crisp bacon, grilled sausage, and shredded pork, you are falling further behind.

2. Shellfish and crustaceans

If you were blown away by my recommendation to strike pork from your diet, I'm not done yet. Atlantic lobster harvested off the east coast of Canada may be called the "king of seafood" and be a dinnertime staple in Nova Scotia, but the crustacean is extremely unhealthy to eat and should be avoided. Even seafood chowder, one of the great "comfort foods" in Canada, shouldn't be eaten because it contains clams, which are shellfish.

I understand how popular lobster, crabs, and clams are in Canada; it's the same in the States. Invariably, whenever I take my wife, Nicki, out to dinner at an expensive seaside restaurant in South Florida, a waiter with a French accent will approach our table and say, "Monsieur et Madame, ze special tonight is pork tenderloin ringed with Alaskan crab and drizzled with a lobster sauce."

But that's not what I heard. His description sounded more like this: *Monsieur et Madame, ze special tonight is fresh garbage, ringed with raw sewage and drizzled with solid waste.*

Stay with me here. Shellfish and crustaceans, as well as fish without fins and scales such as catfish, shark, and eel, were also declared to be "detestable" back in Moses's day. The reasons are similar to those that make pigs out of bounds: lobsters, crabs, shrimp, and catfish are bottom-feeders. They troll along the seabed or lakebed, sustaining themselves with fish waste. The physiology of crabs, clams, and lobsters means that whatever they consume goes straight into their system, which is why scientists can measure water pollution by checking the flesh of shellfish and crustaceans for toxin levels. While all this "clean up" is great for water quality and one of nature's ways to scrub the aquatic environment, eating shellfish and crustaceans is not good for your bodies or your health.

3. Processed meats and hydrolyzed soy protein

The quintessential processed meat of all time is Spam, a syllabic abbreviation of "**S**houlder of **P**ork and h**AM**." Actually, Spam's name should be an acronym for "**S**pecially **P**rocessed **A**merican **M**eat," because it deserves Hall of Fame status in the pantheon of faux foods. Spam is one of those mystery meats sold in Canadian supermarkets alongside tins of Klik, Prem, Holiday, Spork, and Kam. When you eat canned luncheon meat or breakfast links, frankfurters, salisbury steaks, bologna, sausages, and salami—where you have *no* idea what part of the steer or pig was used. You can figure, though, that you're eating ground-up stomach, snout, intestines, spleens, edible fat, and even lips.

One thing you can be sure of is that processed meats contain nitrates to convey flavour, give meats their blood-red colour, and resist the development of botulism spores. Nitrates can convert to nitrites, which have been studied for decades in public and private settings and found to cause cancer and tumours in test animals. While we're on this unpleasant topic, I would also steer clear of processed turkey and chicken luncheon meat for the same nitrate reasons.

You may be wondering what hydrolyzed soy protein is all about. Have you ever substituted imitation crab for the real stuff when making a pasta dish for the family? Sprinkled imitation bacon bits on their salad? Ordered inexpensive sushi at a restaurant? All these foods, which are not part of the Perfect Weight Canada program, are forms of hydrolyzed soy protein.

Hydrolyzed soy protein usually contains a significant amount of genetically modified soy as well as compounds that closely mirror the dangerous monosodium glutamate, or MSG. Hydrolyzed soy protein is also a known excitotoxin, which means it has the potential to cause neurological disturbances. It's not fish or fowl, and it's not real food.

4. White flour

One major reason why we have an obesity epidemic is because the standard North American diet is weighted way too heavily with sketchy foods containing refined grains where the wheat has been stripped of wheat germ, bran, and half of the healthy fatty acids during the milling process. The end result is something called "enriched white flour," but the only reason why enriched flour is bright white is because the wheat stalks are rinsed with various chemical bleaches that sound like a vocabulary test from a high school biology class: nitrogen oxide, chlorine, chloride, nitrosyl, and benzoyl peroxide. The "enriched" adjective comes from the millers adding a few isolated and synthetic vitamins and minerals back into the nutritionally stripped flour, but that's like dressing a play doll in tattered clothes.

Enriched flour, the main ingredient in nearly all the bread and buns on supermarket shelves as well as a zillion other food items baked in commercial bakeries, is easy to spot on the list of ingredients: it's usually the first item listed. The healthy alternative is purchasing or making your own whole-grain bread from unprocessed whole-grain flour.

5. Hydrogenated oils

Pick up a loaf of white bread at the supermarket, and you will notice that hydrogenated oils or partially hydrogenated oils are usually recorded right after enriched white flour on the ingredient list. If you see any words with the "hydro-" prefix or "partially" on a package or box, don't buy it. If a friend offers you a packaged doughnut or cupcake, don't eat it.

During the hydrogenation process, hydrogen gas is injected into the oil under high pressure to make the oil solid at room temperature and prevent the oil from becoming rancid too quickly, but as mentioned earlier, this hydrogenation process produces an ugly stepchild: trans fats. Research shows that trans fats by far are the most dangerous for your heart. They lower the good HDL cholesterol, increase the bad LDL cholesterol, and increase triglycerides as well as another dangerous fat called lipoprotein (a).

As mentioned earlier, if the ingredient list includes the words "shortening," "partially hydrogenated vegetable oil" or "hydrogenated vegetable oil," then the food contains trans fat. Even if the ingredients label says "zero trans fat," that doesn't mean what you think it does; the FDA allows food manufacturers to have any amount less than 0.5 grams of trans fat in the food (per serving) and still legally say "zero trans fats" on the packaging.

It's a good idea when you're eating in a restaurant to ask the server if the kitchen is using partially hydrogenated oil for frying, baking, or cooking their dishes. Ask about salad dressings as well.

6. Pasteurized, homogenized skim milk

When it comes to dairy products, the conventional wisdom in the diet world can be summed up in this way: whole milk, bad; skim milk, good.

Whole milk is loaded with fat and calories, right? But removing the fat to make 2 percent or skim milk makes the milk less nutritious and less digestible as well as cause allergies. Yes, whole milk has more calories, but I've seen research suggesting that the mix of nutrients found in milk, such as calcium and protein, may improve the body's ability to burn fat, particularly around the midsection. Besides, the thought of a cow naturally delivering reduced fat or fat-free milk is "udderly" ridiculous, but I'm going to milk this topic for all it's worth because milk does a body good. (End of cliché alert.)

The richest food sources of calcium are milk and milk products, but I don't recommend drinking any commercially homogenized and pasteurized milk. The pasteurization process alters vital amino acids, which reduces your ability to access the proteins, fats, minerals, and great vitamins like vitamin A, vitamin B_{12}, vitamin D, and folic acid found in raw, unpasteurized milk. The homogenization process may be even more dangerous as it alters the fat globules and creates a compound known as XO, or xanthine oxidase, which is believed by some to cause damage to the arterial walls and may lead to an increased risk for cardiovascular disease.

I recommend drinking unpasteurized milk from grass-fed animals instead of homogenized, pasteurized milk. Unfortunately, raw milk can be dangerous if it comes from a farm that lacks sanitary practices, which is why it's not available in Canada. Farmers that sell unpasteurized milk face stiff fines and even jail time—even if they give it away! Since raw milk is viewed as a risk to human health, the only way to purchase raw dairy is go underground. A farmer interviewed by CTV News said that according to a government document, 250,000 Canadians drink unpasteurized milk, and some travel more than 200 kilometres to buy their illegal milk.[32]

The only good news is that Canada permits the sale of raw milk cheese that is aged for at least sixty days. The next best thing is finding cultured or fermented dairy whole-milk products, such as yogurt and kefir, which are produced from pasteurized, nonhomogenized milk.

If you can get used to its "goaty" smell and taste, goat's milk is naturally homogenized, less allergenic, and more rapidly absorbed in the digestive tract. Goat's cheese, which has become widely available in the last few years, is very healthy, as is cheese made from raw cow's milk. My favourite dairy products are made from sheep's milk, which are easy to digest and more nutritious than dairy products made from cow's or goat's milk. I find the creamy taste wonderful. Look for sheep's milk yogurt and cheese at your local natural foods grocery, although I'm not so sure how widely available these dairy products are in Canada.

I don't believe commercial organic milk is the answer, however. Some companies with organic brand names you would recognize produce pasteurized and homogenized milk.

7. White sugar

I'll bet you a loonie or two that any food with enriched flour also contains sugar or one of its sweet relatives—high-fructose corn syrup, fructose, and sucrose. You'll find these sugars among the first ingredients listed in candy bars, pastries, snack cakes, cookies, and ice cream. You will also find plenty of sugar in foods you might think are healthy, like "natural" breakfast cereals, energy bars, raisin bagels, certain whole-wheat breads, hot dog buns, salad dressing, steak sauce, ketchup—the list is endless.

Sugar is so omnipresent that most people don't realize they eat sugar with every meal: their breakfast cereal is frosted with sugar; break time is soda or coffee mixed with sugar and a Danish; lunch has its cookies and treats; and dinner could be sweet-and-sour ribs, sweet potatoes covered with marshmallows, a garden salad doused with artificially sweetened dressing, and a sugary parfait for dessert. Talk about adding a sweet exclamation point to the day! Statistics Canada estimates that Canadians eat about 23 teaspoons of added sugar each day, a total that includes refined sugars, honey, and maple syrup. Those twenty-three teaspoons don't include all the other added sugars that Canadians received from the consumption of high fructose corn syrup, the main ingredient in soft drinks.[33]

If you're looking for a guilty party to blame for the bellies hanging over beltlines, then look no further than King Sugar, which takes sugarcane or sugar beets from the fields and processes it 99.9 percent before it's dumped into 5-pound bags of bleached white sugar. (I'm sure research scientists are working overtime to remove the last one-tenth of 1 percent in sugarcane that's healthy.)

According to Ann Louise Gittleman, author of *How to Stay Young and Healthy in a Toxic World*, "Sugar is not an innocent substance that gives us pleasure and causes no harm. Quite the contrary; there is perhaps nothing else in the diet that promotes disease and aging more over the long term than excess sugar."[34] She says that more than sixty ailments, ranging from allergies to vaginal yeast infections, have been associated with this dietary demon.

"Without a doubt the biggest change in our diets has been our sugar consumption—in the forms of refined white sugar known as sucrose, brown sugar, corn sweeteners, high-fructose corn syrup, dextrose, glucose, lactose and maltose," said Ann Louise Gittleman. "Over the past two centuries, we have literally shocked our bodily systems with outrageous and ever-growing amounts of nutrient-robbing sugar."[35]

Attention: that the national obsession for sugar makes for a pounding headache when you cut it from your diet. When you change your diet and cut out drastic amounts of sugar, you can expect to experience withdrawal-like symptoms like less energy, gyrating mood swings, and monster cravings.

8. Soft drinks

A 12-ounce, sugar- or high-fructose corn syrup–sweetened beverage contains nearly 9 teaspoons of sugar and 150 calories—empty calories that provide little or no nutritional value. If you drink one can of soda per day and don't change anything else about your diet or exercise regimen, you will consume 55,000 extra calories in one year, which adds up to fifteen pounds of weight gain.

Soft drink manufacturers know that once teenagers leave the adolescent years, they become more health conscious, or at least more aware of how bad sweetened soft drinks are for them, so that's why they try to hook 'em young. Nicki swore off soft drinks during her senior year of high school, but not because she wanted a better fit in her prom dress. Her epiphany came after conducting an experiment in her science class. One day her teacher informed the class that they were going learn about acidic reaction. He dramatically dropped a galvanized construction nail into a glass of Coke to see what would happen overnight. The nail didn't dissolve—that was an old wives' tale—but the red rust encrusting the galvanized nail blew Nicki away. She hasn't had another soft drink since then.

9. High-fructose corn syrup

High-fructose corn syrup, or corn sweetener, is more than plain bad for you—it's horrible for your health and the worst form of sugar. The United States and Canada are the only countries with significant consumption of high-fructose corn syrup, which is a major contributor to weight gain because foods with fructose may not turn off your hunger signals. You get hungry *after* eating a snack containing high-fructose corn syrup because you're not satiated. Your appetite is saying, "Nice try, but I'm still famished!"

With such a high-falutin' name, you'd think that a sweetener with the word *corn* in it wouldn't be as bad for you as regular white sugar, but it is. With high-fructose corn syrup (HFCS), research scientists invented an enzymatic processing method that begins with milling corn to produce cornstarch, which is then made sweeter by chemically converting some of the glucose to fructose. The more fructose in the end product, the sweeter it is. A widely used variety of HFCS, known as 55-HFCS, consists of 55 percent fructose and 42 percent glucose. Thanks to a system of price supports and sugar quotas established in Ottawa and Washington DC, sugar imports have become cost-prohibitive, which has opened up a huge market for companies manufacturing high-fructose corn syrup.

Coca-Cola and Pepsi dumped the sugar from their carbonated soft drinks back in 1984, substituting cheaper HFCS in its place. These days you'd be hard-pressed to walk into a 7-Eleven and find a soda pop sweetened with sugar. The only holdout I could find was Goose Island sodas, although Jolt Cola did use sugar one time with the following marketing slogan: "All the sugar and twice the caffeine." But the makers of Jolt Cola reformulated their product with high-fructose corn syrup, no doubt to make the product less expensive in the stores. I'm sure the opportunity to lower costs is the reason why high-fructose corn syrup has become the principal sweetener in fruit juices, baked goods, canned fruits, dairy products, cookies, gum, and jams and jellies.

So what makes high-fructose corn syrup such an unhealthy, fat-promoting form of sugar?

The body handles fructose differently than it does other sugars. For starters, the body metabolizes fructose into triglycerides more than other sugars, which raises blood triglycerides significantly and increases the risk of heart disease. (Triglycerides are the body's storage form for fat and are found in fat tissues.) Unlike glucose, fructose does not stimulate leptin, the hormone that tells you "I'm full," but reduces ghrelin hormone levels, which tell you "I'm still hungry." Consumption of fructose from corn sweeteners comes with no enzymes, vitamins, or minerals, so it cheats the body of micronutrients. HFCS is different from the natural fructose found in whole fruit because with fruit, the body gets the enzymes, vitamins, and minerals to help with digestion and utilization of the fructose.[36]

King Corn

I like to pick up a freshly cooked ear of fresh, organic corn and dig in at a summer picnic, but I'm having some trouble digging up some sympathy for this simple vegetable—or grain. (Corn should be considered a vegetable when consumed raw and a grain when cooked.) Economists say that we can blame corn for the sharp spike in Canadian grocery prices in the last year, and that's likely to continue as an ever-increasing amount of corn is being diverted to make ethanol to mix with gasoline. In the United States, ethanol now gobbles up 18 percent of the domestic corn supply, up from 10 percent in 2002, an increase no doubt mirrored in Canada.[37] As corn prices move up to meet the demand for ethanol, this raises production costs for all sorts of foods: dairy cows eat corn to make milk, hens consume corn to lay eggs, and cattle, hogs, and chickens are fattened on corn before slaughter. I've already detailed how corn syrup is the main sweetener of soda pop and thousands of other food items.

Future outlook: look for King Corn to tighten its grip over its subjects.

The liver cannot handle fructose very well. When fructose reaches the liver, says Dr. William J. Whelan, a biochemist the University of Miami School of Medicine, "the liver goes bananas and stops everything else to metabolize the fructose." The fructose propels the liver into a fat-promoting mode by activating the formation of enzymes that lead to elevated levels of "bad" cholesterol and triglycerides.[38]

The consumption of high-fructose corn syrup in beverages has certainly left its fingerprints vis-à-vis our nation's obesity epidemic. In the United States, the consumption of high-fructose corn syrup increased 1,000 percent between 1970 and 1990, far exceeding the changes in intake of any other foods or food group.[39] Juice drinks like Minute Maid's Hi-C are among the worst offenders: despite flavours like Blazin' Blueberry and Orange Lavaburst, Hi-C lists pure filtered water and high-fructose corn syrup as its first and second ingredients.

At least they're filtering the water!

10. Artificial sweeteners

Dieting and artificial sweeteners go together like…ham and eggs? *Mea culpa* for the jarring simile, but the huge demand for low-calorie and sugar-free foods and beverages by those seeking to consume fewer calories has created a $6 billion market for artificial sweeteners. Aspartame, saccharin, and sucralose are found in umpteen thousands of foods as well as in blue, pink, and yellow packets of Equal, Sweet'N Low, and Splenda found on restaurant tables.

I will fully address the safety of artificial sweeteners in chapter 10, "Reduce Toxins for Your Perfect Weight" (sneak preview: they're toxic and dangerous), but if you have always thought that artificial sweeteners will help you lose weight, you might want to rethink your position. Researchers at Purdue University say these sugar substitutes could interfere with the body's natural ability to count calories based on a food's sweetness. In other words, drinking a diet soft drink instead of the full-octane sugar version will reduce your caloric intake, but it could also trick the body into thinking that other sweet items don't have as many calories either. This sort of thinking gives weight-conscious people another mental alibi for overindulging in sweet foods and beverages.[40]

I understand the rationale behind drinking low-cal or no-cal drinks—lower total caloric intake—but sipping artificially sweetened drinks is not the solution. Sweeteners like aspartame are addicting, but as bad as sugar and high-fructose corn syrup can be for your body, I'd rather you consume them than artificial sweeteners. They're that bad for you.

11. Artificial flavours and artificial colours

The dictionary definition of *artificial* refers to something not made by human beings or a copy of something natural. Since the goal of Perfect Weight Canada is to eat natural foods, anything containing artificial flavours or artificial colours will be naturally unhealthy as well as increase the toxic load on the body.

Take the recipe for Waldorf-Astoria Red Velvet Cake—please! The cooking instructions for this ooh-la-la confection, which originated at the iconic Manhattan hotel, calls for squeezing two bottles of FD&C Red No. 40 into a mixing bowl filled with the requisite shortening, flour, eggs, and sugar. Pastry chefs say they have to wear gloves to keep the shameful dye off their skin or rub nail polish remover if any red spots appear on their double-breasted white jackets.

"Why should a dose of Red No. 40 turn Betty Crocker into Hester Prynne?" asked Slate.com writer Daniel Engber, referring to the fictional colonial woman forced to wear a scarlet letter "A" for committing adultery. "Ask a gourmand, and you're likely to hear three specious answers. First, Epicurean: *Artificial color tastes bad*. Second, Hippocratic: *It's bad for your health*. And third, Platonic: *It makes food unnatural*."[41]

Don't purchase foods that list artificial flavours and colours on the packaging. These additives have been linked to behavioural problems in children and increase the body's toxic load. They have also been associated with allergies and skin rashes.

12. Beer, wine, and alcoholic drinks

If you like to watch a hockey game with a beer in hand or dine with a glass of fine wine, I have some troublesome news for you: during the first three phases of the Perfect Weight Eating Plan in chapter 7, I'm asking you not to drink any alcohol.

Although I'm a teetotaller who may enjoy a glass of organic wine a couple of times a year, I recognize that there have been studies pointing out the benefits of drinking modest amounts of red wine for cardiovascular health. The "French Paradox," so called for the observation that the French typically suffer low rates of heart disease despite having a diet rich in saturated fats, was attributed to alcohol and olive oil intake. The "French Paradox" is only a paradox if you assume that saturated fat is the cause of obesity and heart disease—something I point out in the next section. No wonder the French—eating all kinds of real food to their hearts' content and toasting family and friends with a glass of *vin rouge*—have that certain *joie de vivre*. (Note to the Québécois: I've now officially used up all the French I know.)

So you're welcome to open a bottle of nice wine in Phase IV of the Perfect Weight Eating Plan, but I balance alcohol's benefits against the downside of excessive drinking, which damages family relationships as well as every organ in the body (especially the liver), promotes depression, causes digestive ailments (ulcers, gastritis, and pancreatitis), and impacts fertility. Alcohol adds weight, a full 7 calories per gram, almost twice that of protein or carbs. That's a significant reason why we see beer bellies in this world.

If you are a regular drinker, see how you feel after you've jumped on the Perfect Weight Canada bandwagon. I'm not saying that you should never have another adult beverage or savour a fine glass of wine with an exquisite meal again, but you may realize that drinking has become a weight-inducting habit that needs to be trimmed back.

The Top Healing Foods

As part of Perfect Weight Canada, the following top healing foods should find a way onto your grocery list.

Grass-fed meat

Let me make another case for staying away from commercially produced beef and chicken and purchasing organic, grass-fed, and pastured cuts of meat. Michael Pollan, author of the excellent book *The Omnivore's Dilemma*, says it's not necessarily our food that's making us sick but what we feed our food.[42] Commercially raised livestock are raised on corn, pumped full of antibiotics, and fattened as fast as possible to get them to market quickly. Seventy-five years ago, steers were four or five years old when they were led into the slaughterhouse. The age fell to two or three years in the 1960s. Today, "production" cattle are fattened up in fourteen to sixteen months before being carved up into roasts, steaks, and hamburger.

"Without cheap corn, the modern urbanization of livestock would probably have never occurred," said Pollan. "We have come to think of 'corn fed' as some kind of old-fashioned virtue; we shouldn't. Granted, a corn-fed cow develops well-marbled flesh, giving it a taste and texture American consumers have learned to like. Yet this meat is demonstrably less healthy to eat since it contains more saturated fat—up to 40 percent. Compare this to the 2 or 3 percent fat found in venison, caribou, or bison.

"A recent study in the *European Journal of Clinical Nutrition* found that the meat of grass-fed livestock not only had substantially less fat than grain-fed meat but that the type of fats found in grass-fed meat were much healthier," Pollan continued. "A growing body of research suggests that many of the health problems associated with eating beef are really problems with corn-fed beef. In the same way ruminants have not evolved to eat grain, humans may not be well adapted to eating grain-fed animals. Yet the USDA's grading system continues to reward marbling—that is, intermuscular fat—and thus the feeding of corn to cows."[43]

I would like to encourage you to step out of your comfort zone and sample grass-fed buffalo, bison, lamb, and venison. Pasture lands in the Canadian prairie are raising meats that aren't "gamy" but rather have delightfully clean, subtle tastes that will please your palate. One of Nicki's signature dishes is a spinach-and-goat-cheese lasagna with ground buffalo meat she cooks whenever we have guests over. Another Rubin family favourite is Nicki's venison meat loaf. My mouth is watering as I type these words.

Grass-fed veal is another meat worth trying. I know that veal has been out of favour ever since the Humane Farming Association spearheaded a national veal boycott back in the 1980s. They purchased advertisements in Canadian and U.S. magazines picturing a frightened calf chained inside a twenty-two-inch crate so small that it could not turn around. The formula-fed veal calves were administered an anemic diet so that the distinctly white meat would retain a mild flavour that epicureans prize.

Seemingly overnight, factory-farm veal was about as socially acceptable as fur coats. Back in the 1960s, Americans ate just under 4 pounds of veal on average, but these days the per capita consumption has levelled off to only half a pound per year.[44] Canadians consume four times as much veal (2.5 pounds per year) as Americans, but that's just a scant amount compared to Canadians' taste for beef (70.3 pounds), chicken (67.7 pounds), and pork (50.5 pounds).[45]

Lately, however, veal has been making a comeback as farmers got the message and made changes in the way they raised their herds. "Unfortunately, I was a sinner," said John Holloway of Misty Morning Farm in Cherry Tree, Pennsylvania. "I did raise factory veal—all the chemicals, antibiotics, steroids I used. We wouldn't let our friends eat what we used to raise." Now all of Holloway's veal is pastured and organic and sold in stores with "Certified Humane" stickers.[46]

Fine meat purveyors and celebrity chefs like Wolfgang Puck say they've noticed the difference: organic veal is more flavourful because it's been allowed to walk around pastures. "If we feed the animals better, treat them better, we will have a better product and a healthier product," said Wolfgang Puck.[47]

Eat More Lamb

It's a shame that Canadians and Americans don't enjoy the taste of lamb. Canadians annual per capita consumption of lamb stands at almost 2.5 pounds, but even that modest amount puts Americans to shame. We consume a measly four-fifths of a pound, not much more than one grand meal a year—Passover or Easter—when you figure a 5-pound leg serves eight people.

I love lamb, and it doesn't have to be a special holiday occasion for lamb to be served at our dinner table. There's something about the golden brown skin and moist pink flesh that resembles beef but is accentuated with a distinctive but pleasing gamy taste. The way to my heart is to serve a lamb roulade—a deboned leg of lamb filled with herbed pesto and crumbled goat cheese, topped with a red wine reduction.

Lamb is high in vitamin B$_{12}$, which supports the production of red blood cells and allows nerves to function properly. The tender meat is also an excellent source of zinc, a mineral critical to immune function and wound healing. Carnitine is great for the heart. We've become big lamb eaters in the Rubin household because of its wonderful flavour. We love all the cuts, especially roasts and barbecued lamb chops. The chops come from the loin muscle, which gets very little exercise and is naturally tender. We also use ground lamb for burgers, meatballs, and meat loaf.

Better yet, more than half of the lamb we eat in the United States is imported from Australia and New Zealand, where herds are raised on dewy grasses found in valley meadows. Domestic lambs are often "finished" on grains, which means they're not grass-fed raised like the little lambs from Down Under and New Zealand.

We've got some catching up to do: Aussies and Kiwis eat more than fifty pounds of lamb per year.[48]

Wild-caught fish

Canadians have greater access to wild-caught fish than nearly any industrialized country in the world. That's great news, but wild-caught fish is more expensive that "farm-raised" salmon and trout, which spend their lives lazily circling around concrete tanks, fattening up on pellets of dubious man-made chow. These "feedlot" fish don't taste as good or pack the same nutritional punch as their cold-water cousins that streak through the Pacific Ocean or ford mountain streams sustaining themselves on small marine life. Fish caught in the wild provide a richer source of omega-3 fats, protein, vitamins, and minerals.

Many popular diets include canned tuna and salad as a lunchtime or dinner staple. I must note, though, that there's canned tuna, and there's *canned tuna*. What I mean is that much of the canned tuna on supermarket shelves comes with something else inside the 6-ounce tin: mercury. You should shop in health food stores for a low-mercury, high-omega-3 tuna that's extremely healthy and safe to consume. For recommended brands, check out the Perfect Weight Canada (PWC) Resource Guide in the back of the book or visit www.PerfectWeightCanada.com, and click on the PWC Resource Guide.

Fermented/cultured dairy products

Fermented? As in fermented cabbage or sauerkraut? Sort of, but not exactly. Dairy products like yogurt, kefir, cottage cheese, and cultured cream (also known as crème fraîche) are examples of lacto-fermented foods and have been around for centuries. Fermentation, also known as culturing, preserves dairy products for longer periods of time. Dairy products are usually stricken from most conventional diets because of the perceived "fat" they contain, but as I've been saying, natural and organic whole-milk dairy products—especially those made from sheep's milk and goat's milk—contain the right fats. I'm also a big fan of strained Greek yogurt, which is high in protein.

I recommend the following dairy products in the Perfect Weight Eating Plan in chapter 7:

- Whole-milk plain yogurt
- Sheep's milk yogurt
- Goat's milk yogurt (plain)
- Whole-milk cheese
- Soft goat's milk cheese
- Sheep's milk hard cheese
- Goat's milk hard cheese
- Feta cheese (sheep's milk)
- Full-fat plain kefir
- Full-fat cottage cheese
- Ricotta cheese
- Full-fat sour cream
- Plain almond milk

- Goat's milk protein powder (substitute for dry milk)
- Buttermilk

Fruits and veggies

Besides being low-calorie foods, fruits and veggies should be eaten in abundance anyway because of all the rich vitamins, minerals, and antioxidants they supply to the body. The government bureaucrats behind the USDA food pyramid came up with a "5 a Day" motto, but that recommendation has fallen on deaf ears as Americans swarm fast-food and sit-down restaurants. (I would imagine the same situation exists in Canada.) Except for salads—which are usually tossed with a chemical-laden dressing to deliver a satisfying "mouth feel"—people don't order many entrees with vegetables. If the main meal does come with any veggies, it's often a few twigs of overcooked and unappetizing broccoli. And fresh fruits just aren't sold in restaurants; the proprietors would rather pad their profits by enticing you to order *mousse au chocolat* or apple pie à la mode.

Rather than counting servings of fruits and vegetables, I would adopt a mind-set that says a meal is not complete without eating some fruits and/or vegetables. I've already mentioned one of my favourite foods—berries. Blueberries, blackberries, raspberries, and strawberries are nutritional powerhouses: low in calories and among the highest antioxidant-containing foods on the planet. I seem to recall that some scientific evidence suggests that blueberries prevent age-related memory loss, but I forget where I heard that. (Just teasing.) Seriously, berries are the unsung heroes of good nutrition.

I'm jealous that Canadians have so many wonderful berries to enjoy. Blueberries, my personal favourite, are native to Canada, and I hear the wild blueberries in Nova Scotia are to die for. Ditto for juniper berries and raspberries.

Figs, whether eaten fresh or dried, are a good source of fibre and potassium, a mineral that helps control blood pressure. If you have blood work done prior to starting Perfect Weight Canada, there's a good chance that you'll have a potassium deficiency, which is a sign that you're not eating enough fruits and vegetables and consuming too much sodium found in processed foods. Upping your intake of organic fruits and veggies will turn these numbers around in a heartbeat.

Also, don't overlook cultured and fermented vegetables such as sauerkraut, pickled carrots, beets, and cucumbers, which are some of the healthiest foods on the planet. If you're not a big fan of sauerkraut or pickled beets, try adding pickled relish atop broiled fish. Fermented foods are excellent sources of digestion-enhancing probiotics and enzymes.

Soups and stocks

There's nothing better than zesty soup made from scratch with fibre-rich vegetables such as celery, carrots, onion, and zucchini, especially when it's freezing outside. I'm thinking of Winnipeg in mid-January. (For more on eating with the seasons, see page 68.)

My grandmother Rose, being of European Jewish heritage, was big on homemade chicken soup, which she called "Jewish penicillin." Countless times she delivered containers of her homemade chicken soup to my bedside when I was hospitalized after those horrible illnesses afflicted me as a college student.

The recuperative effects of chicken soup date as far back as the twelfth century when the Jewish physician and philosopher Moses Maimonides recommended its use for the treatment of respiratory infections. When you're hacking away and battling a cold, chicken soup acts as an anti-inflammatory, meaning that sipping chicken soup reduces the inflammation that occurs when coughs and congestion strike the respiratory tract. In addition, chicken soup keeps a check on inflammatory white blood cells, also known as neutrophils, which are produced by the onset of cold symptoms.

While a hearty soup is good for the soul when there's a raging blizzard outside, I've found that I like a hot soup during Florida's frigid months, like when the highs barely get past 15°C. Seriously, when a cold snap sweeps through, I like to roll up my sleeves and make a soup from scratch. My specialty is Thai Coconut Chicken Soup, a spicy hot soup that dazzles the palate with subtle flavours. The unsweetened coconut milk is a flavourful counterbalance to the Thai chilies and stalks of lemon grass.

Thai Coconut Chicken Soup, like many soups, starts with a stock, which is also called broth. Stocks are extremely nutritious and swimming with minerals, cartilage, collagen, and electrolytes. Meat, fish, chicken, and turkey stocks also contain generous amounts of natural gelatin, an odourless, tasteless substance extracted by boiling bones and animal tissues. Easy to digest, gelatin aids in overall digestion. So the next time you bake a whole chicken or serve a holiday turkey, don't throw those bones in the trash. Use them to make a healthy stock that can form the basis of many great soups.

Extra-virgin coconut oil
Speaking of coconuts, organic extra-virgin coconut oil can be a wonderful ally in your quest to reach your perfect weight. Extra-virgin coconut oil has been the recipient of some great press the last few years for its ability to help balance the thyroid, aid in metabolism, and help the body with energy production. Some experts recommend that people with thyroid and weight troubles should consume as many as 2 to 4 tablespoons of coconut oil per day.

A balanced thyroid plays a vital role in your metabolism. Mary Shomon, author of *The Thyroid Diet*, says that certain foods high in tyrosine assist the body in the production of the thyroid hormone T3, which helps you utilize more oxygen and burn more calories.[49] Besides extra-virgin coconut oil, foods high in tyrosine are cottage cheese, egg whites, safflower seeds, and meats such as turkey, antelope, quail, and buffalo.

One way to add coconut oil to your diet is add some to a saucepan whenever you cook scrambled eggs; need to glaze diced onions, peppers, or other vegetables; or heat up leftovers. When I make smoothies, I often add a teaspoon of extra-virgin coconut oil among the ingredients. Coconut oil is one of those healthy fats that provide satiety and slow the absorption of sugar into the bloodstream, thereby keeping blood sugar and insulin levels on an even keel.

How to Be a Good Shopper

I know what you're thinking: "All those top healing foods sound fantastic, Jordan, but I can't afford to buy them."

The cost of organic foods is a barrier for many. It does cost more to shop in natural food stores, a 20 percent to 200 percent bigger bite out of the family food budget. The situation should improve as market forces and increasing consumer demand drive down prices. But here are some steps you can take in the interim:

- Realize that eating organic food prepared at home is far cheaper than taking the family out to eat at a sit-down family restaurant or even a fast-food joint. If you're a family of four, it costs anywhere from twenty dollars for burgers and fries to sixty-plus Canadian dollars or more for an Applebee's-type dining experience. For those amounts, you can eat *really* well at home for the same amount if you cook for yourself and your family.
- Eating the foods recommended in the Perfect Weight Eating Plan (see chapter 7) cost half as much as following a special diet or dietetic meal plan like Jenny Craig, CarbControl, or Weight Watchers.
- Keep in mind that those "convenience" foods—frozen pizza, Lunchables, Eskimo Pie ice cream bars—are more expensive than you think. A fresh peach is cheaper than peach low-fat yogurt. A banana is cheaper than a candy bar.

Build family dinners around:

- Healthy salads (romaine lettuce, radicchio, escarole, and endive) with tomatoes, celery, red onions, peppers, and avocados
- Healthy grains like amaranth, millet, buckwheat, and quinoa
- Healthy vegetables like spinach, broccoli, cauliflower, onions, sweet potatoes, and white potatoes
- Grass-fed meat, free-range chicken, and wild-caught fish, all served as a vital ingredient, not necessarily the main course

Look for deals when you shop—and stock up. Even the natural foods stores have "loss leaders" designed to get you in the store, where they figure you'll do the bulk of the family grocery shopping that week.

Where We Go From Here

Phew! This was our longest chapter, but eating the wonderful foods found in nature in a form healthy for the body is the key linchpin undergirding Perfect Weight Canada. In our next chapter, we'll turn our attention to liquid refreshments and how you can drink for your perfect weight.

Perfect Weight Recap: Eat for Your Perfect Weight

- Change the way you shop for food by purchasing fresh organic foods at a natural food or health food store or local farmer's market, if possible.
- Understand that processed foods are practically a foolproof guarantee that you'll be consuming genetically modified and refined flour, along with a variety of sweeteners, including bleached white sugar and high-fructose corn syrup.
- Look for ways to add fibre-rich foods such as nuts, seeds, beans, whole-grain sprouted breads, green peas, carrots, cucumbers, zucchini, tomatoes, and baked or boiled unpeeled potatoes to your diet. Foods high in fibre slow down the digestive process and satiate longer.
- Take the nutritional type test and determine whether you are a meat or potato type. Eat a diet based on your nutritional type and see how much better you feel.
- Eat healthy fats such as saturated fats, omega-3 polyunsaturated fats, and monounsaturated (omega-9 or oleic) fatty acids, which are abundant in salmon, lamb, goat's and sheep's milk and cheese, coconut, walnuts, olives, almonds, and avocados.
- Change the way you eat meat. Choose cuts from grass-fed and pastured cattle, not grain-fed cattle raised conventionally. For fish, purchase only fish that have been caught in oceans and rivers, not raised in concrete-lined "fish farms."
- Don't eat any more pork, shrimp, lobster, or other shellfish, which contain many more toxins in their flesh than beef and chicken.
- Double-check the "Dirty Dozen" list and take steps to cross off each of those foods from your shopping list.
- Realize that the best dairy products come from organic grass-fed cow's milk, goat's milk, and sheep's milk. When consuming dairy products, always choose whole-milk or full-fat varieties.

Chapter 4

Drink for Your Perfect Weight

Bob DeMoss, an accomplished writer who just turned fifty, has always had to watch his weight since he began tipping the scales in the 225-pound range back in his college years. So he started drinking Diet Coke to save calories without sacrificing his morning caffeine buzz.

Yup, I said *morning*. On a typical weekday around 7:00 a.m., Bob would cruise into Daily's, a gas-'n'-go mini-mart in Franklin, Tennessee, while chauffeuring his daughter to school. Then he'd carry out a Paul Bunyan–sized plastic cup topped off with 44 ounces (or 1.3 litres) of sugar-free Diet Coke, or what he called his first "44" of the day. "It had to be Diet Coke," he said. "If Daily's was out of Diet Coke, I'd go somewhere else."

Bob, who works out of his home on collaborative book projects, would nurse his "44" throughout the morning, then return to Daily's at lunchtime for a refill. "Since I always kept the cup, my refill price was considerably cheaper," he said. "A buck-fifty a day, seven days, worked out to ten dollars a week. As liquid treats go, that's not that bad, especially when compared to what you pay at Starbucks for one coffee drink." Because he was such a faithful customer, the friendly clerks at Daily's would occasionally wave him off and not charge him.

After finishing his second "44" in the mid-afternoon, Bob would mosey over to his private stash of Diet Coke two-litre bottles stacked up in the garage. "Whenever the price dropped from $1.29 to 89 cents, I would buy a stockpile of them," he said. It was time for another refill.

For thirty years, Bob figures that he consumed around 100 ounces of Diet Coke a day, which, according to my math, means he drank the equivalent of 9 12-ounce cans a day, 56 cans a week, 270 a month, 3,285 a year, or at least 98,550 Diet Cokes in his lifetime. But here's where Bob's story takes a twist: his Diet Coke fix came to a sudden halt in 2007 when he walked into his local Publix, strolled over to the soft drink aisle, and, as his hand reached for a two-litter, a voice in his head said, "No, don't do it."

Diet Coke has legions of fanatics just like Bob DeMoss. Florida State University football coach Bobby Bowden says that half his diet is drinking Diet Coke and the other half is eating peanuts. Victoria Beckham, married to British soccer celebrity David Beckham, claims to hate the taste of water and drinks nothing but Diet Coke.[1]

Diet Coke is the most popular diet soft drink in the world. As sales of diet drinks keep climbing (30 percent of the U.S. soda market in 2007, up from 25 percent in 2000[2]), Coke rolled out a new version of Diet Coke in the summer of 2007 with added vitamins and minerals called Diet Coke Plus. The blue-capped bottles contain 10 to 15 percent of the daily requirement of niacin, zinc, magnesium, and vitamins B_6 and B_{12}.

Whoop-de-doo. We fail to see the point, unless it's to fool heavy Diet Coke drinkers to actually think they're drinking something healthy. You're still ingesting aspartame, an artificial sweetener that has sparked debate for decades. H. J. Roberts, MD, an authority on artificial sweeteners, testified at U.S. congressional hearings that artificial sweeteners like aspartame, saccharin, and sucralose can be highly addictive and trigger toxic substances to cross the blood-brain barrier, causing neurological problems.[3]

Diet and "lite" beverages featuring industrial nonnutritive chemical sweeteners have been touted as the answer to the obesity epidemic for decades. Even people with diabetes could supposedly satisfy their sweet tooth. Saccharin—the chemical in Sweet'N Low—was the first artificial sweetener to market, and the compound is up to 700 times sweeter than table sugar. Since its introduction in the 1960s, though, saccharin has created a string of never-ending debates and fights over its safety, especially since laboratory experiments linked it to bladder cancer in rats.

Probably because of its slight metallic aftertaste, saccharin has been supplanted in popularity by aspartame—sold under the brand names NutraSweet or Equal—which has equally evoked controversies over its safety, including a possible link with brain tumours. Aspartame's breakdown products—methanol and formic acid—are known toxins in high concentrations. Aspartame and another popular sweetener, acesulfame K (marketed as Sweet One or Sunett), are up to 200 times sweeter than table sugar.

Sucralose, known commercially as Splenda, came out in 1998 and immediately made a splash by attempting to distance itself from the chemical aftertaste of popular artificial sweeteners. "Made from sugar, so it tastes like sugar" became its slogan. Clearly, this marketing strategy was designed to wrap Splenda in the cloak of being "natural," which is what the manufacturers of artificial sweeteners want you to believe.

"My wife, Leticia, has been after me for ten years to give up Diet Coke," Bob said. "Frankly, she was always lecturing me about it, and, admittedly, I should have listened a long time ago, but Diet Coke was my one little treat. I thought when I squeezed lemon into my Diet Coke that I was adding nutritional value to it."

Bob replaced his addiction for Diet Coke with…bottled water. Sure, there were some tough moments while he retrained his taste buds, but eventually his body accepted the "boring" taste of water. During a weak moment or two, however, Bob returned to his Daily's for a "44," but the icky-sweet chemical aftertaste now grossed him out. "It was interesting how quickly I lost desire for my favourite diet soft drink." These days Bob says he's a "water fiend." He now buys a thirty-four pack of bottled water at Sam's Club and keeps them stashed in the garage—where his Diet Cokes used to sit. Whenever he takes a drive, Bob brings two half-litre bottles of water for the road.

What was also interesting was how two other "significant events"—Bob's words—happened after he stopped drinking Diet Coke like it was coming out of a drinking fountain. First, his blood pressure dropped twenty points from a moderately high 149/96 to a nearly normal 130/70. "I wasn't expecting that," Bob said, but the second event surprised him even more. "When I stopped drinking all that Diet Coke, I felt less on edge. What I mean is that when I was drinking 44s and one of my children made the smallest infraction, I'd lose it and overreact. I wouldn't totally blow a gasket, but I'd be quicker to bark. Now I'm a different person. I have a much more even temperament. I don't know if it's caffeine or the artificial sweetener aspartame in Diet Coke, but definitely I seem to have a brighter outlook on life and feel more upbeat."

Bob says he's also moving in the right direction on his weight, and you will, too, when you stop drinking colas, diet soft drinks, "energy" drinks like Red Bull, and sports drinks like Gatorade and POWERade. Replacing your old ways of drinking liquid refreshments with water, green tea, certified organic coffee, fresh fruit and veggie juices, and lacto-fermented beverages will do wonders for your health *and* your perfect weight.

Nothing Like Water

Let's turn our attention first to plain old water, which is often overlooked as a weight-loss tool because it's so...ordinary. Any fluid replacement that's odourless and colourless seems downright boring compared to the sexier "fitness waters" and candy-coloured sports drinks you can buy at a Daily's convenience store, for example. Yet regular ol' water can play a significant role in losing weight because of the way it revs up your metabolism and hydrates cells so that they can process carbohydrates and fat more efficiently. When your body's cells are well hydrated, you accelerate the liver's ability to convert stored fat into usable energy and help your kidneys flush out toxins. If you substitute water for soft drinks—and ignore everything else written in *Perfect Weight Canada*—you'll still lose three pounds in short order, according to a study at Children's Hospital and Research Center in Oakland, California.[4]

Water is the ultimate calorie-free and sugar-free substance, the perfect libation. Only water is the perfect fluid replacement to regulate body temperature, carry nutrients and oxygen to the cells, cushion joints, protect organs and tissues, remove toxins, and maintain strength and endurance. Even when bottled, water is still a good deal—unless you're into an imported natural spring water from Tennessee called Bling H_2O, which comes in wine-sized frosted bottles embedded with Swarovski crystals spelling out its name and going for forty dollars a bottle. Bling, as you would imagine, is big with the Hollywood set, where the entertainment media reports that Paris Hilton fills her dog's water dish with the ultra-expensive couture water.

And I thought San Pellegrino was a treat.

Whenever I leave home for my office, I carry a half-gallon polycarbonate plastic container filled with fresh water that's run through my home filtration system. My goal is to drink the same amount of water daily that Bob DeMoss used to drink in his Diet Coke heyday—at least 100 ounces.

I'm a big water drinker because I know that H_2O hydrates my cardiovascular system, irrigates my digestive tract, keeps my body cool in the stifling Florida heat, and helps eliminate waste products from my body. Regularly sipping on my water bottle means I have to visit the restroom more often, but that's a small inconvenience for participating in one of the healthiest practices available to us. You honestly can't improve on plain water.

If you're looking to slim down, drinking plenty of water is just as important as choosing the right foods to eat. The most rigorous and challenging part of the Perfect Weight Eating Plan happens in the first week or two, when the body goes through a "purification" stage. When you suddenly stop eating foods with white sugar, artificial sweeteners, and preservatives, you may experience temporary withdrawal-type symptoms such as headaches, carbohydrate cravings, less energy, mood swings, or even changes in your bowel habits. These "detox" reactions are indications that the body is making adjustments while working to cleanse toxins from the system. Your body needs streams of water during this season of the "blahs." When the body is properly hydrated, the kidneys function normally, effectively removing waste from the body.

You can drink your water cold or lukewarm, as suits your personal taste, but don't drink water with added carbonation, like Perrier. Drinking still or natural sparkling spring water is the best, and consuming water before and during your meals will help you digest your food efficiently and prevent constipation.

How much water should you be drinking? A good rule of thumb is a half-ounce of water for every pound of body weight. As an example, since I weigh between 185 and 190 pounds, that means I should drink 95 ounces (or 2.8 litres) of water per day, or around twelve glasses. I know that's a lot of water—nearly 3 litres—but I usually reach my goal of 100 ounces since I carry my 64-ounce plastic container wherever I go. I try to consume around 32 ounces (nearly a litre) of water before I leave for the office, which is pretty easy for me since I exercise in the morning and guzzle water during my FIT exercise session. (You'll read more on FIT in chapter 9.)

Whenever I travel, I would carry my water jug right onto the plane, but that practice ended when the airport security screeners banned liquids and gels in carry-on baggage during the summer of 2006. These days I either buy a bottle of water before I board, or I ask the flight attendant for two cups (or a bottle) of water each time the beverage cart passes by. Flying is dehydrating due to the extremely dry cabin air, so I try to drink 8 to 16 ounces (around a third of a litre) of water each hour I'm in the air to maintain water levels in my radiator.

What's on Tap?

I mentioned that before I go to work in the morning, I fill a 64-ounce (nearly two litres) container with filtered water that comes directly from a water dispenser at my kitchen sink. The clear liquid comes from a municipal source responsible for making sure my family's water is safe for public consumption. While dependable and germ-free, municipal water still needs to be filtered before it can become a good source of hydration for you. Most drinking water straight from the tap contains over 700 chemicals, including excessive levels of lead.[5]

Municipal water, be it a major metropolis like Toronto to smaller centres and rural areas, undergoes a series of filtration steps to remove fine microorganisms and dissolved inorganic and organic materials. Throughout Canada, nearly all of the water used by municipal water systems comes from lakes and rivers, while the remainder (12 percent of the total) comes from groundwater. Often times, those living in remote areas have individual groundwater supplies.

But for sake of argument, the vast majority of Canadians drink municipal water, as is the case in the States. Even though Canadian water is known for its great taste and for being from pristine sources, it still must be disinfected at the treatment plant to destroy any pathogens that somehow made it through the filtration process. The most common disinfectant is chlorine or its chemical cousins—chloramines and chlorine dioxide.

Chlorine...yes, I'm talking about the granular white stuff the pool guy dumps into swimming pools so that nobody gets sick when the kiddies urinate in the pool. Chlorine is the disinfectant of choice for North American municipalities because it's cheap and doesn't seem to harm humans, but it's still a highly toxic substance. (Just ask Iraqi insurgents why they use chlorine bombs.) If your tap water is treated with chlorine—and it probably is—then I recommend you install water filters at your kitchen sink and between the water line and the refrigerator. A cheaper alternative costing less than thirty dollars would be purchasing a countertop water pitcher with a built-in carbon-based filter.

I went whole hog during the construction of our new home in Florida recently. I asked the contractor to install a whole-house filtration system using ultra filtration and reverse osmosis that would remove the chlorine and other impurities before the water entered our household pipes. Now, before I leave in the morning, I can fill my half-gallon container with filtered water and confidently know that I'm hydrating my body with the best refreshment resource available to me—right from my home.

You should always have a glass of water nearby as well. Reaching for a sip every now and then may not seem like a big deal, but if you don't keep yourself properly hydrated, reaching your perfect weight becomes that much harder.

What About Other Liquids?

I know that every diet book worth its salt—I hope saying "salt" makes you thirsty—encourages readers to drink at least the proverbial "eight glasses of water each day." I've read, however, that medical experts like the National Academy of Sciences' Institute of Medicine believe that the long-held recommendation to drink eight glasses of water is an old wives' tale. After reviewing more than four hundred studies, the National Academy said the majority of Americans already get enough fluids from the orange juice and coffee they drink, the milk on their breakfast cereal, the juicy orange they eat as a snack, the chicken soup they eat at lunch, and the ice-cold beer they slam down during happy hour.[6] (Just kidding about the last one.)

While I agree that drinking coffee counts some toward your hydration totals—as well as the body producing some water from the foods we eat—I don't think munching on a bowl of cereal topped with milk or slurping chicken soup is the same as drinking pure water. Since many more people are *not* properly hydrated than those who are, my gut says that's because they aren't drinking enough water. Having a bowl of cereal, drinking orange juice, or sipping on soup is not the same as drinking water. Your body tells you there's a difference. When I recommend drinking eight glasses of liquids, I'm talking about pure water. Any other beverages should not count toward that total.

Besides, the state of orange juice and other fruit juices in Canada is not good. Most juices are full of concentrated sugars with a loss of nutrients from pasteurization and concentration, which makes them as nutritionally void as refined white flour. I recommend that you stay away from OJ and fruit juice while following the Perfect Weight Eating Plan unless you can somehow buy a fresh-squeezed variety made from organically grown fruit. Fresh-squeezed orange juice should be diluted with purified or naturally carbonated mineral water so that you won't ingest more fruit sugar than you would normally receive when eating a piece of fruit.

In the latter stages of the Perfect Weight Eating Plan, it's OK to drink raw vegetable and raw fruit juice, if you use a juicer to make your own. Stay away from canned vegetable juice, especially tomato juice, which tends to be high in sodium and preservatives. Juicing fruits and vegetables yourself gives you all the nutrients nature has provided without anything artificial.

Water Retention

Then there are those who believe that if they drink too much water, they'll gain weight because of water "retention." Unless there is an underlying medical problem, such as liver or kidney failure, just the opposite occurs. Drinking extra water seems to *boost* metabolism, which promotes weight loss, albeit modest. Michael Borschmann, MD, and colleagues from Franz-Volhard Clinical Research Center in Berlin, Germany, tracked energy expenditures from seven men and seven women—

healthy and not overweight—who drank 17 ounces of water. This was followed by testing their metabolic rates to see how fast they burned calories.

Within ten minutes of consuming a large glass of water, the test subjects' metabolism increased by 30 percent for both men and women and reached a maximum after thirty to forty minutes. The German researchers estimated that over the course of a year, a person who increased his water consumption by 1.5 litres a day (around 50 ounces) would burn an extra 17,400 calories, which translates into a weight loss of approximately five pounds.[7]

F. Batmanghelidj, MD, and author of *Water: For Health, for Healing, for Life*, contends that sipping on a water bottle will act like a governor on an overheated engine to dampen hunger pangs and prevent you from overeating or cheating. He recommends drinking a glass of water before sitting down for breakfast, lunch, and dinner. "You will feel full and will eat only when food is needed," he said. "The volume of food intake will decrease drastically. The type of craving for food will also change. With sufficient water intake, we tend to crave proteins more than fattening carbohydrates.... If you think you are different and your body does not need this amount [eight to ten glasses per day] of water, you are making a major mistake," notes Dr. Batmanghelidj, who believes that many dieters confuse hunger and thirst, thinking they're hungry when actually they're dehydrated.[8]

The sensation of thirst and hunger is generated simultaneously to indicate the brain's needs, but many do not recognize the sensation of thirst and assume both "indicators" to be the urge to eat. Thus, they reach for a bag of chips when they should have been reaching for a glass of water. Dr. Batmanghelidj says that when people reach for water first, they manage to separate the two sensations, which stops them from overeating and taking one step back on their way to reaching their perfect weight.

One way to know if you're properly hydrated is looking at the colour of your urine. If your urine is consistently yellow, then you're not drinking enough water. Clear or light yellow urine is the best indicator that you're drinking enough water throughout the day. Cloudy urine, no matter what the colour, can indicate dehydration.

When you're at work, keep a water bottle or glass of water nearby. Drinking more water than you're used to will be one of the most important things you can do to reach your perfect weight. Filtered water is preferable to "fitness" waters like Propel, which contain sucrose syrup and a bevy of additives. Glacéau Vitamin Water, a trendy "nutrient enhanced water beverage" that sounds Canadian but isn't, is sweetened with crystalline fructose, which, like sucrose syrup, is a variation of high-fructose corn syrup. Depending on what Glacéau Vitamin Water "flavour" you pull from the shelves, a 20-ounce bottle contains 100 to 125 calories and between 20 and 32 grams of sugar, nearly the equivalent of a 12-ounce can of the real thing—Coke. Fresh water has zero calories.

"It is primitive and simplistic thinking that one could easily lace water with all sorts of pleasure-enhancing chemicals and substitute these fluids for the natural and clean water that the human body needs," said Dr. Batmanghelidj. "Some of these chemicals—caffeine, aspartame, saccharin, and alcohol—through their constant lopsided effect on the brain, single-mindedly program the body chemistry with results contrary to the natural design of the body.... The intake of wrong fluids will affect the life of anyone who continually consumes them."[9]

Not to mention reaching your perfect weight.

Tea Time

I have good news to report: drinking tea in moderation—two to three cups a day—certainly contributes to the body's hydration. A published review of tea research conducted at King's College in the United Kingdom—where Dr. Bulwer studied nutrition—showed that tea hydrates the body as effectively as water. "Drinking tea is actually better for you than drinking water," said Dr. Carrie Ruxton, one of the coauthors of the King's College report. "Water is essentially replacing fluid. Tea replaces fluids and contains antioxidants, so it's got two things going for it."[10]

Globally, tea is the most widely consumed beverage, after water. All true varieties of tea come from the leaves of a single evergreen plant, Camellia sinensis. (Herbal teas such as chamomile and peppermint should really be called herbal infusions as they are not true teas.) During harvest time, tea leaves are picked, rolled, dried, and heated. The type of tea depends on how the leaves are processed. Green and white teas are nonoxidized and are the freshest. Black or oxidized teas are the most fermented. Oolong or partially oxidized teas are in between.

Green tea accounts for 20 percent of the global tea market, while black tea (or green tea that has been subjected to additional processing that ferments and oxidizes the leaves) accounts for about 78 percent.[11] I recommend green tea because of less processing and its higher levels of antioxidants than black tea.

As far as caffeine is concerned, I believe that tea's benefits are better delivered in teas containing caffeine, which has a mild diuretic effect. Since tea leaves naturally contain caffeine, I believe it's healthiest for us to consume tea in its most natural form. Obviously, if caffeine tends to keep you up at night, you should avoid consuming caffeinated teas in the late afternoon or in the evening.

Even better news is that new evidence is emerging that green tea can help you reach your perfect weight. The *American Journal of Clinical Nutrition* published the results of a study at the University of Geneva in Switzerland in which men given a combination of caffeine and green tea extract burned more calories than those given only caffeine or a placebo, meaning that green tea accentuates the stimulant properties of caffeine, which raises the metabolic rate.[12] The clinical trials conducted at the University of Geneva also revealed that the catechins in green tea raised the body's thermogenesis rate (amount of calories burned), which, in turn, increased energy expenditure.

What makes green tea so special? The secret behind green tea lies in its high content of a class of health-promoting agents collectively known as polyphenols or flavonoids—specifically the group known as catechins. Epigallocatechin gallate, or EGCG, comprises up to 40 percent of the dry weight of green teas and has a knack for improving the flow of blood through the vessels, which is good for cardiovascular health. EGCG is a powerful antioxidant ("anti-rust" agent) that kills many types of cancer cells in vitro without harming healthy tissue; it is also effective in lowering the bad LDL cholesterol levels, which clog our arteries.

Green tea—I also recommend a traditional type of Chinese tea known as oolong tea—should come from organic sources. Some of the best natural, organic teas I've found are imported from the pristine Wuyi Mountains of China, where tea leaves are harvested by hand and not subjected to pesticides and chemical fertilizers. Japan is also a major producer. Unlike conventional produce, you cannot wash herbicide residue off tea leaves, so stick to boxes marked "Organic Tea." Many organic teas are "Fair Trade" certified, which guarantees that workers picking the leaves receive fair wages for their efforts.

There's a different type of tea drink I want to introduce you to, and it's called kombucha, or mushroom tea. Kombucha (pronounced *kom-BOO-cha*) is a fermented beverage made from black or green tea and a fungus culture. Sounds awful, but I have been known to drink several of these exotic beverages a week. They're not cheap, though, at three or four loonies a bottle, but if you look online, you can find ways to order a kombucha culture and make this sweet-and-sour drink at home.

Many cultures around the world consume lacto-fermented beverages like kombucha for their wonderful health benefits, but it's a beverage unlike anything tasted in this country. One reviewer, Siobhan Roth of the *Pittsburgh Post-Gazette*, compared kombucha to old sweat socks with a lemon twist.[13] I don't think kombucha tastes that bad. Kombucha has a cidery flavour and a definite fizziness, but I like the way the beverage boosts my energy and lightens my mood. My favourite flavour is grape, but you can find flavours like raspberry, mango, and lemon ginger.

Low in calories and sugar—just 8 grams per 8 ounces—you'll find statements like "sparkling Himalayan tonic" or "handmade Chinese tea" on the labels, but kombucha is distinctly Russian in origin. One brand, Kombucha Wonder Drink, started appearing in U.S. and Canadian health food stores several years ago and has developed a cult following. Kombucha is not a drink you guzzle down like a cold bottle of water after playing two sets of tennis. Kathy O'Brien of the Weston A. Price Foundation, which disseminates the research of nutrition pioneer Dr. Weston A. Price, said that you should go slow when drinking this fizzy lacto-fermented beverage—no more than 4 ounces at a time.

Lacto-fermented beverages are very healthy as they're high in lactic and gluconic acids, as well as enzymes and probiotics that are good for digestion. Don't let the pungent aroma or cloudy appearance stop you from trying this healthy drink.

A Jag for Coffee

Although I'm a kombucha fan, I don't see the tart-tasting beverage becoming as popular as the sugared coffee drink you can order at Starbucks and other trendy coffee bars. Any time a barista whips up a coffee confection, you're drinking the equivalent of a liquefied candy bar. Grande sizes of mocha, vanilla, white chocolate, orange mocha, hazelnut, dulce de leche, java chip, and caramel-flavoured coffees top 400 calories per serving and over 50 grams of sugar.

So you'll have to put aside your mocha-flavoured fixes during Perfect Weight Canada, but that doesn't mean you can't drink coffee. It's fine to consume fresh ground organic coffee flavoured with organic cream, honey, or stevia, but exercise moderation, meaning one cup per day or every other day. And just as with tea, I believe coffee is best consumed as it was created—fully loaded. Decaffeinated coffee is highly processed and removes some of the antioxidant benefits contained in the beans.

Personally, I'm not a huge fan of coffee or a coffee drinker myself, but I'm aware that caffeinated coffee, as well as tea, has been consumed for thousands of years by some of the world's healthiest people. As long as your coffee comes from organic sources, you'll be OK. You should buy whole beans, freeze them, and grind them yourself when desired, but you'll be even better off if you put aside coffee until you complete the Perfect Weight Eating Plan.

Caution: you should stay away from so-called "slimming" coffees, which are typically a combination of regular ground coffee, herbs, and supplements touted as appetite suppressants, such as hoodia, guarana, hydroxycitric acid, and guar gum, a type of fibre.

Perfect Weight Recap: Drink for Your Perfect Weight

- Make your No. 1 beverage purified, nonchlorinated water, consuming around eight to twelve cups a day, even during the freezing winter months.
- If you drink natural sparkling water, don't choose brands with added carbonation, such as Perrier.
- Install carbon-based filters at the kitchen faucet and refrigerator, or purchase countertop water pitchers.
- Brew green tea, or consume pre-steeped liquid teas (preferably organic), which may be sweetened with a small amount of honey or stevia.
- Take a step on the wild side and try lacto-fermented beverages like kombucha.
- If you're a coffee drinker, switch over to certified organic coffee, which can be flavoured with organic cream and a small amount of honey or stevia.

Chapter 5

Snack for Your Perfect Weight

BACK IN THE early 1990s, Melissa Gertz was a missionary in India with Youth With A Mission. After living with and ministering to the Indian people for six years, she returned to the United States and eventually settled in Findlay, Ohio, after marrying her husband, Jeff.

Starting an office job was a bit of a cultural shock for Melissa, who weighed 145 pounds at the time. For one thing, the Ohio diet—heavy on fried foods, light on vegetables, and topped off with sweets—was much different from Indian cuisine, characterized by its extensive use of spices and herbs as well as scintillating vegetarian dishes and flat breads like *roti* and *paratha*. But it didn't take long for Melissa to adapt again to American ways. Monday through Friday, her co-workers would bring boxes of chocolate-glazed doughnuts to work, tempting Melissa until she reached for one or three.

After work, Melissa and Jeff liked to visit Findlay's famous ice cream emporium, Dietsch Brothers, where Melissa would order a sugar cone packed with three scoops of her favourite ice cream—Moose Tracks, heavily ribboned with chocolate. "I became a real chocoholic," she said. "Whenever I wanted a snack, I would hide Dove chocolate in between the seat cushions of my couch and eat them while I watched TV. Within a year or so, my weight ballooned to way over 200 pounds."

I'm pleased to say that Melissa's waistline has greatly improved—she got back down to 180 pounds by following the Perfect Weight America program during the Healthy Toledo campaign—but all that harmful noshing nearly did her in. Until she turned her health around, Melissa—and many like her—don't know what constitutes healthy snacking, nor are they aware that you often *should* eat something between meals. Reason: the body's metabolism resembles a furnace that must be stoked at regular intervals. That's why snacking is an important part of the Perfect Weight Eating Plan. Personally, I like to snack, but my in-between treats are healthier—and yummier—than anything Dietsch Brothers' ice cream parlour could serve.

I'm pro-snacking because denying yourself food for long stretches sets you up for three things:

1. Misery
2. Depression
3. Failure

We certainly don't want any of those conditions colouring your experience with Perfect Weight Canada. (Melissa said her out-of-control snacking made her feel very depressed, as if she were being controlled.) Snacking wisely can help you satisfy hunger pangs before they become overwhelming. When blood sugar levels fall, you don't want to reach for one of the bad old snacks—honey-roasted peanuts, mesquite-flavoured potato chips, crème-filled cookies, vanilla ice cream bars dipped in chocolate, and store-bought snack cakes. These commercially produced snack foods are loaded with refined sugar, chemical preservatives, artificial sweeteners, and processed ingredients that rob your health and set you back two steps after making a stride forward.

To stay one step ahead of hunger, you need to arm yourself with SREs—snacks ready to eat, just as U.S. servicemen and servicewomen carry MREs (meals ready to eat). I'm talking about keeping on hand snacks like whole-food nutrition bars or even healthy cacao (chocolate) snacks. Drinking a delicious and satisfying high-protein and high-fibre meal supplement will keep you feeling satiated for up to four hours between meals.

Let's talk about the high-protein and fibre meal supplement drink first because I was involved with the development of this great product called Perfect Meal, which is designed to dampen the munchies an hour or two before lunch or dinner. When you mix a serving of Perfect Meal into water, you are receiving two key ingredients to slow the digestion of carbohydrates in your digestive tract: Fibertrol and native whey protein. Fibertrol is a fibre blend that includes glucomannan derived from konjac root, a traditional Japanese food. It helps you feel full longer, reducing unnecessary food cravings that can lead to overeating during meals and overindulging on unhealthy snacks between meals.

Native whey comes from the milk of free-range, grass-fed cattle that graze on pesticide-free pastures. Normally, whey products are by-products of cheese devoid of vital immune and regenerative components that were destroyed during commercial processing. Perfect Meal's native whey is minimally processed to preserve more of the natural factors, including cysteine, which, Dr. Bulwer says, is an important amino acid with a crucial role in the body's production of glutathione (GSH)—a major antioxidant indispensable for healthy functioning of all body cells, with special protective roles in the liver, the cardiovascular and immune systems, and red blood cells. Laboratory studies have demonstrated that glutathione has the potential to greatly improve many aspects of our health.

Another great thing about Perfect Meal is that it contains probiotics, which are live bacteria cultures shown to enhance the natural flora in the gut. Probiotics increase the number of beneficial or friendly microorganisms present in the digestive tract while improving digestive efficiency. By enhancing the good bacteria, probiotics help drive out bad bacteria, yeasts, viruses, and parasites. Dr. Bulwer says that doctors routinely prescribe probiotics like Lactinex and Florastor to help maintain intestinal balance due to antibiotic use.

As a snack, Perfect Meal helps you stay satiated due to a very low glycemic index of 14. The glycemic index (GI) ranks carbohydrates according to their effect on your blood glucose levels. Any number below 55 is considered a low GI food, so drinking a glass of Perfect Meal will help you maintain healthy blood sugar levels instead of spiking them, like Melissa's Moose Tracks ice cream, for instance. As you would expect, sugary desserts and refined foods have a high glycemic index, which means they are digested very quickly, leaving you hungry in a short time. When you keep nibbling sugary treats to satisfy your sweet tooth, the downward spiral continues.

Perfect Meal can break the cycle. The Perfect Meal powder comes in two natural flavours: creamy vanilla and milk chocolate. Just add water, and you're drinking something that will satisfy your cravings for a sweet treat. With 3 grams of sugar and 200 calories, one serving is packed with protein and fibre. You can purchase Perfect Meal in a small tub or in handy packets, perfect for tucking into a purse as an SRE (snack ready to eat).

Checking Out the Bar Scene

Next on my list of healthy snacks are whole-food nutrition bars, which are commonly known as nutrition or energy bars. If you stroll through a warehouse club these days, you're apt to find a "food demo" for a popular energy bar. Dice-sized squares of various flavours are set on a tray, free for the taking. Energy bars are marketed as a nutritious meal supplement—a candy-bar sized alternative to packing a lunch or purchasing a Snickers from a vending machine. In many ways, energy bars are the perfect snack food for today's grab-and-go lifestyle—portable, nutritious, and tasty.

No longer a niche product for endurance athletes, energy bars have gone mainstream. Energy bars no longer taste like cardboard and sawdust covered with chocolate. Today, you can choose from flavours like Chocolate Raspberry Fudge, Cookie Dough, Dulce de Leche, and Devil's Food Cake, to name a few. They really do taste like a candy bar, except for a certain aftertaste. So are they healthy?

I think you already know my answer: most energy bars are not the nutritional powerhouses they are purported to be, nor are they a great meal replacement for those trying to lose weight and stay healthy. These energy bars are a highly processed mix of protein powders (soy or milk), sugars and/or artificial sweeteners, chemicals, preservatives, and synthetic ingredients.

Take soy protein, for example, which is often the first ingredient listed. Most soy protein comes from genetically modified soybeans. Soybeans are high in phytic acid, which can block absorption of essential minerals like calcium, magnesium, copper, iron, and zinc from the intestinal tract. Soy protein must be processed at high temperatures to reduce phytic acid levels, which pretty much destroy the "important proteins" in soy, such as lysine.

The reason why most energy bars taste so sweet is because they're full of high-fructose corn syrup, sucrose, or corn syrup, which are forms of refined sugar and contribute to weight gain and blood sugar imbalances. In my mind, energy bars are nothing more than glorified candy bars. I mean if it looks like a candy bar, tastes like a candy bar, and has many of the same ingredients as a candy bar...then it's a candy bar and not a nutritious snack for someone trying to lead a healthy lifestyle.

In preparation for the launch of Perfect Weight Canada, my research and development team and I set out to develop a whole-food nutrition bar—I prefer the term "food bar"—that wasn't sweetened with high-fructose corn syrup and that would diminish hunger for those seeking a meal replacement or a snack. After much testing and many revisions, my team and I formulated a pair of truly healthy and great-tasting food bars, sweetened with raw honey and produced entirely from whole foods containing native whey protein, an organic fibre blend, and omega-3 fats.

We call these Perfect Weight America bars (sorry, there's no Canadian version), and they come in two delicious flavours: Peanut Butter fücoProtein and Chocolate MacNut Crunch fücoProtein, the latter containing healthy "real" chocolate called Rainforest Cacao. (I describe the health benefits of Rainforest Cacao later in this chapter.)

There's another ingredient in Perfect Weight America bars that I'm excited about, and it's called fucoxanthin (pronounced *FEW-co-zan-thin*), a carotenoid from brown seaweed that's showing tremendous fat-burning potential. Fucoxanthin can accelerate weight and fat loss, when combined with a calorie-conscious diet, according to a clinical study that I'll tell you about in chapter 6, "Supplement for Your Perfect Weight."

Last but not least, Perfect Weight America bars contain a superstar ingredient called chia. I know that when some people hear the word *chia* they think of "chia pets"—those kitschy animal figurines with green chia sprouts growing where their hair should be. The chia I'm talking about come from an edible seed that grows abundantly in desert plants found in southern Mexico and parts of South America. The seeds of the chia plant have long been consumed in Central and South America for use both as food and a medicine. The seeds are oil-rich, about one-third of the entire seed, of which 60 percent is alpha-linolenic acid (ALA), thereby giving chia's fibre-rich seeds the highest percentage of omega-3 fatty acids of any plant, including flaxseeds. Because chia seeds have much higher antioxidant levels than flaxseeds, chia seeds don't go rancid as easily as flax.

Best of all for those seeking to lose weight, chia is very filling. Chia seeds swell from seven to nine times inside the stomach, which will pack your tummy in a hurry. You can see why when you mix a small amount of chia in a glass of water. After swirling the water for a few moments, the mixture turns gelatin-like and soon has the consistency of tapioca pudding. We're talking thick, but oh-so-nutritious for you.

I made sure during the formulation process that chia was part of the Perfect

Weight America food bars as well as other Garden of Life Organic Living Food bars, which is another snack ready to eat that you could try. Organic Living Food bars come in four varieties:

- Organic Super Seed Whole Food Fibre Bar, which has an apple-cinnamon taste and twice as much fibre as two apples, which keeps you feeling full longer.
- Organic Fruits of Life Whole Food Antioxidant Matrix Bar, which is a mouthful to say and a great-tasting mouthful to eat. These purple-coloured, summer berry-flavoured bars are made with six organic fruits and have more fibre than one cup of blueberries and the antioxidant equivalent of over four servings of fruits and vegetables.
- Organic Perfect Food Whole Foods Greens Bar, which is packed with twenty-one organic vegetables and has as much fibre as five heads of romaine lettuce.
- Organic Perfect Food Chocolate-Covered Greens Bar, which is also packed with twenty-one organic vegetables but is coated with a layer of chocolate for those looking to enjoy a chocolaty taste.

I suggest that you eat a Perfect Weight America or Organic Living Food bar or drink a Perfect Meal shake as an in-between meal snack once or twice each day, especially during Phase I of the Perfect Weight Eating Plan. Each of these two snacks contains 5 or more grams of fibre and is the answer to a growling stomach in mid-afternoon.

Other Great Snacks

I'm a constant snacker, one of those who can't go much longer than a couple of hours without eating. I'm not sure why, but when I'm not fasting or on a ten-day "detox" cleanse (as I'll describe in chapter 8, "Cleanse for Your Perfect Weight"), I get hungry quickly and often.

When it comes to whole foods, vegetables and vegetable dips make for fantastic snacks. For instance, you could dip organic baked chips into organically made salsa. A guacamole dip can be made fresh with organic avocados, lemon, cilantro, and sea salt. Carrots and celery can be eaten raw or dipped in hummus.

Fresh fruit and dried fruit are also nutritious snacks. Take a handful of dried raisins, figs, dates, prunes, pineapple, and papaya and combine them with some raw or soaked nuts or seeds. Make sure there is no sugar added or any sulfites. It's very easy to throw some dried fruit, nuts, and seeds into a bag and carry the mixture with you throughout the day for a quick snack.

Also keep in mind that there are many healthy snack and dessert recipes using organic ingredients you can make on your own, like whole-grain blueberry muffins, banana bread, and coconut almond fudge. Popcorn is another popular snack that can be healthy if prepared right. Use this recipe: First, melt some extra-virgin coconut oil in a pan, pour in organic popcorn kernels, and cook them until popped. Pour some melted organic butter over the popped kernels, and sprinkle with your favourite organic seasoning. *Voila!*

For a list of delicious, healthy recipes, see the Perfect Recipes and Perfect Snacks appendices in the back of this book, or visit www.PerfectWeightCanada.com.

Some of the most convenient and healthiest snacks are nuts and seeds, which are great sources of fibre, healthy fats, and nutrients. If properly prepared, they are extremely nutritious. "Properly prepared" means raw, soaked, or even dry-roasted nuts and seeds not roasted in vegetable oil. Just make sure they are organic and without added salt. Try almonds, walnuts, cashews, pecans, pumpkin seeds, and sunflower seeds, or make your own healthy trail mix.

Raw nut butters, made from almonds, cashews, and sunflower seeds, are something worth checking out. They're special because they're unheated, not roasted, so their delicate oils haven't been damaged, and they still have their vitamins, minerals, and enzymes intact. Nut butters can be used as a veggie dip or spread onto sprouted bread or fresh fruit. Organic peanut butter is also recommended and can be found in natural food stores, supermarkets, and even warehouse clubs these days.

The Case for Chocolate

Back in 1830, British candy makers J. S. Fry and Sons developed the world's first chocolate bar by roasting fermented cacao pods and then grinding them into a fine paste that could be separated into either cacao solids (also known as cocoa powder) or cocoa butter. When they blended the cocoa solids and cocoa butter with refined sugar, the result was chocolate—the "nectar of the gods," as the confection came to be known in Europe.

Canadians developed a taste for chocolate when Arthur Ganong introduced the "nickel" bar in 1910, the first Canadian chocolate bar for the masses. As chocolate became popular on both sides of the border throughout the rest of the twentieth century, some chocolatiers discovered they could substitute cocoa butter with cheaper emulsifying agents and gain a price advantage.

These days it's not unusual to see chocolate made with soy lecithin—don't forget that soybeans are a heavily genetically modified crop—or an artificial emulsifier derived from castor oil. This allows manufacturers to reduce the amount of the more expensive cocoa butter while retaining the same melt-in-your-mouth sensation when taking a bite. Chocolate connoisseurs, though, can easily tell the difference between the "real stuff" and heavily processed chocolate in a single bite.

High-quality chocolate creates a taste sensation so intense that people get more excited from eating chocolate than they do when they passionately kiss their lovers, according to recent research carried out by Dr. David Lewis, formerly with the University of Sussex but now with the Mind Lab.[1]

Like most Americans, Canadians have a thing for chocolate: you consume 5.4 kilos per capita each year, according to the International Cocoa Organization, a hundred-gram bar more than Americans, who eat 5.3 kilos of chocolate each year. That works out to around a bar of chocolate every other day.[2]

As with anything in the food industry these days, manufacturers can take a perfectly great natural product and completely mess it up. In my country, the Chocolate Manufacturers Association, a Washington DC trade organization whose members include Hershey, Nestlé, Guittard, and World's Finest Chocolate, lobbied the U.S. Food and Drug Administration (FDA) in 2007 for permission to substitute partially hydrogenated vegetable oils for cocoa butter as well as the right to use artificial sweeteners and milk substitutes. (Can you believe it? Partially hydrogenated vegetable oils are a major source of dangerous trans fats!) Currently, the FDA stipulates that candy makers must call their products "chocolate flavoured" or "chocolaty" if the product contains any of these ersatz ingredients. They can't call their confection "chocolate."

I have found a chocolate that's nutritionally miles ahead of the mass-produced chocolate bars and peanut butter cups found on supermarket store aisles and checkout stands. It's a dark organic chocolate derived from the seeds of the fruit of cacao trees, which are native to the rainforest regions of South America. When I sampled some of the rich chocolate from this jungle plant, the perfect balance of bitter and sweet as well as cacao's healthy properties were a rush. Real chocolate from cacao beans is:

- Super-rich in antioxidant flavonols
- One of nature's best sources of magnesium (a nutrient that supports the heart, increases brainpower, and causes bowel movements)
- High in phenylethylamine (PEA), which is thought to help create feelings of attraction and excitement
- High in fibre, which is great for the heart as well as the gut

Dark chocolate also releases both serotonin and endorphins, which act as anti-depressants.[9] Chocolate can lift a dark mood rather quickly, and it diminishes the appetite.

I asked my team at Garden of Life to find an organic chocolate that was delicious, portable, and would make a great snack or dessert-time treat. The result was Rainforest Cacao Chocolate, which comes from all-natural, roasted cacao beans from the Ecuadorian Amazon region. We purchase fresh-picked cacao beans directly from a village in Ecuador at Fair Trade prices during the March-to-July harvest. After the cacao beans dry out in the sun, they're slowly roasted and lightly sweetened with a touch of sugar cane syrup.

Rainforest Cacao Chocolate is an awesome snack and comes in three flavours: Raisins & Coconut; Macadamia Nuts; and Brazilian Nuts & Coffee. Just be sure to enjoy in moderation. A small handful—an ounce—contains 100 calories, so it remains a treat, not a cheat.

Slowly roasting the cacao beans and allowing them to ferment brings out the rich chocolate taste of Rainforest Cacao, but raw foodists sing the praises of having their chocolate "naked" by peeling and eating raw cacao beans. Raw food enthusiasts David Wolfe and Shazzie (she goes by one name, just like Cher) call the raw cacao bean one of nature's most fantastic superfoods.

"Typical commercial chocolate will contain a mixture of alkalized cacao powder, cacao butter, genetically modified soy lecithin, vanilla extract, and refined sugar," they write in their book, *Naked Chocolate*. "Milk chocolate contains powdered milk with its harmful antioxidant-blocking properties and a vast array of pesticide residues and artificial hormones that have been fed to the animal. After all this, no wonder people want the real thing."[4]

Eating the real thing can be part of a weight-loss program. Wolfe and Shazzie point out that no scientific evidence implicates chocolate consumption with obesity. "In fact," they say, "the reverse seems to be the case. Eating cacao helps one to lose weight. This is why seemingly every weight-loss product on the market contains cocoa powder, which decreases appetite. Diet companies hint they are doing you a favour by providing chocolate weight-loss products, when in fact they use chocolate because it works!"[5]

You can purchase raw cacao "nibs" in health food stores. This raw chocolate, however, is bitter-tasting and not sweet at all. Our Rainforest Cacao Chocolate is lightly sweetened with sugar cane syrup, which I think is a happy and healthy compromise.

When a Treat Turns Into a Cheat

Lifetime habits are hard to change. Many cannot quit eating junk food cold turkey; they often feel like they "deserve" a nutritional indulgence for even trying. Others chafe at restrictions or being told what to do. Indeed, we live in a culture that trumpets the breaking of rules. At one time Burger King told us, "Sometimes you gotta break the rules," while Outback Steakhouses ("No rules. Just right."), Neiman Marcus ("No rules here"), Don Q rum ("Break all the rules"), and even an NFL video game ("No refs, no rules, no mercy") expound the antisocial theme that rules are a drag on life. I could make a joke about hockey and rules, but I won't.

At any rate, I'll go with the flow: you have my official permission to cheat.

Why am I giving you my OK to eat a prodigal meal? Because I've learned that allowing people to cheat results in better compliance with the overall Perfect Weight Eating Plan. Cheat meals give people a greater feeling of control over their lives. They look forward to their preset cheat meals, when they can feel "normal" again.

I recommend that you cheat on the weekends. That's when most families and couples socialize anyway, so if you want to go for it—just two meals per week, remember—do so sometime between Friday evening and Sunday night. My one request is that you don't eat any of the foods I listed in the Dirty Dozen.

Now I know this will be a problem for some. You're thinking, "Jordan, everything I ate before I started Perfect Weight Canada was one of the Dirty Dozen.

Are you telling me that cocktail wienies, Boston Crème Rolls, chocolate-covered pretzels, and Lucky Charms cereal are off limits?"

Yes, if at all possible. You begin by taking steps to remove temptation from your path. You'll find the route to weight loss easier if your pantry isn't stocked with snack cakes, chocolate-covered candy bars, or all your old favourite breakfast cereals. Toss that junk food into the trash. Clean out your cupboards. Scour through the deep recesses of your freezer. Rummage through your refrigerator.

Then replenish your pantry with organic treats purchased at the health food store: dates rolled in coconut, flaxseed crackers, cashews, and rice chips, to name a few items. Dried fruits such as apricots, peaches, prunes, and raisins are known as "nature's candy" and are ready to eat at any time. These convenient, healthy snacks pack almost as much a nutritious punch as their fresh counterparts.

What about those occasions when you're invited over to a friend's barbecue or Stanley Cup playoff party, and all the old pleasure foods are beckoning from the buffet table? Your resistance melts like a Hershey chocolate bar in the warm sun. Within minutes, you're filling a paper plate with hogs in a sleeping blanket, gooey nachos dripping in melted cheese sauce, and Swedish meatballs drowning in a pool of sweet molasses sauce. You know you're cheating, but you can't stop yourself.

Well, I have good news for you. If you're going to cheat in the scenario I just described, just make sure you do all your cheating in a one-hour time frame.

Why sixty minutes? The husband-and-wife team of Richard and Rachel Heller, PhDs and retired professors from the Mount Sinai School of Medicine in New York, say that when the body has been deprived of insulin-triggering foods high in carbohydrates for two or more consecutive meals—which happens when you're following the Perfect Weight Eating Plan—the body makes adjustments. The body learns to release less insulin because it figures that fewer carbohydrates will be coming its way in the future. Since less insulin is released, less fat is stored and more fat is burned up. "The lowered level of insulin also allows the brain chemical serotonin to act as it should—as an appetite regulator," the Hellers write in *The Carbohydrate Addict's Diet*. "You will probably eat far less than you would if you have been eating three consecutive carbohydrate-rich meals."[6]

When you keep eating after halftime of the big football game, the body responds to this onslaught of crummy foods by releasing a second phase of insulin, which produces more fat. Not good. This second insulin phase usually kicks in, say the Hellers, between seventy-five and ninety minutes after you begin eating. If you stop eating those cheesy chips and Swedish meatballs *before* sixty minutes are up, however, the second phase of insulin release stays much lower. That's why it's important to keep your cheating within a sixty-minute time window.

Summertime barbecues, when the twilight lingers, can be worse than Stanley Cup parties. The cheeseburgers might not come off the grill for a couple of hours, leaving your growling stomach plenty of time to graze on sour cream chips and imitation dip while sipping a sugared iced tea. After a leisurely meal with friends, you may wait until you have "more room" for the brownie and ice cream dessert, but eating a rich trifle more than an hour *after* the finger foods and main meal will push your insulin readings over the edge. Result: you've taken *three* steps backward, maybe four. Again, try to keep the cheating within a one-hour time period.

If you are home with your family but absolutely, positively have to cheat at dessert time, munch on cookies made with organic ingredients. In our home, we have tins of Jennies Macaroons available for those times when my sweet tooth wants to be pleased. I like that Jennies Macaroons are made with only three ingredients: coconut, honey, and egg whites. I'm also partial to the aforementioned homemade blueberry muffins and banana bread—both healthy, organic delights. (For more recommended brands, check out the PWC Resource Guide on page 322.)

"Jordan, what about ice cream?" you may be asking. *We all scream for ice cream!* OK, if you have a craving for a delicious frozen dessert, you can shop for delicious organic ice cream in the freezer case of progressive health stores. Another option is to make your own ice cream or frozen yogurt, which I do a couple of times per month. I use a Vita-Mix blender to make the best ice cream and frozen yogurt east of the Mississippi River, using all organic ingredients.

A final thought regarding cheating: nighttime isn't the best time to let yourself have a dessert. You'll be better off cheating in the morning since this will give you extra time to work off those extra calories. No matter what time you cheat, though, you should consume a high-fibre food or beverage to fill up that tummy before the cheat. This would be a good time to drink a glass of your Perfect Meal, with the idea of cleansing the system and getting right back on track.

Whether you cheat a little or a lot, you can bolster your health by taking nutritional supplements, including an exciting new product made from fucoxanthin. Our next chapter, "Supplement for Your Perfect Weight," is a primer on the importance and benefits of taking nutritional supplements, especially in relation to weight loss.

Perfect Weight Recap: Snack for Your Perfect Weight

- Drink Perfect Meal shakes as a meal supplement to take the edge off between-meal hunger.
- Look for whole-food nutrition bars with native whey protein and chia, which are extremely high in omega-3 fatty acids and very filling as well.
- Keep a variety of SREs on hand—snacks ready to eat. Fresh fruit, dried fruit, nuts, seeds, and vegetables like baby carrots can hold you over until dinnertime.
- Enjoy chocolate produced from cacao beans grown in South American rainforests—the healthiest chocolate and a real tasty treat.
- Be aware of the difference between a treat and a cheat. You're allowed two cheat meals a week during the sixteen-week Perfect Weight Eating Plan, but don't eat any of the Dirty Dozen foods.
- Limit your cheating to a sixty-minute time period since eating for a longer period causes the body to raise insulin levels, which makes you gain weight.

Chapter 6

Supplement for Your Perfect Weight

DURING SIGNUPS FOR the Healthy Toledo program, the Perfect Weight America pilot campaign, each participant completed a two-page health questionnaire, penned a five-hundred-word essay describing the state of their health, signed the perquisite release forms, and submitted to a battery of health tests: blood pressure, heartbeat rate, body fat composition, as well as the dreaded weigh-in and full-body photos. I salute this "first graduating class" for putting it all on the line.

The Healthy Toledo participants also put their money where their mouths were. What I mean is that we requested that each pay a sign-up fee to cover the cost of the nutritional supplements that I wanted everyone to take. For the Winzeler family— Alan and Patti along with their nineteen-year-old daughter, Tanae—the amount represented a tangible investment in their health. Following their weigh-ins, the Winzelers carried home three cardboard boxes, each containing four different nutritional supplements from Garden of Life, a health and wellness company I founded.

Of the four products I recommended to the participants of Healthy Toledo, I was betting that a brand-new supplement called fücoTHIN (pronounced *FEW-co-thin*) would make the biggest difference when the Toledans submitted to the final weigh-in eleven weeks from the start date. The fücoTHIN supplement was seven years in the making and not even in many stores yet. Characterized as a nonstimulant weight-management supplement with a thermogenic effect for fat metabolism, fücoTHIN had shown an ability to break down belly fat by raising the body's metabolic rate without causing jitters, an increase in heart rate, or lost sleep. I was confident that fücoTHIN would accelerate weight loss for Healthy Toledo participants, although research showed that fücoTHIN wouldn't "kick in" for five or six weeks.

Before we go much further, there's a fascinating backstory to fücoTHIN that I have to share. About seven or eight years ago, I was introduced to a Russian biochemist named Zakir Ramazanov, PhD, a classically trained biochemist and plant physiologist who graduated from the Soviet Union's North Caucasian State University in 1978 at the top of his class.

While serving with the Soviet army in Afghanistan in the late 1970s, Dr. Ramazanov discovered a tonic that boosted his mental and physical energy—a tea made from the golden yellow roots of a Siberian plant called *Rhodiola rosea*. It seems that a Siberian soldier in Dr. Ramazanov's company received packets of Rhodiola rosea in the care packages sent from home, so Dr. Ramazanov decided to give the special tea a try. Rhodiola rosea, he learned, was a perennial plant that grows in dry, sandy ground at high altitudes in the Siberian arctic, and this herbal tonic would become a research focus after his return to civilian life.

Following his stint as a Soviet soldier, Dr. Ramazanov became the head engineer at the Institute of Solar Energy, where he designed and constructed solar batteries and solar energy stations. It was there that he began experimenting with solar bioreactors and how they affected the cultivation of certain marine vegetables and algae, including spirulina and chlorella.

As his career advanced, Dr. Ramazanov left the Soviet Union in 1989 and eventually made his way to the United States, where he accepted a research fellowship at Louisiana State University at Baton Rouge before he founded a company called National Bioscience Corp., headquartered in Chester, New York.

Dr. Ramazanov's specialty was insolating phytonutrients and antioxidants found in land and ocean plants. For instance, the Russian scientist applied innovative technology to the extraction of lycopene, beta-carotene, and lutein from tomatoes, mushrooms, and algae; the extraction of antioxidants from fruits and vegetables; and the intensive biotechnological cultivation of health-promoting marine plants or seaweed. Dr. Ramazanov helped introduce the healing properties of Rhodiola rosea to an American audience by serving as an essential contributor to *The Rhodiola Revolution: Transform Your Health with the Herbal Breakthrough of the 21st Century* by Richard P. Brown, Patricia L. Gerbarg, and Barbara Graham.

But Dr. Ramazanov's real passion was research into sea vegetables, particularly brown seaweed, because epidemiological data from some of the longest living and healthiest cultures on the planet—most notably the Japanese—showed that the human consumption of brown seaweed portended tremendous health benefits. Dr. Ramazanov informed me early on—this had to be around 2002 or so—that he was having success isolating a carotenoid called fucoxanthin from brown seaweed. Carotenoids are a class of natural pigments found principally in plants and algae. Acting as biological antioxidants, carotenoids protect cells and tissues from the damaging effects of free radicals.

Fucoxanthin, Dr. Ramazanov explained, was the carotenoid—or pigment—that turned brown seaweed "brown." This pigment prevented seaweed floating on the ocean surface from being scorched by the sun. Called *wakame* by the Japanese and a part of Asian diets for centuries, about the only time we're served brown seaweed in this country is when we enjoy a bowl of miso soup or seaweed salad in a Japanese restaurant. Although fucoxanthin was found in abundance in several different types of brown seaweed, the carotenoid was present in far lesser amounts in green and red sea vegetables.

Dr. Ramazanov told me that he believed fucoxanthin could regulate a protein called uncoupling protein 1, or UCP1, which controls the amount of fat stored in the body. UCP1, which regulates the activity of a key gene responsible for maintaining the body's temperature, is found in white adipose tissue, or visceral fat.[1] This type of fat, which usually surrounds the internal organs and sits under our bellies, is one of the major causes of "middle-age spread." White adipose tissue isn't that white; it more resembles a disgusting yellowish glob of tissue. This type of fat gathers toxins, leads to low-level inflammation, and harms people's hormonal health.

Dr. Ramazanov kept me posted on the latest research regarding fucoxanthin after moving his operation to the Canary Islands off the coast of Spain, where he served as director of science for the Institute of Technology and Marine Sciences. In the summer of 2006, he passed along news of a study coming out of Hokkaido University in Sapporo, where Japanese researchers studied the effects of fucoxanthin on more than two hundred laboratory animals. The Japanese study found fucoxanthin effective in fighting flab stimulating the UCP1 protein, which caused stored fat to break down.[2] In tests on the laboratory animals, fucoxanthin resulted in a 5 percent to 10 percent reduction in weight. The Japanese researchers said that since the abdominal area contains white adipose tissue, the compound might be particularly effective at shrinking oversized midsections.

Could fucoxanthin do the same for humans? That became the $64,000 question. Study leader Dr. Kazua Miyashita said his team hoped that fucoxanthin could be developed into a nutritional supplement that targeted harmful fat.[3] Professor Miyashita said that their testing was the first to find that a natural food component had been shown to reduce fat by targeting the UCP1 protein, but dieters shouldn't eat a lot of miso soup or toss strands of brown seaweed in their salad (yuck!) to lose weight. Indeed, Professor Miyashita advised against the consumption of massive amounts of seaweed to lose weight because fucoxanthin was not easily absorbed from whole seaweed.[4]

On the heels of the Japanese study came word from Dr. Ramazanov's Russian sources regarding the results of two double-blind, randomized, placebo-controlled clinical trials involving 150 obese women. These studies (pending publication), a collaboration of multiple organizations including the Center of Modern Medicine and Russian Academy of Natural Sciences in Moscow, involved having overweight women follow a meal plan of 1,800 calories a day while taking fucoxanthin or a placebo. The two key results:

1. Those who received fucoxanthin lost an average of 14.5 pounds in just sixteen weeks, versus those who received the placebo pill, who lost only 3 pounds.
2. Participants taking fucoxanthin raised their metabolic rate an average of 18.2 percent.

In addition, body fat loss was 11.8 pounds in the fucoxanthin group, compared to 2.8 pounds in the placebo group. That's a 450 percent greater weight loss and 422 percent greater fat loss, respectively. The women taking fucoxanthin also received reductions in liver fat, blood pressure, triglycerides, and C-reactive protein (CRP).

What the Russian scientists hypothesized was that fucoxanthin possessed strong thermogenic—or fat-burning—properties. Thermogenesis is defined as a process in which the body generates internal heat and thereby increases its metabolic rate, which in turn requires the utilization of internal stores of energy, such as fat. Translation: thermogenesis raises the temperature of the body's calorie-burning furnace, which burns fat. It's the reason why hibernating bears don't freeze to death during a long, hard winter. Their bodies spend the entire winter burning up stored fat that they accumulated during the feeding season. The same principle could be applied to humans: when stored fat begins burning up, the weight will start coming off.

Another way to explain the thermogenic process is by starting with mitochondria, which are the cells' powerhouses. What the fucoxanthin compound does is increase the UCP1 protein (also known as *thermogenin*) by boosting the metabolic rate within the fat cell so that it burns more fat. In fact, the research showed that users of fucoxanthin increased their metabolic rate by 18.2 percent to 24 percent, depending on the dosage. Participants who consumed the amount of fucoxanthin in three capsules had an average increase in their metabolic rate by 18.2 percent and began to notice results in five to six weeks, while those who took the equivalent of ten capsules increased their metabolic rate by nearly 24 percent and began to see results in two to three weeks. By contrast, green tea—which is known for providing an increase in metabolism—has been shown in clinical studies to raise the metabolic rate by only 4 percent. Taking fucoxanthin is literally like charging your fat-burning batteries, supporting the metabolism, or breakdown, of fat in white adipose tissue.

The clinical research also indicated that the metabolic boost from taking fucoxanthin did not stimulate the central nervous system, meaning it didn't cause the jitters or lost sleep like caffeine, nicotine, or thyroid hormones. Dr. Ramazanov reported that the fucoxanthin was safe with no side effects, and it even provided other health benefits, including improved cardiovascular health, reduction of inflammation (a major cause of heart disease), healthy cholesterol and triglyceride levels, improvements in blood pressure levels, and healthy liver function. As a carotenoid, fucoxanthin was a powerful antioxidant that protected cells from free-radical damage.

After learning of the incredible results of the clinical study on fucoxanthin, my colleagues at Garden of Life worked with Dr. Ramazanov and his team to introduce fucoxanthin into the marketplace, employing the same doses as used in the Russian clinical research. The result was fücoTHIN—a combination of fucoxanthin from two species of brown seaweed—*undaria* (wakame) and *laminaria* (kombu)—and pomegranate seed oil.

By harvesting the brown seaweed at a young age, fücoTHIN delivers fucoxanthin in a concentration 250 to 500 times greater than by consuming sea vegetables alone. You'd have to drink miso soup by the gallon or use your chopsticks on bowl after bowl of seaweed salad to get a fraction as much of fucoxanthin.

Garden of Life released fücoTHIN just before we launched Healthy Toledo, great timing for the participants and great news for those following the Perfect Weight America program. What we told Healthy Toledo participants is something I need to say here: all the research we viewed showed that fücoTHIN's fat-burning results took about five to six weeks to react after you started taking one capsule with each meal. The effects seemed to be gradual and measurable, providing a steady metabolic boost, but research suggested that by taking an advanced dosage of nine to ten capsules per day in divided doses, results could be noticed as early as two or three weeks. Either way, don't buy a bottle and think it's going to work right away. It takes time for your metabolism to shift.

There Are No Magic Pills

Toss a basketball into a storefront vitamin store, and I'll guarantee that you'll knock dozens of weight-loss supplements boasting about their thermogenic properties off the shelves. The Natural Medicines Comprehensive Database lists more than 50 individual supplements and 125 proprietary products being marketed as weight-loss products, although their efficacy and long-term safety are question marks. For example, guar gum, produced from Indian cluster beans, and chitosan, extracted from shellfish, are sold as "fat blockers."

Hoodia, the extract of a South African cactus, is the rage in some weight-loss circles because of the way it purportedly dampens hunger. The supplement "is not thermogenic, so it does not speed up metabolism," explained Fred Pescatore, MD, and author of The Hamptons Diet. "It is simply an appetite suppressant. It does work, but it's not a superstar."[5]

Hoodia is mild stuff compared to ephedra, one of the most famous—or infamous— "fat-burner" supplements in the last ten years. Dietary aids containing the herbal supplement ephedra were huge sellers until they were linked to 155 deaths in the United States earlier this decade, including that of Baltimore Orioles 6-foot, 2-inch, 249-pound pitching prospect Steve Bechler, who died of a heatstroke during a spring-training workout in 2003. Bechler's body temperature rose to 108 degrees, causing his major organs to fail. Toxicology tests on Bechler revealed significant amounts of ephedra in his blood. The Broward County medical examiner in South Florida declared that ephedra was a factor in causing the heatstroke that led to his death.[6]

Following the rash of bad publicity, the U.S. Food and Drug Administration reacted by banning ephedra, but a federal judge threw out the FDA ban in 2005. The FDA appealed the ruling, and in 2006, the U.S. Court of Appeals for the Tenth Circuit upheld the FDA's ban of ephedra. The sale of ephedra-containing dietary supplements remains illegal in the United States. Canadian authorities were on the ball earlier in the game; they banned ephedra weight-loss products in 2001.

Colour me a skeptic. Believe me, I know that there are still hundreds of weight-loss products that tout their ability to burn fat or raise your metabolism. The vast majority of them don't work or, as in the case of ephedra, are extremely dangerous.

For the last half-dozen years, I've resisted the urge to launch a fat-burning product until Dr. Ramazanov and fucoxanthin came along. The clinical trials with the 150 obese Russian women sealed the deal for me because the overweight Russian women took the concentrated fucoxanthin developed by Dr. Ramazanov, whom I trusted. I'm confident that fücoTHIN will be one of the greatest fat-loss breakthroughs in the last decade.

What Dr. Bernard Bulwer and Dr. Joseph Brasco Have to Say

I asked my coauthor Bernard Bulwer, MD, and Joseph Brasco, MD, my coauthor on other books I've published, to read Dr. Ramazanov's research on fucoxanthin as well as a pair of double-blind, randomized, placebo-controlled clinical trials authored by Dr. Musa Abidov, professor of medicine at the Russian Academy of Natural Sciences in Moscow, and others on his team. These were the studies involving 150 obese women. Here's what my medical colleagues had to say:

Bernard Bulwer, MD, Cardiology (Noninvasive)/Echocardiography, Harvard Medical School

It appears, from my reading of the research data, that we have a promising weapon to help fight the battle of the bulge. I don't like to use the phrase "the next big thing," but fucoxanthin is a potentially powerful tool in our quest for improved health of Americans.

Many "fat loss" products have come and gone. A number—both prescription and nonprescription varieties (for example, fen-phen and ephedra)—proved risky, even fatal, and were banned by the FDA. The findings from the Moscow fucoxanthin/pomegranate seed oil study of 150 obese women—which appears to be a carefully crafted study pending publication—indicated that in addition to losing the unhealthiest form of body fat (abdominal and visceral fat), fucoxanthin did not increase heart rate or cause jitters.

I noted with keen interest that fucoxanthin helped to maintain good C-reactive protein (CRP) levels, an indicator of inflammation within our bodies that, when elevated, is a strong and independent predictor of cardiovascular disease. Recent Japanese laboratory experiments in animals showed that fucoxanthin promoted the production of DHA—a healthy omega-3 fat found in fatty fish—that lowers CRP.

Consumption of brown seaweed and pomegranate are age-old practices by some of the world's longest-lived and leanest cultures. Judging from its long history of consumption and safety, and the evidence from published laboratory and animal experiments, and now this first recent clinical trial in humans—and there is even a buzz about fucoxanthin on WebMD.com—I have little doubt that this supplement will receive a lot more attention in the near future.

Joseph Brasco, MD, Board Certified, Internal Medicine and Gastroenterology

Most weight-loss products offer a multitude of claims with little scientific evidence to back them up, so it was exciting to read a well-designed study that had a reasonable amount of patients and a valid statistical model.

Fucoxanthin doesn't appear to be a cosmetic, shed-a-few-pounds type of supplement. It really seems to have profound health benefits. Not only will I be recommending it to my patients, but I am also planning on conducting a clinical study in my own clinic. When asked who should take fucoxanthin, my answer is: *Who shouldn't?* In fact, as an avid outdoorsman and triathlete, I use the product myself and have lost those last few stubborn pounds. I'm proud to say that I have a six-pack at age forty-seven!

Whole-Food Supplements

I'm confident that when you consume the right foods, exercise, and take *füco*THIN, you pose a triple threat against fat. While consuming the right foods is the foundation of overall wellness, you could be missing out on nutrients essential to good health for the following reasons:

- Reducing calories
- Disliking certain foods
- Losing nutrients from cooking
- The variable quality of food supply
- Lack of knowledge, motivation, or time for healthy meals
- Nutrient depletion from farming and processing, stress, lifestyle, pollution, and toxins

If you have been a yo-yo dieter for many years—and eaten nothing but cabbage soup or grapefruit for weeks on end, followed by months of junk food—you have deprived your body of vitamins and minerals that it needs to function at its best. If you found yourself nodding your head as you read those bullet points, then I would like you to consider how a couple of key whole-food nutritional supplements can fill the nutritional gaps in your diet.

I believe supplements are needed more than ever, and it's because of the less nutritious foods we eat. First, a history class: Thousands of years ago, our hunter-gatherer ancestors functioned healthily on the "caveman diet," which was comprised of wild plants, foraged fruits, plant roots, mushrooms, nuts, eggs, fish, local game, and honey for dessert. This "Stone Age diet" ended years ago with the development of agricultural practices—the farming of grains and cereals; domesticating cattle, goats, sheep, and lamb; and the development of fermented foods like cultured dairy, relish, and wine. Life on the farm, so to speak, remained this way until the onset of the Industrial Age in the late 1800s and early 1900s, which led to the introduction of manufactured processes that "refined" foods like grains, cereals, and sugar. The fourth and final trend—the one we're living in today—began in the 1950s with the rise of agribusiness, fast-food restaurants, and convenience foods—fast, nutritionally low, highly processed foods.

I believe we need supplemental vitamins, minerals, and antioxidants because our bodies do not produce these nutrients, so they must come from an outside source. Our modern foods have been stripped of many of their healthy components and are devoid of many vitamins and minerals. Today's conventionally grown food is usually low in antioxidants and can cause free-radical damage that can compromise cellular health.

Many overweight people are starved of nutrients because their diets contain mostly "empty" calorie foods. If you begin each day by gulping a multivitamin or two with your orange juice, I have a question for you: Have you checked the label of your multivitamin lately? If you see ingredients such as sucrose, cornstarch, thiamine mononitrate, pyridoxine hydrochloride, or sodium metasilicate listed, your multivitamin is produced from isolated and synthetic materials. When you look on the packaging and see the letters *dl* in front of an ingredient—like "dl-alpha tocopheryl," for example—your multivitamin is using a synthetic version of vitamin E. Again, not all vitamin E is created equal.

Synthetic or isolated multivitamins are never going to be as good or potent as the ones produced from natural sources; studies show that synthetically made vitamins are 50 percent less biologically active than vitamins made from natural sources.[7] So when you introduce nutritional supplements produced from whole foods and other natural sources into your body, you'll double the nutrients available to the body.

I wanted the Healthy Toledo participants to take a natural source, whole-food multivitamin containing important compounds—organic acids, antioxidants, and key nutrients—that would be essential to their health during the campaign. Each participant received three bottles of Garden of Life Living Multi, a whole-food nutritional supplement made with antioxidant-rich fruits and vegetables as well as nutrient-rich cereal grasses, which are super foods. Cereal grasses are the only foods in the vegetable kingdom that, even if consumed alone, enable animals to continually maintain weight, strength, and optimal health.

Grass is richer in nutrients than spinach, broccoli, eggs, and chicken in virtually all categories, including protein. Grass abounds in unidentified growth factors, powerful antioxidants, immune boosters, and many other health-supporting nutrients. Cereal grasses, including the green leaves of wheat, barley, rye, oat, and kamut, are nutrient-dense foods. Wheat and barley grasses are high in chlorophyll, beta-carotene, vitamins C and E, and are among the best plant sources of protein.

Among the seventy-six whole food concentrates in Living Multi are a pair of ingredients provided to us by associates of Dr. Ramazanov: sea vegetables and microalgaes. *Chlorella, spirulina*, and *dunaliella* (golden algae) are common microalgae and provide many of the nutrients the body needs. Chlorella contains an enormous amount of readily available chlorophyll, protein, carbohydrates, all of the B vitamins, vitamins C and E, amino acids, and additional rare trace minerals.

Living Multi is a broad-based whole-food vitamin and mineral supplement containing a potent blend of antioxidant-rich ingredients derived from naturally grown and organic fruits as well as vegetables, tonic mushrooms, sea vegetables, and botanicals, plus trace minerals that supply nutrients important for general health and well-being. Living Multi is made with "living nutrients" containing necessary cofactors required for proper absorption and utilization by the body, including amino acids, antioxidants, probiotics, and organic acids. This multivitamin provides a range of nutrients to support immune function, which is valuable to good health.

Cod Liver Oil

I don't know any hockey analogies, but in baseball terms, fücoTHIN is like a hot-hitting rookie who takes the major leagues by storm right from opening day. But there's a veteran performer—a solid .300 hitter—that I want to tell you about, and it's omega-3-rich cod liver oil, which has been around since Abner Doubleday allegedly invented baseball in 1839.

The benefits of cod liver oil were discovered in the fishing communities dotting the coasts of Norway, Scotland, and Iceland in the nineteenth century. In these remote outposts, taking a spoonful of golden oil pressed from the livers of cod fish carried all sorts of health advantages.

Cod liver oil is a superstar because it contains four nutrients that we hardly get enough of: eicosapentaenoic acid (EPA), docosahexaenoic acid (DHA), vitamin A, and vitamin D. EPA and DHA are long-chain polyunsaturated fats known as omega-3 fatty acids, which are found in cold-water fish and eggs from chickens that run around and eat worms. The omega-3 fatty acids are wonderful not only for maintaining your immune system but also for their ability to promote healthy blood lipids since omega-3 fatty acids can lower blood triglyceride levels. They also support neurological and brain function.

The vitamin A in cod liver oil supports eye health, normal skin and hair structure, and the health and integrity of mucosal lining of the body, such as the gastrointestinal tract and lungs.

The vitamin D in cod liver oil builds strong bones, which can prevent bone deterioration in adults. In addition, vitamin D is suggested to play a pivotal rule in supporting muscle tone and strength.

Each Healthy Toledo participant received three 8-ounce bottles of Garden of Life's Olde World Icelandic Cod Liver Oil with instructions to take between 1 teaspoon and 1 tablespoon a day. Our cod liver comes in a lemon mint flavour to mask the "fishy" odour, but for the uninitiated, cod liver oil can be daunting at the outset.

Well, I don't think cod liver oil tastes *that* bad, but then again, I've been either sipping a spoonful or taking easy-to-swallow liquid capsules of cod liver oil for more than a decade. I'm so used to the fishy taste that I could sip the stuff right out of the bottle.

Don't let the fishy taste keep you from introducing this Hall of Fame nutrient into your diet. Cod liver oil helps prevent bone deterioration in adults, improves cardiovascular function, and contributes to long life—great reasons to get cod liver oil off the bench and into the game.

Q&A Time

I'm going to answer some common questions about the use of nutritional supplements during Perfect Weight Canada:

1. Should all the supplements recommended in this chapter be taken together?
It's OK to take fücoTHIN, Living Multi, and cod liver oil all at the same time. Supplements can also be taken between meals if you missed them at breakfast or lunch, and they can be swallowed with a Perfect Meal shake.

2. What if I feel worse after I start taking supplements?

When starting a healthier diet and lifestyle, you should start slowly, and then gradually work up to the recommended amounts. More importantly, check with your health professional to rule out any other reason for these issues. If issues persist and interfere with daily activities, stop supplementation and build up slowly when feeling better.

3. If I'm eating all these healthy foods, why do I need to take so many Living Multi vitamins?

Taking Living Multi is a wonderful way to ensure that you're getting all the needed nutrients daily. Since it's a whole-food supplement, the dosage amount that satisfies the recommended levels will be higher. They are more like taking concentrated food with your meals than pills. Although they can be taken on an empty stomach with good results, it's better to take them with meals because of the benefits of breaking down foods and carrying nutrients through the bloodstream.

4. After I finish the Perfect Weight Canada sixteen-week plan, do I still need to take all the required supplements daily?

After the completion of the Perfect Weight Eating Plan, it's entirely up to you whether or not you continue taking the supplements. If possible, though, you should continue taking them since they can help optimize your health.

5. Is there a difference in which supplements you should take based on age? What about children?

No, there isn't a difference, but it's always a good idea to check with your primary care physician before starting a supplement program. Every individual is unique, especially when you consider differences in age and fitness level. As for children, we do not have a suggested usage for those under the age of sixteen. Suggested use is based on a 150-pound individual. Please contact your pediatrician for any recommendations.

6. Can I take supplements with my medication?

As you might anticipate, we are not able to provide medical advice. Please ask your doctor or pharmacist if you can take the recommended supplements with your medication.

Perfect Weight Recap: Supplement for Your Perfect Weight

- Support your body's own breakdown of fat and increase your metabolism with fücoTHIN. Take this supplement for at least two or three months since research shows that fücoTHIN doesn't start kicking in until forty-five days have passed.
- Cover your bases with Garden of Life Living Multi.
- Even if you have to hold your nose the first time or two, take 1 teaspoon to 1 tablespoon of cod liver oil. (I recommend Olde World Icelandic Cod Liver Oil, as I know where and how this is prepared.) Or, if you're traveling or just can't handle taking oil off the spoon, try Garden of Life's CODMega omega-3 cod liver oil capsules.

Chapter 7

The Perfect Weight Eating Plan

Now that we've talked about how you can eat, drink, snack, and supplement for your perfect weight, I'd like to present you with the sixteen-week Perfect Weight Eating Plan that's broken down into four phases. Each phase offers approved foods while restricting others. Phase I is the most challenging and requires the most discipline. But, as in life, the more you put in, the more you get in return. If you follow Phase I to the best of your abilities, you should receive excellent results and lose between six and sixteen pounds. The following three phases get progressively easier as certain foods are reintroduced to your diet.

In Chapter 15, "The Perfect Weight Daily Health Plan," you will find four different Perfect Weight Nutritional Type Wellness Plans, which are based upon your answers to the nutritional type questionnaire in chapter 3, "Eat for Your Perfect Weight," on page 64. These health and wellness plans are divided by gender and whether you're a meat type or a potato type.

You'll notice that under the listing for "Get FIT for your perfect weight," I've given you rigorous functional interval training (FIT) exercise instructions that you can follow. If you feel the physical demands are too great, then pick and choose the exercises you can perform.

For a more personalized sixteen-week eating and lifestyle plan, visit www .PerfectWeightCanada.com and take your online personal health assessment. Once you complete this short questionnaire, you will receive daily e-mails and a customized eating, supplementation, and exercise plan that includes daily menus, shopping lists, and many additional features to help you achieve your perfect weight. Best of all, a one-year subscription to PerfectWeightCanada.com is free. Log on to www.PerfectWeightCanada.com today.

Phase I (Week 1–Week 4)

This sixteen-week program begins with Phase I, the "purification" phase, which is the most rigorous and challenging part of Perfect Weight Canada but also the most rewarding. You'll see in the approved foods lists that white sugar, artificial sweeteners, and preservatives are forbidden. Not eating these foods often causes temporary withdrawal-type symptoms such as headaches, carbohydrate cravings, less energy, mood swings, or even changes in your bowel habits. These "detox" reactions are indications that the body is working to cleanse toxins from the system. When you have the "blahs," increase water intake and rest.

Phase I is designed to stabilize blood sugar levels, reduce inflammation, enhance digestion, and balance hormone levels in the body. This phase restricts disaccharide-heavy carbohydrate foods such as pastas and breads but makes up for it in the variety of delicious, high-nutrient, high-fibre foods you can enjoy. You are more likely to see significant weight loss during this phase due to the consumption of higher amounts of protein and healthy fats and less carbohydrates. There is also the added benefit of improved digestion, smoother skin, and increased energy levels.

During Phase I, I recommend that you not drink any alcohol—wine, beer, or mixed drinks—but you are allowed two "cheat" meals per week. The best time to cheat is on the weekend, but do not eat, if possible, any of the "Dirty Dozen" foods listed in chapter 3, "Eat for Your Perfect Weight." Organic treats such as dates rolled in coconut, flaxseed crackers, rice chips, and dried fruits—"nature's candy"—make up "good" cheats.

Try to keep your cheating within a sixty-minute period so the body doesn't release more insulin into the bloodstream.

PHASE I FOODS: WEEKS 1–4	
MEAT (GRASS-FED/ORGANIC IS BEST)	
Approved	Avoid
Goat	Alligator
Beef or buffalo sausages or hot dogs (no pork casing—natural nitrite/nitrate free is best)	Bacon
Veal	Emu
Elk	Frog
Lamb	Ham
Bone soup/stock	Imitation meat products (soy)
Liver and heart (must be organic or grass fed)	Ostrich
Beef	Pork
Venison	Sausage (pork)
Buffalo	Turtle
	Veggie burgers
FISH (WILD FRESHWATER/OCEAN-CAUGHT FISH IS BEST; MAKE SURE IT HAS FINS AND SCALES)	
Approved	Avoid
Salmon	Fried, breaded fish
Tuna	Eel
Scrod	Shark
Halibut	Catfish
Cod	Squid
Grouper	All shellfish (crab, clams, oyster, mussels, lobster, shrimp, scallops, and crawfish)
Haddock	
Pompano	
Trout	
Orange roughy	

Snapper	
Herring	
Whitefish	
Sardines (canned in water or olive oil only)	
Salmon (canned in spring water)	
Tuna (canned in spring water)	
Mahi mahi	
Wahoo	
Tilapia	
Sea bass	
Mackerel	
Sole	
Fish bone soup/stock	

POULTRY (PASTURED/ORGANIC IS BEST)

Approved	Avoid
Chicken	Fried, breaded chicken
Guinea fowl	Processed lunch meats
Duck	
Chicken or turkey bacon (no pork casing—organic and nitrite/nitrate free is best)	
Natural chicken or turkey hot dogs	
Cornish game hen	
Turkey	
Bone soup/stock	
Natural deli meats, including chicken, turkey, and roast beef	
Chicken or turkey sausage (no pork casing—natural and nitrite/nitrate free is best; use sparingly in Phase I)	
Liver and heart (must be organic or grass fed)	

EGGS (HIGH OMEGA-3/DHA OR ORGANIC ARE BEST)

Approved	Avoid
Chicken eggs (whole with yoke)	Imitation eggs (such as Egg Beaters)
Duck eggs (whole with yolk)	

DAIRY (ORGANIC IS BEST)

Approved	Avoid
Whole-milk yogurt (plain)	Soy milk
Sheep's milk yogurt (plain)	Rice milk
Goat's milk yogurt (plain)	Cow's milk and ice cream
Whole-milk cheese	Processed cheese food
Soft goat's, cow's, or sheep's milk cheese	Flavored, low-fat, or fat-free cheese, yogurt, and kefir
Sheep's milk hard cheese	Dry milk (many processed foods contain this ingredient)
Goat's milk hard cheese	
Feta cheese (sheep's milk or goat's milk)	
Full-fat plain kefir	

Full-fat cottage cheese	
Ricotta cheese	
Full-fat sour cream	
Plain almond milk (unsweetened)	
Goat's milk protein powder (for smoothies)	
Cultured buttermilk	

FATS AND OILS (ORGANIC IS BEST)

Approved	Avoid
Flaxseed oil (not for cooking)	Lard
Butter oil (ghee)	Margarine
Hemp seed oil (not for cooking)	Shortening
Avocado	Soy oil
Cow's milk butter	Safflower oil
Goat's milk butter	Sunflower oil
Expeller-pressed sesame oil	Cottonseed oil
Coconut milk/cream (canned or fresh)	Canola oil
Extra-virgin coconut oil (best for cooking)	Corn oil
Extra-virgin olive oil (not best for cooking)	Any partially hydrogenated oil
Peanut oil (cold-pressed and unrefined)	

VEGETABLES (ORGANIC FRESH OR FROZEN ARE BEST)

Approved	Avoid
Squash (winter or summer)	Corn
Asparagus	Sweet potatoes
Cauliflower	White potatoes
Cabbage	
Celery	
Eggplant	
Garlic	
Okra	
Peas	
String beans	
Lettuce (all varieties)	
Artichoke (French, not Jerusalem)	
Leafy greens (kale, collard, broccoli rabe, mustard greens, etc.)	
Sprouts (broccoli, sunflower, pea shoots, radish, etc.)	
Sea vegetables (kelp, dulse, nori, kombu, hijiki, etc.)	
Raw, fermented vegetables (lacto-fermented only, no vinegar)	
Broccoli	
Beets	
Brussels sprouts	
Carrots	
Cucumber	
Pumpkin	
Onion	

Mushrooms	
Peppers	
Tomatoes	
Spinach	

BEANS AND LEGUMES (SOAKED OR FERMENTED ARE BEST)	
Approved	**Avoid**
Small amounts of fermented soybean paste (miso) as a broth	Soybeans
Lentils	Tofu
Black beans	
Navy beans	
Garbanzo beans	
Lima beans	
Tempeh (fermented soybean loaf)	
Kidney beans	
White beans	
Pinto beans	
Split beans	
Black-eyed peas	
Red beans	
Broad beans	

NUTS AND SEEDS (ORGANIC, RAW, OR SOAKED ARE BEST)	
Approved	**Avoid**
Almonds/almond butter	Honey-roasted nuts
Hemp seeds/hemp seed butter	Peanuts/peanut butter
Sunflower seeds/sunflower butter	Cashews
Tahini/sesame butter	
Macadamia nuts	
Hazelnuts	
Pecans	
Walnuts	
Brazil nuts	
Chia seeds	
Pumpkin seeds/pumpkin seed butter	
Flaxseeds	

CONDIMENTS, SPICES, SEASONINGS, COOKING INGREDIENTS, AND SALAD DRESSINGS (ORGANIC IS BEST)	
Approved	**Avoid**
Ketchup (natural or organic)	All spices that contain added sugar
Salsa (fresh or canned, organic)	Commercial ketchup with sugar
Hot sauce (preservative-free)	Commercial barbecue sauce with sugar
Tomato sauce (no added sugar)	White wine vinegar
Soy sauce (wheat free), tamari	
Herbamare seasoning	
Omega-3 mayonnaise	

Homemade salad dressing and marinades using Phase I–allowable ingredients	
Guacamole (fresh)	
Apple cider vinegar	
Mustard	
Celtic Sea Salt	
Umeboshi paste	
Bragg salad dressings	
Bragg Liquid Aminos	
Balsamic vinegar	
Red wine vinegar	
Herbs and spices (no added stabilizers)	
Pickled ginger (no preservatives or color)	
Wasabi (no preservatives or color)	
Organic flavoring extracts (alcohol-based, no sugar added, vanilla, almond, etc.)	
Cooking wine (organic red and white)	
Capers	

FRUITS (ORGANIC FRESH OR FROZEN IS BEST)

Approved	Avoid
Blueberries	Bananas
Blackberries	Mangoes
Cherries	Dried fruit
Lemons	Canned fruit
Pomegranates	
Apples (with skin)	
Melons	
Apricots (not dried)	
Peaches	
Grapes	
Oranges	
Pears	
Papayas	
Kiwi	
Nectarines	
Strawberries	
Raspberries	
Grapefruit	
Limes	
Cranberries (not dried)	
Olives	
Pineapple	
Plums	
Fresh figs	

BEVERAGES

Approved	Avoid
Purified, nonchlorinated water	Alcoholic beverages of any kind

Natural sparkling water, no carbonation added	Preground commercial coffee
Herbal teas (preferably organic)—unsweetened or with a small amount of honey or stevia	Sodas
Raw vegetable juice (beet or carrot juice—maximum 25 percent of total)	Fruit juices
Lacto-fermented beverages	Chlorinated tap water
Certified organic coffee—buy whole beans, freeze them, and grind them yourself when desired; flavor only with organic cream and a small amount of honey	

SWEETENERS	
Approved	**Avoid**
Unheated, raw honey in very small amounts (2 tablespoons per day maximum)	Sugar (including organic sugars, all-natural cane sugar, and organic brown sugar)
The herbal supplement stevia in small quantities	Maple syrup
Lo Han Guo in small quantities	Fructose or corn syrup
Xylitol in small quantities or in mints and gum	All artificial sweeteners, including aspartame, sucralose, and acesulfame K
	Sugar alcohol, including sorbitol and malitol

MISCELLANEOUS	
Approved	**Avoid**
Perfect Meal	Milk or whey protein powder from cow's milk
Goat's milk protein powder (for recommendations, see the PWA Resource Guide)	Soy protein powder
Native whey protein	Rice protein powder

GRAINS AND STARCHY CARBOHYDRATES	
Approved	**Avoid**
Arrowroot powder (as a substitute for cornstarch)	All grains and starchy foods
	Bread
	Pasta
	Cereal
	Rice
	Oatmeal
	Pastries
	Baked goods
	Corn tortillas

Phase II Foods
Weeks 5–8

Phase II allows for a greater variety of foods, but weight loss is not as rapid during this phase. The most important point of Phase II is to maintain blood sugar levels and create and instill healthy eating habits that can last a lifetime. During Phase II, you're cleared to eat all the foods listed in Phase I, plus the foods listed below. Remember, you should still not drink any alcohol: wine, beer, or mixed drinks. Keep your cheat meals to a minimum; no more than one or two a week.

Dairy

- Cow's feta cheese
- Blue cheese
- Parmesan cheese

Eggs

- Fish roe or caviar (fresh, not preserved)

Fruits

- Bananas and mangoes
- Dates and dried figs

Avoid canned fruit and dried fruit, including raisins, dates, figs, prunes, bananas, mango, and papaya.

Fats and oils

- Expeller-pressed peanut oil or coconut oil, both good for cooking

Vegetables

- Sweet potatoes and yams
- White potatoes and corn

Beans and legumes

- Tofu and soybeans (endamame)

Avoid garbanzo beans and lima beans.

Nuts and seeds

- Peanuts, peanut butter, and cashews

Avoid honey-roasted nuts and any nuts or seeds roasted in oil.

Condiments, spices, and seasonings

- Healthy salad dressings

Avoid canola oil, fat-free dressings, and dressings with chemicals.

Beverages

- Raw vegetable juice (beet or carrot—maximum 50 percent of total)
- Coconut water

Sweeteners

- Unheated, raw honey (no limitation on amount)
- The herbal supplement stevia in small quantities

- Lo Han Guo in small quantities
- Xylitol in small quantities or in mints and gum

Avoid maple syrup, heated honey, fructose or corn syrup, and sugars like all-natural cane sugar, organic white sugar, and organic brown sugar.

Snacks/miscellaneous

- Organic whole food bars (naturally sweetened)

Phase III Foods
Weeks 9–12

Phase III allows you to increase the varieties of foods as well as more carbohydrates into the diet. You may be wondering, "Can I maintain weight loss by eating carbohydrates again?"

The answer is yes! Carbohydrates do have a place in our diets and bodies, but the carbs must be in their natural and unrefined state. Fuel your body with simple whole fruits and honey, complex sprouted grains, delightful beans, and healthy vegetables. Supplying your body with these excellent and natural carbohydrates will help you to balance the chemical processes in your body and keep you healthy.

In addition to the approved foods in Phase I and Phase II, you can add the following foods in Phase III:

- Dairy such as raw cow's or goat's milk, or organic nonhomogenized cow's and goat's milk
- Dried fruit with no sugar or sulfites, and canned fruit in its own juices
- Grains such as sprouted Ezekiel-type bread, sprouted Essene bread, fermented whole-grain sourdough bread, quinoa, amaranth, buckwheat, millet, brown rice, sprouted cereal, oats, kamut, spelt, barley, bulgur wheat, and whole-grain kamut or spelt pasta in small quantities
- Sweeteners such as sucanat, Rapadura, agave nectar, and unrefined maple syrup (but don't consume organic sugars like all-natural cane sugar, organic white sugar, and organic brown sugar)
- Miscellaneous snacks such as healthy trail mix, Jennie's Macaroons, organic chocolate spreads, and healthy popcorn

I still recommend that you not drink any alcohol, but if it's a special occasion, organic red wine is preferred. Organic white wine is OK, but it contains less of the antioxidant benefits of organic red wine. As for beer, an unpasteurized organic beer is the best choice. I don't recommend mixed drinks at all.

By now, your desire to "cheat" should have waned considerably.

Phase IV Foods
Weeks 13–16

Phase IV is the "lifestyle" phase that will allow you to maintain your perfect weight. As you approach your perfect weight, you should notice significant improvements in your health. If you're feeling great and feeling like you're reached your perfect weight, then continue on this lifestyle phase.

Phase IV also provides you the opportunity to step back and ask some questions: Have you reached the goals you've set for yourself? Do you feel and look the way you want? If you are still suffering from symptoms related to insulin resistance or you feel like you've gotten off track, then use this time period to implement Phase I or Phase II again.

You're cleared to resume drinking alcohol, but in moderate amounts. Remember: organic red wine is best, followed by organic white wine and unpasteurized organic beer. Skip the Cosmopolitans and other mixed drinks that use hard spirits. Don't forget that alcohol has twice as many calories per gram as protein or carbohydrates. Cheat meals should be a thing of the past, as well as your cravings for junk food.

Eat meals balanced with whole foods and healthy proteins and fats, watch your portion size, continue to eliminate refined foods, and maintain regular exercise into your week. Also, don't forget that you can receive a daily eating plan complete with menus, recipes, and shopping lists that are appropriate for the eating phase that you're on, as well as recipes, a personal exercise program, and daily health tips by visiting www.PerfectWeightCanada.com and filling out your personal health assessment.

I've provided four different health and wellness plans based on your nutritional type, which was determined by your answers to the nutritional type questionnaire in chapter 3, "Eat for Your Perfect Weight" on page 64. You will find these four plans in chapter 15, "The Perfect Weight Daily Health Plan," on page 224. No matter what you eat or what meal plan you follow, however, it's imperative to think about cleansing your body, which is the topic of our next chapter.

Perfect Weight Recap: The Perfect Weight Eating Plan

- Phase I, or the "purification" phase, of the Perfect Weight Eating Program is designed to stabilize blood sugar levels, reduce inflammation, enhance digestion, and balance hormone levels in the body.
- Phase II allows for a greater variety of food, and although weight loss is not rapid, it does help maintain blood sugar levels and create lifelong healthy eating habits.
- Natural, unrefined carbohydrates fuel your system and balance the chemical process in your body and keep you healthy. Phase III incorporates a larger, delicious variety if carbohydrates.
- In Phase IV, or the "lifestyle" phase, you will have the opportunity to step back and ask yourself questions to pinpoint areas where you may have gotten off track.

Section III
Change Your Life

Chapter 8

Cleanse for Your Perfect Weight

WHAT GOES INTO the body must come out.

Alimentary, my dear Watson, but all too often, everything *doesn't* come out, which is why cleansing is an important part of Perfect Weight Canada.

The gastrointestinal tract, elementarily known as the alimentary canal, is expertly designed to help the body break down food and absorb its nutrients as well as eliminate unwanted waste products. Not that anyone would want to, but if you stretched your digestive tract from end to end, it would measure 25 to 35 feet—around the width of a singles tennis court.

The digestive tract needs that much length to completely break down the food's nutrients and distribute them throughout the body by way of the bloodstream. Anything that's left over is expelled from the body either through urine or fecal elimination. (The body also eliminates wastes and toxins through exhalation and sweating, but the heavy lifting is performed by the digestive tract.) During your lifetime, sixty tons of food will pass through the gastrointestinal system, making for a lot of…elimination.[1]

When you grab a forkful of pasta or bite into a delicious apple, you begin a physiological process that you have taken for granted since your mother spoon-fed you Gerber's yams in a high chair. Every time you take a bite of food into your mouth, the salivary glands begin their work, filling your mouth with mucus-like saliva that adheres to the food. After you're finished chewing and are ready to swallow, the tongue pushes the soft mass—called the *bolus*—to the back of the mouth and into the pharynx, which is the cavity between the mouth and the windpipe that serves as the body's alimentary passageway to the stomach via the esophagus.

How long your food spends in the esophagus before reaching the stomach depends on how well it was chewed. Food that has been chewed well—properly masticated, as they say in jolly old England—makes the journey in just seven seconds. Food that's dry or not properly chewed can take a full minute to wend its way through the esophagus, which is not good for the delicate tissues lining this 10-inch tube between the throat and the stomach. Improperly chewed food that reaches the stomach takes longer to digest, which creates acute, temporary stress on the entire gastrointestinal process.

129

Chewing foods properly, however, allows enzymes in your saliva to turn the food into a near liquid form before swallowing, allowing it to shimmy down the esophagus like a fireman sliding down a slick pole to answer an emergency call. The act of working your jaw also sends a neurological message to your stomach and pancreas to increase acid and digestive enzyme production because food's on the way.

Regarding the chewing end of the deal, I'm figuring you've never heard of Horace Fletcher, an American health-food faddist during Victorian times who was known as "The Great Masticator." A raconteur, world traveler, millionaire businessman, amateur painter, speaker, and author, Fletcher tirelessly promoted his theory of good chewing: he recommended that food be chewed thirty-two times—which works the jaw one hundred times per minute—before being swallowed. "Nature will castigate those who don't masticate," he warned. Followers of "Fletcherism," as his doctrine became known, included industrialist John D. Rockefeller and authors Upton Sinclair and Henry James.[2]

I understand that chewing your food many times will seem like an arduous task, but masticating your food thoroughly—especially foods high in carbohydrates—enhances the digestive process and reduces post-meal bloating. More importantly, as it relates to Perfect Weight Canada, chewing your food slowly and thoroughly can help you reach your perfect weight since the brain will have more time to register the amount of food you are consuming—and perhaps make you eat less. In other words, chewing well will give you time to set your fork down and come to a stop when the stoplight flashes yellow, signalling you're full and it's time to shut down the eating express. Chewing your food thirty-two times before swallowing may be a bit much, but can you chew each bite fifteen or twenty times before gulping and swallowing?

Dr. Fletcher would be proud of me. I've become a much better "chewer" over the years, especially compared to my college days at Florida State, where I wolfed down double cheeseburgers bite-for-humongous-bite with the best of my fraternity buddies. In fact, if you were to dine with me today, you'd be surprised at how long I take to chew my food. It has taken some effort to reprogram the way I eat, but I know that chewing food slowly ensures that plenty of digestive juices are added to each bite before it begins its long, winding journey through the digestive tract.

The reason I'm making a big deal about this mastication business is because properly chewing your food is the first step in cleansing your body as you march toward your perfect weight. Speaking as someone who nearly died from horrible digestive problems, I can assure you that the health of the gastrointestinal tract is imperative for overall wellness. Unfortunately for many of us, the typical modern diet never allows the body to cleanse itself properly. Eating the wrong foods—I'm thinking greasy chicken and sticky sweets—is like filling your car's fuel tank with crude oil rather than 93-octane fuel.

Furthermore, a diet heavy in processed foods does not provide the deep-seated nutrition the body needs to build and repair muscles, grow strong bones, or keep things moving where it counts. Processed foods strain the gut, causing the digestive system to work harder to extract nutrients. This explains why many North Americans feel "down in the dumps" after they eat; they feel stuffed, bloated, or constipated. When an overloaded gastrointestinal system gets backed up, fecal matter can ferment in the colon and cause painful bowel problems. The colon wall absorbs the remaining water in the feces, turning the stool hard as stone pebbles. The harder the feces, the more difficult it is to eliminate.

The goal is for the digestive tract to run like a Swiss train: everything leaving the station on time. Under ideal conditions—and the consumption of whole foods—twelve to twenty-four hours should pass between the moment the meal is finished until the moment waste is eliminated at the other end. The amount of time that foods stay in the digestive tract before you have to go to the bathroom is called "bowel transit time." Food that leaves the body in less than twelve hours—which happens when you have diarrhea—cannot be adequately absorbed. The body cannot extract the nutrients it needs in such a short time, which is one reason why you feel weak and uneasy after a bout of diarrhea.

On the other hand, those who munch throughout the day on glazed doughnuts, french fries, pretzels, and snack cakes present the body with *too many* carbohydrates to digest. Leftover undigested carbs camp in the gut longer than twenty-four hours and impair digestion. Instead of everything being eliminated on time, the substances linger inside the intestines, causing an overgrowth of harmful bacteria and yeasts, which can lead to abdominal discomfort and mischief.

In addition, those who consume too many desserts with refined sugars unwittingly feed the "bad" microorganisms in the intestines. Sugary foods feed harmful bacteria that irritate and unbalance the delicate flora lining of the gastrointestinal or GI tract. Sugary foods also encourage specific kinds of intestinal bacteria to flourish at the expense of others. More than four hundred different types of bacteria or "gut flora" live inside our intestines, and what we eat influences the ratio of "good" versus "bad" gut flora by allowing some kinds to out-compete others.

Habitual intake of a diet high in refined and highly processed foods leads to accumulation of toxins, increased contact time, and damage to the lining of the gut due to constipation and higher pressures developing inside the bowel. In plain language, such foods gunk up the digestive tract like a mass of cookie dough in a garbage disposal.

Enough already! That's what the body is saying after years, if not decades, of abuse. If the digestive system isn't given a chance to restore itself—through body therapies known as cleansing and fasting—then digestive-related disorders and diseases can and will occur, affecting the very core of how the body grows, repairs itself, gains energy, and reaches its perfect weight.

The famous British surgeon Sir Dennis Burkitt, who worked in Africa during the World War II and for decades afterward, remarked that he rarely saw the "diseases of civilization"—constipation, hemorrhoids, diarrhea, etc.—among the African people. As for the British and Americans he treated, he concluded that the West's highly refined diet resulted in hard, dry stools that passed sluggishly through the intestine and required a large increase in luminal pressure for their evacuation.

The longer toxins hang around your body, including inside your gut—the greater their potential for discomfort and problems. From where do these toxins arise? Toxins are literally everywhere in our environment. No food is guaranteed 100 percent safe. We live on a fallen planet. We drink, eat, inhale, and produce toxins. This is not an alarmist statement.

Don't believe me; check out the facts yourself. The foods we eat contain untold numbers of agents that are *not* food: pesticides, additives, colourants, extraneous hormones, chemicals, and heavy metals, not to mention prescription and nonprescription drugs—which our bodies, especially the liver, are forced to detoxify, which is why we have elimination systems, especially in our urine and stool.

This is why I strongly recommend that you embark on something I call the Perfect Cleanse—a ten-day detoxification and cleansing system I recommend be done four times a year. The Perfect Cleanse combines a revolutionary ten-day detoxifying eating plan and a ten-day, three-step cleansing supplement system aimed at purifying, capturing, and removing toxins from the body. Toward the end of this chapter, I give a complete hour-by-hour road map of the Perfect Cleanse, broken down by the seasons, that you can follow.

What the Perfect Cleanse Is All About

The Perfect Cleanse is a ten-day detoxification cleanse that should be done quarterly in January, April, July, and October. During your ten-day Perfect Cleanse, you will eat five times a day, every two to three hours. Most people eat breakfast around 7:30 a.m., followed by a second meal at 10:30 a.m., lunch at 1:00 p.m., a mid-afternoon meal at 3:30 p.m., and dinner at 6:00 p.m. The first day of each seasonal detox cleanse is crucial.

Winter Perfect Cleanse

For the Winter Perfect Cleanse, you should consume only homemade chicken soup (or a broth from a vegetable soup) for all five meals on the first day. My wife, Nicki, who's a wonderful cook, and I have come up with an excellent recipe that we call, tongue in cheek, "Cleansing Chicken Soup." This recipe was inspired by my late grandmother Rose:

Cleansing Chicken Soup	
1 whole chicken (free range, pastured, or organic chicken)	3–4 quarts filtered water
1 Tbsp. raw apple cider vinegar	4 medium-sized onions, coarsely chopped

8 carrots, peeled and coarsely chopped	6 celery stalks, coarsely chopped
2–4 zucchinis chopped	1 pound green beans
4 Tbsp. extra-virgin coconut oil	1 bunch parsley
½ cup fresh or frozen green peas	5 garlic cloves
4 inches grated ginger	2–4 Tbsp. Celtic Sea Salt
¼–½ tsp. cayenne pepper	

If you are using a whole chicken, remove fat glands and gizzards from the cavity. Place chicken or chicken pieces in a large stainless steel pot with the water, vinegar, garlic, ginger, salt, cayenne pepper, extra-virgin coconut oil, and all vegetables except parsley. Let stand for 10 minutes before heating. Bring to a boil, removing the scum that rises to the top. Cover and cook for 8–12 hours. The longer you cook the stock, the more cleansing it will be. About 15 minutes before finishing the stock, add parsley. This will impart additional mineral ions to the broth.

Remove from heat and take out the chicken. After it cools, remove chicken meat from the carcass, discarding the bones. Drop the meat back to the soup. You may purée for even easier digestion.

On days 2–4, consume Cleansing Chicken Soup during the four daytime meals, followed by a healthy salad for dinner containing all the coloured vegetables you can think of. Greens and sprouts are wonderful high-fibre foods, but be sure to add slices of cucumbers, carrots, red onion, cabbage, tomatoes, and celery. Garnish with half an avocado, and add 2 tablespoons of a healthy raw salad dressing. (Please see the PWC Resource Guide on page 322 for recommended brands.) You can also make your own dressing from the following ingredients:

- Extra-virgin olive oil
- Apple-cider vinegar or lemon juice
- Some of your favourite herbs, spices, and seasonings
- A dash of sea salt, liquid aminos, or soy sauce

You can eat as much salad as you want, limiting the avocado to one-half and the dressing to 2 tablespoons, but make sure you finish eating by 7:00 p.m. After that, I'm afraid, you're done eating for the day, and that's the toughest part, especially for those used to a bowl of Ben & Jerry's ice cream or a handful of chocolate chip cookies before going to bed.

On days 5–7, you can add raw nuts and seeds to your salad after eating Cleansing Chicken Soup throughout the day.

On days 8–10, eat Cleansing Chicken Soup for the first four meals, but you may add 4 ounces of plain whole-milk yogurt or kefir and 1 tablespoon of raw honey for your third and fourth meal.

For your fifth meal, it's advisable to add some fatty fish (salmon, mackerel, herring, sardines, or tuna) and raw cheese to your salad, which will help you transition into the Perfect Weight Eating Plan once the Perfect Cleanse is over. In addition to the five meals, it is important to drink ¾ of an ounce of water per pound of body weight per day.

Spring and Fall Perfect Cleanses

For the Spring and Fall Perfect Cleanses, the first two meals of the day are fruit. Be sure to eat only one type of fruit—1 or 2 cups—at each meal. Try to eat high-sugar fruit like mangoes, pineapple, and papaya early in the day rather than late. Lower-sugar fruits are apples, cantaloupe, watermelon, berries, grapefruit, oranges, peaches, plums, and tangerines.

The lunch and mid-afternoon meals are Cleansing Chicken Soup, and your fifth meal is a salad. As with the Winter Cleanse, you can make your salad with your favourite greens and vegetables. Garnish with half an avocado, and add 2 tablespoons of a healthy raw salad dressing or make your own. Follow this regimen for the first four days.

On days 5–7, you can add raw nuts and seeds to your salad after eating fruit for the first two meals and Cleansing Chicken Soup for the third and fourth meal.

On days 8–10, during your fruit meals (meals one and two), add 4 ounces of whole-milk plain yogurt or kefir and 1 tablespoon raw honey. Consume Cleansing Chicken Soup for meals three and four. At your last (fifth) meal, add cheese and fatty fish (like wild-caught salmon) to your salad, which will help you transition into the Perfect Weight Eating Plan once the Perfect Cleanse is over.

As mentioned earlier, you can eat as much salad as you want, but make sure you finish eating by 7:00 p.m.

Summer Perfect Cleanse

For the Summer Perfect Cleanse, the first day is a mono diet where you will eat the same fruit at each meal for the entire day, marked by five fruit servings (1 or 2 cups of fruit for each serving). The best fruits for cleansing have a lot of water: watermelon, grapes, apples, and oranges. Bananas don't have nearly as much water.

On days 2–4, eat four servings of fruit during the day, separated by two to three hours, followed by a healthy salad for dinner containing all the vegetables you can think of. Greens and sprouts are wonderful high-fibre foods, but be sure to add slices of cucumbers, carrots, red onion, cabbage, tomatoes, and celery. Garnish with half an avocado, and add 2 tablespoons of a healthy raw salad dressing or make your own.

On days 5–7, follow the same regimen, but now you can add raw nuts and seeds to your salad.

On days 8–10, eat one serving of fruit during the first two meals of the day. For your third and fourth meal, eat one type of fruit, 4 ounces of whole-milk plain yogurt or kefir, and 1 tablespoon of honey. Add raw cheese and fatty fish (like wild-caught salmon) to your salad meal, which will help you transition into the Perfect Weight Eating Plan once the Perfect Cleanse is over.

OK, it was a publicity stunt, but nine Brits pitched a tent at Paignton Zoo in Devon, right next to the monkey exhibit. Their goal: cast aside processed foods in favour of a twelve-day "Evo Diet," consuming up to 5 kilos (12 pounds) of raw fruits and vegetables a day. TV cameras were on hand twenty-four hours a day to film their exploits for a reality show.

Dieticians from King's College Hospital devised a three-day rotating menu of fruit, vegetables, nuts, and honey. In the second week, standard portions of cooked oily fish were added to their diet. Water was the only liquid refreshment allowed.

The cleansing diet provoked significant weight loss (4.4 kilos or 9.7 pounds), dramatic drops in cholesterol (23 percent) and blood pressure levels (an average of 140/83 to 122/76), and odorous flatulence inside the tent (no comment). One volunteer, Jon Thornton, a thirty-six-year-old driving instructor, explained that he hadn't eaten vegetables since he was a very young child. Following his "release" from the zoo, Mr. Thornton said he had vegetables with his Christmas dinner for the first time in thirty-six years.[3]

Although the Perfect Cleanse may seem similar to the Evo Diet, I won't ask you to camp out next to the ape house.

During each of these seasonal cleanses, you should increase your water consumption to ¾ ounce per pound of body weight, compared to the ½ ounce I recommended earlier. That means, for a 160-pound person, drinking 3.5 litres of filtered water. That's a lot of water, but if you start sipping in the morning, you can make it. You need these liquids to really flush the system.

I've been asked why I don't recommend drinking vegetable and fruit juice during a cleanse. While vegetable and fruit juices are great sources of nutrients, they are quickly absorbed and are often times higher in sugar, which leaves you feeling hungrier than when you started. When you eat whole fruits and their fibre, however, you shouldn't get as hungry, especially if you're eating every two to three hours or so. Don't drink any Perfect Meal shakes, however, because the first seven days of the cleanse should be dairy-free to help your body get rid of any allergens.

While cleansing, you should take the recommended Perfect Weight Canada supplements, which you learned about in chapter 6, "Supplement for Your Perfect Weight." The supplements included in the Winter, Spring/Fall, and Summer Perfect Cleanses are a whole-food multivitamin, a fucoxanthin supplement, and omega-3 cod liver oil.

I realize that doing a Perfect Cleanse four times a year is asking a great deal and that not every reader will attempt this (some of you are wimps). But how about giving it a try? Even if you don't make it past the fourth day of a ten-day cleanse, you'll still be better off for having made the attempt. I did two of these cleanses while writing *Perfect Weight Canada* and keeping up with my other responsibilities. I wasn't able to go the full ten days on each occasion because I was traveling, but the results were super.

After my second cleanse, I began an intense exercise program I call Functional Interval Training (FIT) (which you'll hear about in chapter 9, "Get FIT for your Perfect Weight") and gained several pounds of muscle.

When you're ready to do the Perfect Cleanse, you can follow an hour-by-hour road map toward the end of this chapter.

Take Your Cleanse to the Next Level

One of the interesting aspects of Healthy Toledo was learning how many participants thought it was normal to have a bowel movement every two or three days. No wonder they felt lousy! You should eliminate every day—and better yet, two or three times a day—just as infants do. If you don't go potty, you have constipation, and the retention of waste inside the colon presents all kinds of health problems: harmful bacteria, intestinal parasites, yeasts, and hemorrhoids.

My bowel consciousness was raised by nutritionist Bernard Jensen, PhD, who owned a health sanatorium in Escondido, California, called the Hidden Valley Health Ranch. Dr. Jensen had become kind of a hero of mine for his pioneering work in digestive cleansing and his book *Tissue Cleansing Through Bowel Management*. Back in 2001, when Dr. Jensen was ninety-two years old and in failing health, a friend and I visited him at his ranch outside of San Diego. I knew he was dying (in fact, Dr. Jensen would pass away three weeks later), but I had always wanted to meet him. He was confined to his bed but willing to see me. After his wife, Marie, made the introduction, Dr. Jensen told me to get my notepad out. I eagerly agreed, feeling like a freshman student sitting at the foot of his professor. Dr. Jensen reminded me that cleansing doesn't just affect your gut but everything in your body.

"What goes in doesn't always come out," he declared. The bowel holds onto waste materials longer than anyone realizes, he said, and the toxic material decaying in the large colon is a good place for health issues to get started. He called chronic constipation a "modern plague" and the greatest present-day danger to health. He blamed America's love for fast food and being clueless about the importance of colonic cleanses. Dr. Jensen urged me—as someone just starting to speak and write books—to carry on the message of good health. I felt humbled that afternoon.

That meeting with Dr. Jensen is one of the major reasons why I asked my team of scientists and physicians at Garden of Life, including board-certified gastroenterologist Joseph Brasco, MD, to design a gentle digestive cleanse that works in synergy with the detoxification process. It's now available as a Garden of Life product called Perfect Cleanse, which works naturally in the digestive track to contribute to overall health and wellness.

I know that when some people hear the phrase "digestive cleanse," they picture themselves taking a harsh laxative that will keep them chained to a porcelain throne for the next week. Maybe your idea of a cleanse is being hooked up to an colonic machine, where a tube is inserted into the rectum and your bowel is flooded with several gallons of water in a matter of seconds. That will get things moving.

Garden of Life's Perfect Cleanse system takes a less painful "Road to Wellville," which was the title of a raunchy 1994 Hollywood film about Dr. John Harvey Kellogg's colon cleanses at the Battle Creek Sanitarium a hundred years ago. Perfect Cleanse is a ten-day internal cleanse program that doesn't disrupt everyday activities. It is not expensive, time consuming, or challenging to perform.

You may think that embarking on a digestive cleanse is one of the wackiest things you could ever do, but I urge you to put away that thinking. If you've never tried this type of cleanse, I urge to view this like a spring cleaning, a chance to complete an—ahem—top-to-bottom scrubbing of every nook and cranny of your digestive tract. You need to reduce the toxic load that has built up over the years from exposure to toxins in the air, water, and food. Excess toxins can make you feel lethargic and impact your health in many ways.

A digestive cleansing reduces the toxic load on your body. Perfect Cleanse uses only the best whole food–based ingredients and botanicals for a natural cleanse without synthetic stimulants or designer chemicals. You will not be introducing additional toxins into the body. Anyone with a medical condition, however, should consult a licensed physician before starting this cleanse.

The Perfect Cleanse system involves following three simple steps:

1. Perfect Cleanse Purify

Your body is constantly working to eliminate toxins via the lungs, kidneys, and particularly the liver. Every minute, around the clock, a properly functioning liver eliminates small amounts of toxins, heavy metals, bacteria, and other impurities from the blood before returning the life-sustaining substance to the rest of the body.

Another liver function is the secretion of about one to two quarts of bile each day to carry processed, nonfunctional, nonnutrient environmental compounds—this is a polite, scientific way of saying "junk food"—to the large intestine, where they are expelled from the body. The liver also carries toxins, metals, microbes, and other metabolic by-products that must be eliminated through the gastrointestinal tract. Perfect Cleanse Purify supports the body's cleansing function, particularly the liver, to help with natural detoxification.

Perfect Cleanse Purify is formulated with natural botanicals and contains chlorella, which is widely studied for its ability to bind with environmental toxins and liver antioxidants that participate in the production of detoxification enzymes. Perfect Cleanse Purify contains milk thistle seed extract, cilantro, yarrow flower extract, probiotic whole-food selenium, cracked-wall chlorella, aged garlic extract, dandelion root extract, and broccoli extract. Three capsules of Perfect Cleanse Purify should be taken thirty minutes before dinner with 8 ounces of water.

2. Perfect Cleanse Capture

Capturing and binding toxins secreted through the bile for transport out of the body is crucial for effective support of the body's normal internal detox and cleansing functions. Normally, eating foods high in fibre—such as green vegetables—help the body capture toxins in the gastrointestinal tract, binding them for transport out of the body. While dietary fibres from edible fruits, vegetables, and grains are capable of absorbing environmental pollutants and other impurities, some types of fibres are easily broken down by intestinal flora.

What is intestinal flora? The normal human gastrointestinal tract contains hundreds of different species of harmless bacteria, otherwise known as intestinal flora. When the normal balance of bacteria is impacted by a poor diet heavy in processed foods, imbalances can occur and may result in occasional constipation or diarrhea.

Perfect Cleanse Capture facilitates the effective elimination of trapped toxins, and these fibres have been combined in a specific ratio to ensure that they are not broken down by your intestinal flora. Another benefit to Perfect Cleanse Capture is that the organic fibres bind toxins for transport and do not bring additional toxins into the body.

Perfect Cleanse Capture helps to trap and bind undesirable compounds in the digestive tract for transport from the body, which is crucial for healthy detoxification. The dietary fibres in Capture have been specifically selected and combined into a patent-pending formulation that optimizes toxin absorption by the fibre. This formula is free of common allergens, including gluten, and is certified organic. Perfect Cleanse Capture contains a certified organic blend of flaxseed, pea hull fibre, alfalfa leaf, barley grass, and chia seed. Perfect Cleanse Capture should be taken thirty minutes after dinner by mixing one scoop of powder into 8 to 12 ounces of water.

3. Perfect Cleanse Remove

The third and final step is Perfect Cleanse Remove, which works by assisting the trapped toxins to move smoothly through the digestive track, gently sweeping the colon of accumulated waste. Perfect Cleanse Remove is a gentle formula with a digestive botanical blend that works while you sleep to promote healthy, comfortable bowel movements. Perfect Cleanse Remove is designed to support effective elimination of intestinal waste and the removal of toxins from the body.

Perfect Cleanse Remove contains natural magnesium, salts, fenugreek seed extract, bishop's weed, peppermint leaf, aloe vera, ginger root, and fennel seed. Three caplets of Perfect Cleanse Remove should be taken before bedtime with 8 ounces of water.

You can expect some changes in your bowel movements when undergoing this type of digestive cleanse. Your stools are likely to become more frequent, softer, and change colour. You may require more sleep, and you may feel tired during certain parts of the day. All of these changes are a result of the body's efforts to eliminate toxins.

So take a load off your digestive tract and cleanse. A ten-day Perfect Cleanse will leave you feeling lighter on your feet and with a brighter outlook in just ten days. This cleanse works in harmony with your body to release and remove toxins naturally so that you will feel like a better you. Again, without getting into too many bathroom details, you will be impressed with the results.

I'm a busy mom and live with my three school-age children and loving husband in the Chicago area. Last New Year's, following my sweet tooth marathon over the holidays, I knew it was time to clean house. Perhaps it was the sugar overload I felt in my system. At any rate, I began doing the Garden of Life Perfect Cleanse.

I had incredible results the first day. By the third day, I felt like a revived person because the toxic build-up in my system was leaving my body. My energy level increased immensely as well as my mental alertness. Trust me, I need to be alert and full of energy every day.

I've recommended Perfect Cleanse to a few of my friends, and they loved the results as well. The simple-to-use directions on the box are great: just follow the 1-2-3 steps on each bottle and you can't mess up. I love that Perfect Cleanse is easy, safe, made with organic ingredients, and is whole-food based. I also love the way it doesn't introduce extraneous toxins back into my system. I even lost my cravings for sweet things, like chocolate, and that's not easy!

(Note from Jordan: I met Duong at my Weekend of Wellness conference while writing this book. At the tender age of six, she was one of the fortunate "boat people" who escaped to the United States after the fall of Vietnam back in 1975. I loved her servant heart.)

The Seasonal Cleanse Protocols

As promised, here's a complete protocol that you can follow during a ten-day seasonal Perfect Cleanse.

Winter Cleanse
Day 1

The mealtimes are approximate; obviously, feel free to adjust the times to eat based upon your schedule. Keep in mind that a single serving of fruit is either one cup (berries, grapes, and cut-up pineapple, for example) or one or two pieces (for example, grapefruit, peaches, plums, apples, or oranges).

Upon waking
Drink for your perfect weight: 16–24 ounces of water
Think for your perfect weight: Perform the Healing Codes Exercise. (You can find out what the Healing Codes Exercise is by turning to page 189. I recommend that you perform the Healing Codes Exercise at least twice a day—once in the morning and once in the evening—but feel free to try this two-minute exercise three, four, or five times a day.)

7:30 a.m.
Cleanse for your perfect weight: Eat one serving (1 or 2 cups) of homemade Cleansing Chicken Soup.
Drink for your perfect weight: 12–16 ounces of water

Supplement for your perfect weight: Take two or three whole-food multivitamin caplets and one to four capsules of concentrated fucoxanthin.

10:30 a.m.
Cleanse for your perfect weight: Eat one serving of homemade Cleansing Chicken Soup.

Drink for your perfect weight: 12–16 ounces of water

1:00 p.m.
Cleanse for your perfect weight: Eat one serving of homemade Cleansing Chicken Soup.

Drink for your perfect weight: 12–16 ounces of water

Supplement for your perfect weight: Take two or three whole-food multivitamin caplets and one to three capsules of concentrated fucoxanthin.

3:30 p.m.
Cleanse for your perfect weight: Eat one serving of homemade Cleansing Chicken Soup.

Drink for your perfect weight: 12–16 ounces of water

5:30 p.m.
Perfect Cleanse: Take three capsules of Perfect Cleanse Purify with 8–12 ounces of water.

6:00 p.m.
Cleanse for your perfect weight: Eat one serving of homemade Cleansing Chicken Soup.

Drink for your perfect weight: 8–12 ounces of water

Supplement for your perfect weight: Take two or three whole-food multivitamin caplets, one to three capsules of concentrated fucoxanthin, and 1 to 3 teaspoons (or three to nine capsules) of a high omega-3 cod liver oil complex. (See the PWC Resource Guide on page 322 for recommended products.)

7:00 p.m.
Perfect Cleanse: Take one scoop of Perfect Cleanse Capture mixed in 8–12 ounces of water.

Before bed
Think for your perfect weight: Perform the Healing Codes Exercise on page 189.

Perfect Cleanse: Take three caplets of Perfect Cleanse Remove with 8–12 ounces of water.

Sleep for your perfect weight: Go to bed by 10:30 p.m.

Days 2–4

Upon waking

Drink for your perfect weight: 16–24 ounces of water

Think for your perfect weight: Perform the Healing Codes Exercise on page 189.

7:30 a.m.

Cleanse for your perfect weight: Eat one serving of homemade Cleansing Chicken Soup.

Drink for your perfect weight: 12–16 ounces of water

Supplement for your perfect weight: Take two or three whole-food multivitamin caplets and one to four capsules of concentrated fucoxanthin.

10:30 a.m.

Cleanse for your perfect weight: Eat one serving of homemade Cleansing Chicken Soup.

Drink for your perfect weight: 12–16 ounces of water

1:00 p.m.

Cleanse for your perfect weight: Eat one serving of homemade Cleansing Chicken Soup.

Drink for your perfect weight: 12–16 ounces of water

Supplement for your perfect weight: Take two or three whole-food multivitamin caplets and one to three capsules of concentrated fucoxanthin.

3:30 p.m.

Cleanse for your perfect weight: Eat one serving of homemade Cleansing Chicken Soup.

Drink for your perfect weight: 12–16 ounces of water

5:30 p.m.

Perfect Cleanse: Take three capsules of Perfect Cleanse Purify with 8–12 ounces of water.

6:00 p.m.

Cleanse for your perfect weight: Mix a large green salad with any of the following: mixed greens; carrots; cucumbers; celery; tomatoes; red cabbage; red onions; red, yellow, and orange peppers; radishes; sprouts; and half an avocado.

Salad dressing: use 2 tablespoons of one of the following:

- Homemade dressing: extra-virgin olive oil, apple-cider vinegar or lemon juice, Celtic Sea Salt, herbs, liquid aminos, and soy sauce
- A healthy store-bought salad dressing (please see the PWC Resource Guide on page 322 for recommended brands)

Drink for your perfect weight: 8–12 ounces of water

Supplement for your perfect weight: Take two or three whole-food multivitamin

caplets, one to three capsules of concentrated fucoxanthin, and 1 to 3 teaspoons (or three to nine capsules) of a high omega-3 cod liver oil complex. (See the PWC Resource Guide on page 322 for recommended products.)

7:00 p.m.

Perfect Cleanse: Take one scoop of Perfect Cleanse Capture mixed in 8–12 ounces of water.

Before bed

Think for your perfect weight: Perform the Healing Codes Exercise on page 189.

Perfect Cleanse: Take three caplets of Perfect Cleanse Remove with 8–12 ounces of water.

Sleep for your perfect weight: Go to bed by 10:30 p.m.

Days 5–7

Upon waking

Drink for your perfect weight: 16–24 ounces of water

Think for your perfect weight: Perform the Healing Codes Exercise on page 189.

7:30 a.m.

Cleanse for your perfect weight: Eat one serving of homemade Cleansing Chicken Soup.

Drink for your perfect weight: 12–16 ounces of water

Supplement for your perfect weight: Take two or three whole-food multivitamin caplets and one to four capsules of concentrated fucoxanthin.

10:30 a.m.

Cleanse for your perfect weight: Eat one serving of homemade Cleansing Chicken Soup.

Drink for your perfect weight: 12–16 ounces of water

1:00 p.m.

Cleanse for your perfect weight: Eat one serving of homemade Cleansing Chicken Soup.

Drink for your perfect weight: 12–16 ounces of water

Supplement for your perfect weight: Take two or three whole-food multivitamin caplets and one to three capsules of concentrated fucoxanthin.

3:30 p.m.

Cleanse for your perfect weight: Eat one serving of homemade Cleansing Chicken Soup.

Drink for your perfect weight: 12–16 ounces of water

5:30 p.m.

Perfect Cleanse: Take three capsules of Perfect Cleanse Purify with 8–12 ounces of water.

6:00 p.m.

Cleanse for your perfect weight: Mix a large green salad with any of the following: mixed greens; carrots; cucumbers; celery; tomatoes; red cabbage; red onions; red, yellow, or orange peppers; radishes; sprouts; half an avocado; and raw or soaked and dried nuts or seeds.

Salad dressing: use 2 tablespoons of one of the following:

- Homemade dressing: extra-virgin olive oil, apple-cider vinegar or lemon juice, Celtic Sea Salt, herbs, liquid aminos, and soy sauce
- A healthy store-bought salad dressing (please see the PWC Resource Guide on page 322 for recommended brands)

Drink for your perfect weight: 8–12 ounces of water

Supplement for your perfect weight: Take two or three whole-food multivitamin caplets, one to three capsules of concentrated fucoxanthin, and 1 to 3 teaspoons (or three to nine capsules) of a high omega-3 cod liver oil complex. (See the PWC Resource Guide on page 322 for recommended products.)

7:00 p.m.

Perfect Cleanse: Take one scoop of Perfect Cleanse Capture mixed in 8–12 ounces of water.

Before bed

Perfect Cleanse: Take three caplets of Perfect Cleanse Remove with 8–12 ounces of water.

Think for your perfect weight: perform the Healing Codes Exercise on page 189.

Sleep for your perfect weight: Go to bed by 10:30 p.m.

Days 8–10

Upon waking

Drink for your perfect weight: 16–24 ounces of water

Think for your perfect weight: Perform the Healing Codes Exercise on page 189.

7:30 a.m.

Cleanse for your perfect weight: Eat one serving of homemade Cleansing Chicken Soup.

Drink for your perfect weight: 12–16 ounces of water

Supplement for your perfect weight: Take two or three whole-food multivitamin caplets and one to four capsules of concentrated fucoxanthin.

10:30 a.m.

Cleanse for your perfect weight: Eat one serving of homemade Cleansing Chicken Soup.

Drink for your perfect weight: 12–16 ounces of water

1:00 p.m.

Cleanse for your perfect weight: Eat one serving of homemade Cleansing Chicken Soup, 4 ounces of plain whole-milk yogurt or kefir (cow's, goat's, or sheep's milk), and 1 tablespoon of raw honey.

Drink for your perfect weight: 12–16 ounces of water

Supplement for your perfect weight: Take two or three whole-food multivitamin caplets and one to three capsules of concentrated fucoxanthin.

3:30 p.m.

Cleanse for your perfect weight: Eat one serving of homemade Cleansing Chicken Soup, 4 ounces of plain whole-milk yogurt or kefir (cow's, goat's, or sheep's milk), and 1 tablespoon of raw honey.

Drink for your perfect weight: 12–16 ounces of water

5:30 p.m.

Perfect Cleanse: Take three capsules of Perfect Cleanse Purify with 8–12 ounces of water.

6:00 p.m.

Cleanse for your perfect weight: Mix a large green salad with any of the following: mixed greens; carrots; cucumbers; celery; tomatoes; red cabbage; red onions; red, yellow, or orange peppers; radishes; sprouts; half an avocado; and raw or soaked and dried nuts or seeds. Add 4 ounces of cold-water fatty fish (salmon, mackerel, herring, tuna, sardines) and 2 ounces of raw cheese (cow's, sheep's, goat's).

Salad dressing: use 2 tablespoons of one of the following:

- Homemade dressing: extra-virgin olive oil, apple-cider vinegar or lemon juice, Celtic Sea Salt, herbs, liquid aminos, and soy sauce
- A healthy store-bought salad dressing (please see the PWC Resource Guide on page 322 for recommended brands)

Drink for your perfect weight: 8–12 ounces of water

Supplement for your perfect weight: Take two or three whole-food multivitamin caplets, one to three capsules of concentrated fucoxanthin, and 1 to 3 teaspoons (or three to nine capsules) of a high omega-3 cod liver oil complex. (See the PWC Resource Guide on page 322 for recommended products.)

7:00 p.m.

Perfect Cleanse: Take one scoop of Perfect Cleanse Capture mixed in 8–12 ounces of water.

Before bed

    Think for your perfect weight: Perform the Healing Codes Exercise on page 189.

    Perfect Cleanse: Take three caplets of Perfect Cleanse Remove with 8–12 ounces of water.

    Sleep for your perfect weight: Go to bed by 10:30 p.m.

The Spring/Fall Perfect Cleanse
Days 1–4

The mealtimes are approximate; obviously, feel free to adjust the times to eat based upon your schedule.

Upon waking

    Drink for your perfect weight: 16–24 ounces of water

    Think for your perfect weight: Perform the Healing Codes Exercise. (You can find out what the Healing Codes Exercise is by turning to page 189. I recommend that you perform the Healing Codes Exercise at least twice a day—once in the morning and once in the evening—but feel free to try this two-minute exercise three, four, or five times a day.)

7:30 a.m.

    Cleanse for your perfect weight: Eat one serving of grapefruit.

    Drink for your perfect weight: 12–16 ounces of water

    Supplement for your perfect weight: Take two or three whole-food multivitamin caplets and one to four capsules of concentrated fucoxanthin

10:30 a.m.

    Cleanse for your perfect weight: Eat one serving of oranges.

    Drink for your perfect weight: 12–16 ounces of water

1:00 p.m.

    Cleanse for your perfect weight: Eat one serving (1 or 2 cups) of homemade Cleansing Chicken Soup.

    Drink for your perfect weight: 12–16 ounces of water

    Supplement for your perfect weight: Take two or three whole-food multivitamin caplets and one to three capsules of concentrated fucoxanthin.

3:30 p.m.

    Cleanse for your perfect weight: Eat one serving of homemade Cleansing Chicken Soup.

    Drink for your perfect weight: 12–16 ounces of water

5:30 p.m.

    Perfect Cleanse: Take three capsules of Perfect Cleanse Purify with 8–12 ounces of water.

6:00 p.m.

Cleanse for your perfect weight: Eat one serving of homemade Cleansing Chicken Soup.

Drink for your perfect weight: 8–12 ounces of water

Supplement for your perfect weight: Take two or three whole-food multivitamin caplets, one to three capsules of concentrated fucoxanthin, and 1 to 3 teaspoons (or three to nine capsules) of a high omega-3 cod liver oil complex. (See the PWC Resource Guide on page 322 for recommended products.)

7:00 p.m.

Perfect Cleanse: Take one scoop of Perfect Cleanse Capture mixed in 8–12 ounces of water.

Before bed

Think for your perfect weight: Perform the Healing Codes Exercise on page 189.

Perfect Cleanse: Take three caplets of Perfect Cleanse Remove with 8–12 ounces of water.

Sleep for your perfect weight: Go to bed by 10:30 p.m.

Days 5–7

Upon waking

Drink for your perfect weight: 16–24 ounces of water

Think for your perfect weight: Perform the Healing Codes exercise on page 189.

7:30 a.m.

Cleanse for your perfect weight: Eat one serving of apples.

Drink for your perfect weight: 12–16 ounces of water

Supplement for your perfect weight: Take two or three whole-food multivitamin caplets and one to four capsules of concentrated fucoxanthin.

10:30 a.m.

Cleanse for your perfect weight: Eat one serving of strawberries.

Drink for your perfect weight: 12–16 ounces of water

1:00 p.m.

Cleanse for your perfect weight: Eat one serving of homemade Cleansing Chicken Soup.

Drink for your perfect weight: 12–16 ounces of water.

Supplement for your perfect weight: Take two or three whole-food multivitamin caplets and one to three capsules of concentrated fucoxanthin.

3:30 p.m.

Cleanse for your perfect weight: Eat one serving of homemade Cleansing Chicken Soup.

Drink for your perfect weight: 12–16 ounces of water

5:30 p.m.

Perfect Cleanse: Take three capsules of Perfect Cleanse Purify with 8–12 ounces of water.

6:00 p.m.

Cleanse for your perfect weight: Mix a large green salad with any of the following: mixed greens; carrots; cucumbers; celery; tomatoes; red cabbage; red onions; red, yellow, or orange peppers; radishes; sprouts; half an avocado; and raw or soaked and dried nuts or seeds.

Salad dressing: use 2 tablespoons of one of the following:

- Homemade dressing: extra-virgin olive oil, apple-cider vinegar or lemon juice, Celtic Sea Salt, herbs, liquid aminos, and soy sauce
- A healthy store-bought salad dressing (please see the PWC Resource Guide on page 322 for recommended brands)

Drink for your perfect weight: 8–12 ounces of water

Supplement for your perfect weight: Take two or three whole-food multivitamin caplets, one to three capsules of concentrated fucoxanthin, and 1 to 3 teaspoons (or three to nine capsules) of a high omega-3 cod liver oil complex. (See the PWC Resource Guide on page 322 for recommended products.)

7:00 p.m.

Perfect Cleanse: Take one scoop of Perfect Cleanse Capture mixed in 8–12 ounces of water.

Before bed

Think for your perfect weight: Perform the Healing Codes Exercise on page 189.

Perfect Cleanse: Take three caplets of Perfect Cleanse Remove with 8–12 ounces of water.

Sleep for your perfect weight: Go to bed by 10:30 p.m.

Days 8–10

Upon waking

Drink for your perfect weight: 16–24 ounces of water

Think for your perfect weight: Perform the Healing Codes exercise on page 189.

7:30 a.m.

Cleanse for your perfect weight: Eat one serving of plums, 4 ounces of plain whole-milk yogurt or kefir (cow's, goat's, or sheep's milk), and 1 tablespoon of raw honey.

Drink for your perfect weight: 12–16 ounces of water

Supplement for your perfect weight: Take two or three whole-food multivitamin caplets and one to four capsules of concentrated fucoxanthin.

10:30 a.m.

Cleanse for your perfect weight: Eat one serving of grapes, 4 ounces of plain whole-milk yogurt or kefir (cow's, goat's, or sheep's milk), and 1 tablespoon of raw honey.

Drink for your perfect weight: 12–16 ounces of water

1:00 p.m.

Cleanse for your perfect weight: Eat one serving of homemade Cleansing Chicken Soup.

Drink for your perfect weight: 12–16 ounces of water

Supplement for your perfect weight: Take two or three whole-food multivitamin caplets and one to three capsules of concentrated fucoxanthin.

3:30 p.m.

Cleanse for your perfect weight: Eat one serving of homemade Cleansing Chicken Soup.

Drink for your perfect weight: 12–16 ounces of water

5:30 p.m.

Perfect Cleanse: Take three capsules of Perfect Cleanse Purify with 8–12 ounces of water.

6:00 p.m.

Cleanse for your perfect weight: Mix a large green salad with any of the following: mixed greens; carrots; cucumbers; celery; tomatoes; red cabbage; red onions; red, yellow, or orange peppers; radishes; sprouts; half an avocado; and raw or soaked and dried nuts or seeds. Add 4 ounces of cold-water fatty fish (salmon, mackerel, herring, tuna, sardines) and 2 ounces of raw cheese (cow's, sheep's, or goat's).

Salad dressing: use 2 tablespoons of one of the following:

- Homemade dressing: extra-virgin olive oil, apple-cider vinegar or lemon juice, Celtic Sea Salt, herbs, liquid aminos, and soy sauce
- A healthy store-bought salad dressing (please see the PWC Resource Guide on page 322 for recommended brands)

Drink for your perfect weight: 8–12 ounces of water

Supplement for your perfect weight: Take two or three whole-food multivitamin caplets, one to three capsules of concentrated fucoxanthin, and 1 to 3 teaspoons (or three to nine capsules) of a high omega-3 cod liver oil complex. (See the PWC Resource Guide on page 322 for recommended products.)

7:00 p.m.

Perfect Cleanse: Take one scoop of Perfect Cleanse Capture mixed in 8–12 ounces of water.

Before bed

Think for your perfect weight: Perform the Healing Codes Exercise on page 189.

Perfect Cleanse: Take three caplets of Perfect Cleanse Remove with 8–12 ounces of water.

Sleep for your perfect weight: Go to bed by 10:30 p.m.

The Summer Perfect Cleanse
Day 1

The mealtimes are approximate; obviously, feel free to adjust the times to eat based upon your schedule.

Upon waking

Drink for your perfect weight: 16–24 ounces of water

Think for your perfect weight: Perform the Healing Codes Exercise. (You can find out what the Healing Codes Exercise is by turning to page 189. I recommend that you perform the Healing Codes Exercise at least twice a day—once in the morning and once in the evening—but feel free to try this two-minute exercise three, four, or five times a day.)

7:30 a.m.

Cleanse for your perfect weight: Eat one serving of grapes—any variety.
Drink for your perfect weight: 12–16 ounces of water
Supplement for your perfect weight: Take two or three whole-food multivitamin caplets and one to four capsules of concentrated fucoxanthin.

10:30 a.m.

Cleanse for your perfect weight: Eat one serving of grapes—any variety.
Drink for your perfect weight: 12–16 ounces of water

1:00 p.m.

Cleanse for your perfect weight: Eat one serving of grapes—any variety.
Drink for your perfect weight: 12–16 ounces of water
Supplement for your perfect weight: Take two or three whole-food multivitamin caplets and one to three capsules of concentrated fucoxanthin.

3:30 p.m.

Cleanse for your perfect weight: Eat one serving of grapes—any variety.
Drink for your perfect weight: 12–16 ounces of water

5:30 p.m.

Perfect Cleanse: Take three capsules of Perfect Cleanse Purify with 8–12 ounces of water.

6:00 p.m.

Cleanse for your perfect weight: Eat one serving of grapes—any variety.
Drink for your perfect weight: 8–12 ounces of water
Supplement for your perfect weight: Take two or three whole-food multivitamin

caplets, one to three capsules of concentrated fucoxanthin, and 1 to 3 teaspoons (or three to nine capsules) of a high omega-3 cod liver oil complex. (See the PWC Resource Guide on page 322 for recommended products.)

7:00 p.m.

Perfect Cleanse: Take one scoop of Perfect Cleanse Capture mixed in 8–12 ounces of water.

Before bed

Think for your perfect weight: Perform the Healing Codes Exercise on page 189.

Perfect Cleanse: Take three caplets of Perfect Cleanse Remove with 8–12 ounces of water.

Sleep for your perfect weight: Go to bed by 10:30 p.m.

Days 2–4

Upon waking

Drink for your perfect weight: 16–24 ounces of water

Think for your perfect weight: Perform the Healing Codes exercise on page 189.

7:30 a.m.

Cleanse for your perfect weight: Eat one serving of mango.

Drink for your perfect weight: 12–16 ounces of water

Supplement for your perfect weight: Take two or three whole-food multivitamin caplets and one to four capsules of concentrated fucoxanthin.

10:30 a.m.

Cleanse for your perfect weight: Eat one serving of watermelon.

Drink for your perfect weight: 12–16 ounces of water

1:00 p.m.

Cleanse for your perfect weight: Eat one serving of pineapple.

Drink for your perfect weight: 12–16 ounces of water

Supplement for your perfect weight: Take two or three whole-food multivitamin caplets and one to three capsules of concentrated fucoxanthin.

3:30 p.m.

Cleanse for your perfect weight: Eat one serving of cherries.

Drink for your perfect weight: 12–16 ounces of water

5:30 p.m.

Perfect Cleanse: Take three capsules of Perfect Cleanse Purify with 8–12 ounces of water.

6:00 p.m.

Cleanse for your perfect weight: Mix a large green salad with any of the following: mixed greens; carrots; cucumbers; celery; tomatoes; red cabbage; red onions; red, yellow, or orange peppers; radishes; sprouts; and half an avocado.

Salad dressing: use 2 tablespoons of one of the following:

- Homemade dressing: extra-virgin olive oil, apple-cider vinegar or lemon juice, Celtic Sea Salt, herbs, liquid aminos, and soy sauce
- A healthy store-bought salad dressing (please see the PWC Resource Guide on page 322 for recommended brands)

Drink for your perfect weight: 8–12 ounces of water

Supplement for your perfect weight: Take two or three whole food multivitamin caplets, one to three capsules of concentrated fucoxanthin, and 1 to 3 teaspoons (or three to nine capsules) of a high omega-3 cod liver oil complex. (See the PWC Resource Guide on page 322 for recommended products.)

7:00 p.m.

Perfect Cleanse: Take one scoop of Perfect Cleanse Capture mixed in 8–12 ounces of water.

Before bed

Think for your perfect weight: Perform the Healing Codes Exercise on page 189.

Perfect Cleanse: Take three caplets of Perfect Cleanse Remove with 8–12 ounces of water.

Sleep for your perfect weight: Go to bed by 10:30 p.m.

Days 5–7

Upon waking

Drink for your perfect weight: 16–24 ounces of water

Think for your perfect weight: Perform the Healing Codes exercise on page 189.

7:30 a.m.

Cleanse for your perfect weight: Eat one serving of papaya.

Drink for your perfect weight: 12–16 ounces of water

Supplement for your perfect weight: Take two or three whole-food multivitamin caplets and one to four capsules of concentrated fucoxanthin.

10:30 a.m.

Cleanse for your perfect weight: Eat one serving of peaches.

Drink for your perfect weight: 12–16 ounces of water

1:00 p.m.

Cleanse for your perfect weight: Eat one serving of raspberries.

Drink for your perfect weight: 12–16 ounces of water

Supplement for your perfect weight: Take two or three whole-food multivitamin caplets and one to three capsules of concentrated fucoxanthin.

3:30 p.m.

Cleanse for your perfect weight: Eat one serving of apples.
Drink for your perfect weight: 12–16 ounces of water

5:30 p.m.

Perfect Cleanse: Take three capsules of Perfect Cleanse Purify with 8–12 ounces of water.

6:00 p.m.

Cleanse for your perfect weight: Mix a large green salad with any of the following: mixed greens; carrots; cucumbers; celery; tomatoes; red cabbage; red onions; red, yellow, or orange peppers; radishes; sprouts; half an avocado; and raw or soaked and dried nuts or seeds.

Salad dressing: use 2 tablespoons of one of the following:

- Homemade dressing: extra-virgin olive oil, apple-cider vinegar or lemon juice, Celtic Sea Salt, herbs, liquid aminos, and soy sauce
- A healthy store-bought salad dressing (please see the PWC Resource Guide on page 322 for recommended brands)

Drink for your perfect weight: 8–12 ounces of water.

Supplement for your perfect weight: Take two or three whole-food multivitamin caplets, one to three capsules of concentrated fucoxanthin, and 1 to 3 teaspoons (or three to nine capsules) of a high omega-3 cod liver oil complex. (See the PWC Resource Guide on page 322 for recommended products.)

7:00 p.m.

Perfect Cleanse: Take one scoop of Perfect Cleanse Capture mixed in 8–12 ounces of water.

Before bed

Think for your perfect weight: Perform the Healing Codes Exercise on page 189.
Perfect Cleanse: Take three caplets of Perfect Cleanse Remove with 8–12 ounces of water.
Sleep for your perfect weight: Go to bed by 10:30 p.m.

Days 8–10

Upon waking

Drink for your perfect weight: 16–24 ounces of water
Think for your perfect weight: Perform the Healing Codes exercise on page 189.

7:30 a.m.

Cleanse for your perfect weight: Eat one serving of kiwi.

Drink for your perfect weight: 12–16 ounces of water

Supplement for your perfect weight: Take two or three whole-food multivitamin caplets and one to four capsules of concentrated fucoxanthin.

10:30 a.m.

Cleanse for your perfect weight: Eat one serving of pears.

Drink for your perfect weight: 12–16 ounces of water

1:00 p.m.

Cleanse for your perfect weight: Eat one serving of blueberries, 4 ounces of plain whole-milk yogurt or kefir (cow's, goat's, or sheep's milk), and 1 tablespoon of raw honey.

Drink for your perfect weight: 12–16 ounces of water

Supplement for your perfect weight: Take two or three whole-food multivitamin caplets and one to three capsules of concentrated fucoxanthin.

3:30 p.m.

Cleanse for your perfect weight: Eat one serving of strawberries, 4 ounces of plain whole-milk yogurt or kefir (cow's, goat's, or sheep's milk), and 1 tablespoon of raw honey.

Drink for your perfect weight: 12–16 ounces of water

5:30 p.m.

Perfect Cleanse: Take three capsules of Perfect Cleanse Purify with 8–12 ounces of water.

6:00 p.m.

Cleanse for your perfect weight: Mix a large green salad with any of the following: mixed greens; carrots; cucumbers; celery; tomatoes; red cabbage; red onions; red, yellow, or orange peppers; radishes; sprouts; half an avocado; and raw or soaked and dried nuts or seeds. Add 4 ounces of cold-water fatty fish (salmon, mackerel, herring, tuna, sardines) and 2 ounces of raw cheese (cow's, sheep's, goat's).

Salad dressing: use 2 tablespoons of one of the following:

- Homemade dressing: extra-virgin olive oil, apple-cider vinegar or lemon juice, Celtic Sea Salt, herbs, liquid aminos, and soy sauce
- A healthy store-bought salad dressing (please see the PWC Resource Guide on page 322 for recommended brands)

Drink for your perfect weight: 8–12 ounces of water

Supplement for your perfect weight: Take two or three whole-food multivitamin caplets, one to three capsules of concentrated fucoxanthin, and 1 to 3 teaspoons (or three to nine capsules) of a high omega-3 cod liver oil complex. (See the PWC Resource Guide on page 322 for recommended products.)

7:00 p.m.

Perfect Cleanse: Take one scoop of Perfect Cleanse Capture mixed in 8–12 ounces of water.

Before bed

Think for your perfect weight: Perform the Healing Codes Exercise on page 189.

Perfect Cleanse: Take three caplets of Perfect Cleanse Remove with 8–12 ounces of water.

Sleep for your perfect weight: Go to bed by 10:30 p.m.

On Deck

We've just addressed the inside of the body and how we can to make it function at its best. In our next chapter, we'll focus on making the outside match how good you feel inside by discussing the importance of getting fit for your perfect weight.

Perfect Weight Recap: Cleanse for Your Perfect Weight

- The next time you're eating alone, count the number of times you chew your food before swallowing. Try to chew your food fifteen to thirty times before swallowing.
- When starting the sixteen-week Perfect Weight Canada program, consider going on the Perfect Cleanse, a ten-day detoxification program. Make this a quarterly routine.
- Concurrent with the Perfect Cleanse eating plan, use the three-part cleansing supplement system called Perfect Cleanse by Garden of Life.

Chapter 9

Get FIT for Your Perfect Weight

I SWIVELLED MY hips to maintain my balance on the stability ball and then gave the 7-kilo medicine ball (15½ pounds) a two-handed chest pass toward my workout partner, Mike Yorkey.

Mike, seated on a stability ball about six feet away, caught the heavy ball and immediately thrust it back into the air in my direction. I deftly caught it and glanced at my watch. "Another minute to go," I huffed.

"You're killing me," a red-faced Mike exerted. "I won't be able to comb my hair tomorrow morning if we keep going."

"Last series," I said. "Not too much longer."

For the last half hour Mike and I had squatted on stability balls and tossed medicine balls back and forth to each other. We started with the lightest ball—a 2-kilo ball about the size of a volleyball—and played toss-and-catch for two timed minutes before taking a break. During each "rest" interval, Mike held the medicine ball with outstretched arms while I reached the next ball—a bit heavier—and cradled it. After one minute of ball holding, it was back to playing catch with the next heavier medicine ball for two minutes.

Mike, who's been my research and writing partner on my last fifteen books, is twenty years my senior. For a member of the Baby Boom generation, he's in good shape. Mike does meaningful exercise five or six days a week, either working out in the gym, playing doubles with his tennis buddies, or bike riding with his wife, Nicole. On this occasion, Mike had flown to Florida from his San Diego home to work on the *Perfect Weight America* and *Perfect Weight Canada* editions with me. When I suggested we take a break from brainstorming and work out together in my home gym, Mike was gung-ho to raise his heart rate with me. "I want to show you some exercises I'm working on for the book," I said.

I told Mike that the exercise chapter would be absolutely crucial to the Perfect Weight campaign, but to issue the standard health-and-fitness book advice—"Start exercising in a gym"—wouldn't cut it. My preference is that you adopt an exercise system that I call FIT—Functional Interval Training—into your daily schedule, or at least four times a week.

Interval training involves alternating short, intense bouts of exercise with brief recovery times. That's why Mike and I "rested" between sessions of tossing the medicine ball back and forth, although holding a 3-kilo medicine ball demanded its own effort. By sharply increasing and decreasing our heart rates, we burned more calories than if we had spent the same amount of time striding on side-by-side treadmills. Interval workout training will improve your resting metabolic rate (RMR) as well as your VO$_2$ max rate, which is the maximum amount of oxygen that can be used by an individual, in millilitres, in one minute per kilogram of body weight.

In addition, FIT exercises that work the body's "core" muscles with dumbbells, resistance bands, stability balls, medicine balls, or even Russian kettlebells are examples of "functional" exercises long on exertion and short on duration. If you will give me twenty minutes of concentrated, huff-and-puff exercise, you will benefit from huge caloric expenditures and continue to burn fat long after I've kicked you out of the gym and told you to take a shower.

You see, you can't lose weight—or at least sustain any weight loss—without stoking the body's furnace to burn up reserves of fat. When you complete a series of FIT exercises, you increase your oxygen intake as well as your heart and lung capacity so that your body turns into a fat-burning engine that incinerates fat cells long after you've stopped working out. You do this by building muscle—or restoring muscle that's been lost over the years—through functional, anaerobic, or, as I like to call them, anabolic (building) exercises. Even if you add a pound or two from gaining muscle, you'll be better off because one pound of muscle burns thirty to fifty calories a day while one pound of fat burns only three calories a day. It goes without saying, but be sure to check with your doctor before starting any fitness program, especially if it's been awhile since you've exercised.

My experience in fitness—I received my certification in fitness training in my early twenties—augurs my belief that engaging in intense workouts designed to deplete oxygen stores will cause the body to switch on the fat-burning cells. In other words, the standard "cardio" exercises—that is, walking on a treadmill like a mind-numbed robot for forty-five minutes—are somewhat helpful; however, intense oxygen-depriving anaerobic exercise does two important things to help you lose weight:

1. Anaerobic exercise increases the percentage of calories and fat burned as compared to the percentage of carbohydrates burned.
2. Anaerobic exercise raises your metabolic rate, which helps you burn off even more calories when you're at rest.

You may be wondering what "anaerobic exercise" is all about. When the body exercises, it works in two basic ways: aerobically and anaerobically. The body is said to be working aerobically when it operates at a pace that allows the cardiorespiratory system—the lungs, heart, and bloodstream—to replenish energy as you exercise. Put another way, aerobic exercise causes the body to utilize oxygen to create energy. This is basically anything that gets the heart going, like walking on treadmills, cycling on stationary bikes, or stepping on stair-stepper machines.

Aerobic exercise is generally associated with nonresistance exercises such as:

- Aerobic classes
- Bicycling
- Dancing
- Golfing
- Ice-skating
- Racquetball
- Snowboarding
- Soccer
- Squash
- Tennis
- Walking

- Basketball
- Calisthenics
- Gardening
- Hiking on level terrain
- Inline skating
- Scuba diving
- Snow skiing
- Softball
- Table tennis
- Volleyball
- Water skiing

In general, aerobic exercise is performed at a low to moderate intensity level. You're said to be exercising aerobically if you can pass the "talk test," meaning you can hold a conversation and exercise at the same time. The fitness bar is raised when you're very proficient at one of the aforementioned sports and can expertly compete against top-flight competition that demands your very best effort. An energetic set of singles between a pair of advanced tennis players can be more anaerobic than aerobic exercise, for example. Ditto for high-intensity "step" aerobic classes or amateur hockey games.

Long-Duration Exercise: Not That Good for Your Health

Low-intensity exercise—like walking on a treadmill or jogging around the neighbourhood—is long on making repetitive steps but short on cardiovascular variation. While we could all afford to walk more each day (the average American accumulates only three thousand to five thousand steps per day, according to researcher David R. Bassett Jr., professor of exercise science at the University of Tennessee[1]), stepping on a treadmill to make up the shortfall is a short-sighted answer.

"Routinely forcing your body to perform the same continuous cardiovascular challenge, by repeating the same movement, at the same rate, thousands of times over, without variation, and without rest, is unnatural," declared Alan Sears, MD, and author of *PACE: Rediscover Your Native Fitness*.[2] Long-duration exercise "downsizes" the heart's capacity to rapidly provide you with big bursts of energy when you need them, increases LDL cholesterol and triglycerides, elevates clotting and inflammation factors, and creates loss of bone density.

We need to look no further than the Pennsylvania Amish for an example on how to meld low-intensity exercise with quick bursts of energy and the great health that results. During his research, Professor Bassett placed pedometers on ninety-eight Amish adults and learned that men averaged an astounding eighteen thousand steps a day, but they also performed ten hours of vigorous physical activity a week—anaerobic activities like heavy lifting, shovelling trenches, and tossing hay bales. Women averaged fourteen thousand steps a day and three and a half hours of vigorous physical activity on the family farm each week.[3] This level of exertion goes a long way toward explaining why obesity in the Amish community ranks at a paltry 4 percent, as compared to 31 percent of American adults.[4]

On the other hand, anaerobic exercise is any form of nonsustained physical activity that typically involves a limited number of specific muscles over a short time, such as strength training or lifting free weights. You're said to be working the body anaerobically when the cardiovascular capacity cannot replenish the muscles with energy—and you're so out of breath that you can't pass the "talk test." In fact, a good test to see if you're in the anaerobic zone during your workout—where you're strengthening your heart and lungs—is the fact that you're panting and sweating between each set. I know during my FIT sessions that I'm certainly doing both.

Anaerobic exercise causes the body to make energy without oxygen because the demand for energy is so fast and huge that the body must create it from numerous body chemicals.

Examples of anaerobic exercise are:

- Lifting weights
- Using strength-training machines such as Nautilus and Hoist
- Jumping rope or jumping on a rebounder
- Sprinting
- Working the body's core muscles through the use of functional exercises with rubber bands, stability balls, medicine balls, and kettlebells

Practice Deep Breathing, Too

I've seen many people forget to breathe when they're exercising—or breathe shallowly and use only the top half of their lungs. When performing FIT exercises, it's imperative that you inhale deeply as you begin the exercise movement and exhale completely, removing the air from your lungs during the eccentric portion where the exertion of the exercise kicks in. When the lungs are fully oxygenated, two things occur:

1. The body receives enough oxygen to nourish the cells.
2. The body expels waste products like carbon dioxide.

When you're tossing the medicine ball to a friend, concentrate on filling the lungs completely as you hold the ball up. Exhale with each toss. When the ball is tossed back to you, hold your breath for several seconds before exhaling again on the toss back. Visualize the diaphragm moving up and down to provide more room for your lungs to expand.

One of my personal trainers, Ron Kardashian, said it takes practice to voluntarily exchange the oxygen within the respiratory system through deep breathing exercises. "The beauty of FIT anaerobic, high-intensity bursts of exercise is that they increase this voluntary exchange," he said. "This creates a utilization of oxygen from the top of your head to the toes of your feet."

Failing to inhale and exhale deep breaths when you exercise can be responsible for restricting the intensity and duration of a workout. Many people stop exercising when they experience an overwhelming feeling of shortness of breath, but doing proper breathing exercises can help you exercise longer and more intensely. I know I get more out of my workouts when I concentrate on my breathing.

I can explain the differences between aerobic and anaerobic exercise further by using a word picture. Let's say you've been exercising on a stationary bike all winter long at your fitness club. Your usual routine is to pedal two or three times a week for thirty-minute stints. Spring is in the air, so you decide to take advantage of the warm sun by going on an outdoor bike ride. The temperature is just right on this Saturday morning—around 20 degrees Celsius. It feels good to pedal briskly in the fresh air on a level bike path. You are performing classic aerobic exercise.

In the distance, you spot a series of hills. You pedal over the first one with little exertion, but you can feel it in your legs on the second hill. The final climb, however, is a killer: to keep up your cadence and speed, you stand on your pedals and give that little extra *oomph* to clear the rise.

What you've just done on that third hill is switch over from aerobic to anaerobic exercise. You handled the first two hills aerobically, but to maintain speed on the final rise, you needed extra help. When you stood on the pedals and pumped those tired leg muscles, you crossed a threshold and began exercising the body *anaerobically*. Chances are you couldn't sustain that type of energy exertion very long since only elite athletes can do *any* form of anaerobic exercise beyond a few moments. Yet anaerobic exercise is the best way to build muscle and lose weight. Many studies have shown that anaerobic exercise burns more calories and thus more fat than aerobic exercise—up to *five* times more, according to this Colorado State University study:[5]

CALORIES BURNED IN SIXTY MINUTES OF EXERCISE			
Exercise	During exercise	Two hours after exercise	Three to fifteen hours after exercise
Aerobic	210	25	0
Anaerobic	650	150	260

As you can see, we're talking about a huge difference in caloric expenditures. What happens is that aerobic exercise typically burns 25 percent muscle and 75 percent fat for body energy, but anaerobic exercise burns 100 percent body fat for body energy.

The dirty little secret in the weight-loss world is that the first thing you lose when you diet—and casually exercise—is muscle tissue. Your body cannibalizes muscle tissue to support your energy needs, but the fat stays on your tummy and hips. Trying to lose weight without exercising anaerobically would be like running a 10K race with ankle weights: it's going to take you a lot longer to reach the finish line. It's extremely difficult to lose fat permanently without exercising anaerobically.

You can achieve your fitness goals as well as drop gobs of weight by incorporating functional interval training exercises into your lifestyle. But first I interrupt this chapter to issue a health advisory: functional interval training is not recommended to those new to exercise or out of shape. You may have to spend the first week or two, maybe your first month, getting your body reacquainted with physical exertion. You should walk on a treadmill, pedal a stationary bike, or jump on a rebounder before tackling intense, interval training.

The sooner you transition into FIT, however, the better, because the benefits become evident almost immediately. You can see results as soon as two weeks, according to a 2005 study published in the *Journal of Applied Physiology*. Six of the eight college-age men and women who were asked to ride a stationary bicycle until they were exhausted doubled their endurance after two weeks of interval training. All eight volunteers in a control group, who skipped interval training but followed their normal "aerobic" training, didn't improve their endurance rates at all. Researchers at McMaster University in Hamilton, Ontario, expressed surprise with the results because the volunteers were already reasonably fit before the study, having jogged, biked, or performed aerobic exercise two or three times a week.[6]

In a similar study at the University of Guelph in Ontario—I salute Canadians for taking the lead in this area of study—researchers had the test subjects alternate short bursts of high-intensity exercise with easy-does-it recovery times. Eight women in their early twenties pedaled a stationary bike for four minutes of hard riding, then rested for two minutes on their way to completing ten sets. After this interval training, the amount of fat burned increased by 36 percent. Jason L. Talanian, the lead author of the University of Guelph study, said it didn't matter how fit the subjects were before because sedentary adults and college athletes both showed similar increases in fitness and fat burning. "Even when interval training was added on top of other exercise they were doing, they still saw a significant improvement," Talanian said.[7]

Get Thee to a Doctor by Bernard Bulwer, MD

What kind of shape are you in? If the last time you exercised was when comedian Jerry Seinfeld was still taping original episodes of *Seinfeld*, then it's incumbent upon you to see a medical physician before embarking on a fitness program. Skipping a medical checkup before attempting to lose a solid amount of weight is foolhardy at best and death-defying at worst, especially if you're over forty.

You can expect your doctor to register some concern if:

- You've been smoking cigarettes or puffing on cigars.
- You're overweight by forty or more pounds.
- You have a history of heart disease or sudden death in the family.
- You have received an abnormal stress electrocardiogram (EKG) test.
- You complain about arthritis in your joints or bones.
- You have suffered a debilitating illness in the last five years.
- You're on medications for diabetes or hypertension.

During a routine physical, your physician will check your eyes, ears, nose, throat, heart, height, weight, blood pressure, abdomen, lungs, neurological and skeletal systems, and urinary tracts.

Ask your doctor how your medications may affect your exercise plan. Drugs for diabetes, high blood pressure, and heart disease, as well as sedatives, antihistamines, and cold medications, can cause hypoglycemia (low blood sugar), dehydration, weakness, impaired balance, and blurred vision; in addition, some medications can affect the way your body reacts to exercise.[8]

Scheduling a physical examination is one of those prevention ideas that's high in common sense, so don't hesitate to see your family physician before engaging in any vigorous physical activity.

Grab a Towel

Every person is different, every person is in different shape, and you know yourself best, but I'd love to get you started with FIT as soon as possible since intense exercise, followed by periods of rest, enhances the body's ability to metabolize both carbohydrates and fat. If you visited me at my home gym, the first thing I'd tell you is that we will be targeting the body's core—the area around your trunk and pelvis—because this is where fat lives, either as subcutaneous fat (which the whole world can see) or visceral fat (which is hidden but is even more unhealthy since it latches onto your vital organs). Working your core muscles also works more muscles at the same time. Toning up your muscles makes them less flabby, which improves your shape and posture.

If you perform these exercises consistently and with determined effort, there's no reason why you shouldn't finish a FIT workout in twenty minutes or so. Feel free to mix and match, but the goal is to exert yourself and raise your target heart rate into the anaerobic zone, which is 80 to 90 percent of maximum heart rate.

Your maximum heart rate is about 220 minus your age, so if your target heart rate is 85 percent, you want to see your heart rate reach the following number sometime during your workout:

Age	Target Heart Rate Zone (85 percent)	Average Maximum Heart Rate (100 percent)
20	170	200
25	166	195
30	162	190
35	157	185
40	153	180
45	149	175
50	145	170
55	140	165
60	136	160
65	132	155
70	128	150

Be advised that you will find it difficult to reach the 85th percentile if you're not in good shape. And I don't want you to die trying. This is just a goal to work toward. What I would like you to do is push yourself for as long as you can, then rest for a few minutes before exerting yourself again. That is one of the fundamental ideas behind FIT.

Start Off Easy

Before starting any moderate to intense physical activity, it's a good idea to warm up your muscles. If you're in a gym, the most obvious method of warming up is stepping on a treadmill. Others prefer to pedal an upright exercise bicycle or a recumbent exercise bike, which is easier on the back than traditional upright bikes. If you're working out at home, a series of stretching exercises will get you limber.

A more anaerobic way to warm up is by using a rebounder (mini-trampoline) or an elliptical machine, which is a cross between an exercise bike and a cross-country ski trainer, with a bit of stair climber thrown in for good measure. Your feet loop forward while your hands grasp the handlebars, which are also known as the pedal arms. You can dial up the pedaling resistance to deplete oxygen in a hurry, which will raise your heart rate quickly into the "target zone." Nearly all elliptical trainers, as well as stair steppers, exercise bikes, and treadmills, have metallic sensors that you can grasp, which allows a heart rate monitor to measure your pulse.

If you have five minutes to warm up, great, but if you're pressed for time, even two minutes will suffice. On page 164 is a list of my favourite exercises that you can pick and choose from to get FIT. Commitment and effort will be the keys to success.

What Personal Trainers Can Do for You

Every club has them—personal trainers who guide, show, exhort, motivate, educate, encourage, and stimulate you to physical levels you never thought possible. I'm a great believer in PTs, or personal trainers, and it's not because I used to be one. A good personal trainer knows dozens of ways to exercise those core muscles by using stability balls, medicine balls, and other toys that you will never think of. A good personal trainer will also be up to speed on the latest fitness innovations to keep your workout fresh and exciting.

The biggest drawback to trainers is cost: most charge between forty and seventy-five dollars an hour, which means if you employ the services of a personal trainer twice weekly, eight times a month at fifty dollars per workout, you'll receive a four hundred dollar add-on to your health club bill. That's more than a nice car payment.

If your budget can handle the extra expense, however, I highly recommend personal trainers, especially if you're walking the fitness comeback trail. Trainers can help you lose weight, reduce chances of injuring yourself, and motivate you in a million different ways. Most personal trainers I know "get it" when it comes to the importance of functional anaerobic training and pushing you with short but intense exercise that helps you burn body fat.

Personal trainers not only will show you how to exercise anaerobically, but they also hold you accountable. You *have* to show up at the appointed time (unless you're willing to forfeit a fifty-dollar cancellation fee for standing up your PT). They won't let you slack off. They put you through a vigorous workout, track your progress, correct your form, come up with new and exciting ways to exercise, and help you accomplish your fitness goals. You get a better workout and end up making more progress than if you were on your own. Personal trainers help prevent injuries since the most common training mistakes are related to technique. Many people have a tendency to use too much weight, resulting in poor form. Incorrect technique decreases the effectiveness of anaerobic training and greatly increases the risk of injury.

A good personal trainer will work muscles you never thought you had, but the soreness will feel good! Personal trainers are knowledgeable about different exercises, how to properly use strength-training equipment, and how to work past your fitness plateaus and avoid boredom.

Please know, however, that all you need to call yourself a personal trainer is a business card. No regulatory or licensing agency governs the industry, and no law demands trainers to be certified, although many gyms require it. If you are a woman, then I understand why you may feel more comfortable having another woman at your side. This is a hands-on profession, so a good personal trainer will be touching and pushing you. On the other hand, some women prefer having a gung-ho guy barking out, "Give me four more reps!"

Finding a personal trainer should be easy. Ask friends for recommendations, and when you get a name, watch that person put someone else through the paces. You should interview your potential personal trainer, asking questions that can reveal why he (or she) got into the field and how he plans to help you reach your perfect weight. Consider the personal trainer's attitude, interpersonal skills, and appearance. Does he practice what he preaches? What are his credentials and educational background? Was he or she certified by the Certified Strength and Conditioning Specialists (CSCS) or the American Council on Exercise (ACE)? Being certified by Young Men's/Women's Christian Association (YMCA/YWCA), Sports Performance Institute (SPI), or the Canadian Personal Trainers Network (CPTN) is acceptable.

I think you would be well served to solicit the expertise of a trainer, especially during the early stages of Perfect Weight Canada. Over the last ten years, I have apprenticed and trained with some of the best personal trainers and strength coaches in the world, including renowned trainers, fitness innovators, and authors Charles Poliquin and Juan Carlos Santana.

I was still putting together my favourite FIT exercises when I put Mike Yorkey through the paces. A couple of months later, a good friend and one of the top trainers in the country, Ron Kardashian, was in town, and I invited him over to the house to see what he thought. Ron was one of three persons nominated for Personal Trainer of the Year by the National Strength and Conditioning Association (out of 26,000 NSCA members!) in 2003 and 2004, and although he didn't receive this prestigious award, he's called the "Fitness Evangelist" in his industry because he is a minister as well as a strength and conditioning coach.

Over the years, Ron has served me as a personal fitness coach, but on this occasion, it was my turn to put this popular trainer—Ron estimated that he's given twelve thousand hour-long sessions since the late 1990s—through the paces. Here's what Ron had to say.

"I had a great time hanging with Jordan in his home gym, but I was critiquing him as he went. As usual, he had an answer for everything. We went through what Jordan called 'The Big 5,' where he introduced me to Russian kettlebells. Believe me, we did a full kettlebell workout. We had such a good time that we did two workouts that day, one in the late morning, the other three hours later. Believe me, these workouts were tough, but afterward I felt phenomenal.

"I would recommend the FIT program to anyone, from the forty-five-year-old female who wants to lose some fat to those muscle heads in the gym who spend all of their time doing bench presses and curls. It's quick, it's easy, and it's highly beneficial."

Ron has trained NFL football players, NBA players, and Hollywood celebrities, so he had to bust my chops a few times, but we had a great workout that day.

Stability Balls

You've probably seen them—giant, soft rubber exercise balls used for strength exercises, improving balance and coordination, and really giving the core muscles a workout. These exercise balls are known as stability balls or Swiss balls, but they aren't made of cheese or chocolate. These jumbo exercise balls have been used for many years in physical therapy and for good reason. Just sitting on the ball places the spine in neutral alignment and targets your core muscles—abdominals, obliques, and back.

Most people should use a 55-cm stability ball. If you've never sat on a stability ball, it may take you a few minutes to find the right balance. Keep your feet wide on the floor and move your hips slightly side to side. This provides you with a "feel" for the ball and the balance needed to stay upright.

Chest exercises

1. Position yourself with your stomach resting on the ball, which is called the plank position. Put your hands on the floor. Roll your body forward until the ball reaches the feet. Then perform a push-up.
2. Start in the plank position and roll your legs until your knees are on top of the ball. Press your knees into the ball, using your abdominal muscles to bring your knees into your chest.

Abdominal muscles

1. Lie on the floor and place your legs on the ball. Put your hands behind your head and perform crunches.
2. Position yourself with your back lying on the ball. Raise your arms and interlock your fingers. After finding the right balance, perform abdominal crunches as your arms reach for the sky.
3. Sit tall on your ball with your feet resting on the floor. Fold your arms across your chest so that your hands are resting on the front of your opposite shoulders. Slowly lean backward until you feel your abdominal muscles kick in. Hold this position for several seconds before returning to the start position.
4. Lie on your back on the floor and rest your legs on top of the ball. Your legs should be hip-distance apart. Squeeze your legs together and raise the ball off the floor. Hold for three deep breaths before returning to the start position.

Leg and calf exercises

1. Trap the ball between the small of your back and a wall. With your arms outstretched for balance, perform deep knee bends.

2. To perfect hamstring stretches, lay on the ball with your stomach. Then raise your right leg and the left arm at the same time, followed by left leg and right arm raises.

Prone back extensions

1. Kneel on the ground behind the stability ball. Slowly lower yourself so that you are lying on your stomach on top of the ball while your knees and feet stay on the ground. Begin by curling your upper body around the ball and placing your hands underneath your chin for support. Lift your upper body backward off the ball in a reverse crunch motion.

Medicine Balls

1. When sitting on the stability ball, hold a medicine ball in front of you. Swing the ball and your body from one side to another, almost like you're a quarterback making a handoff.
2. If you have a training partner, toss a medicine ball back and forth to each other. Toss the ball back and forth to each other for one minute; then rest for one minute. If you feel up to it, go for two minutes before resting for one minute. Use heavier medicine balls if they're available.
3. Stand with your feet hip-width apart. While holding a medicine ball in your hands, make a backward lunge with your right foot. Lower your body by bending at the hip while keeping chest upright. Return to start position, but don't let the right foot touch the ground. Bounce the medicine ball off your knee and then make another backward lunge.
4. Lie on your back with your arms at the side with palms down on the floor. Raise your legs with your knees bent. Place the medicine ball between your knees and rotate your legs from one side to the next.
5. With the medicine ball still between your knees, bring your knees toward your abdominal area, raising your glutes (butt) off the floor.

Russian Kettlebells

Ron Kardashian's eyes popped out when I introduced him to Russian kettlebells. Hefting these kettlebells—which look like oversized cannon balls with handles—are one of those old-school workouts that's been around so long that it's new again.

The Pied Piper for kettlebells is Pavel Tsatsouline, a Red Army Special Forces trainer back in the USSR days, who immigrated to the United States with a half-dozen kettlebells in his suitcase (that's a joke). He opened his first gym in an abandoned bank vault (that's not a joke), which was perfect, he said, because you could drop the kettlebells without problems and "nobody could hear my victims' screams."[9] No wonder he was given the nickname "The Evil Russian." Tsatsouline began advising elite units of the U.S. Marine Corps and various law enforcement agencies on how to develop overall strength and fighting capability as well as writing books like *Enter the Kettlebell!* and *From Russia With Tough Love* for the comrade ladies. CNN and *FOX News* gave him airtime because he was different: a muscular, well-cut fitness instructor with a Russian accent swinging kettlebells every which way.

All the publicity has helped put Russian kettlebells on the map, and more fitness gyms are stocking cast iron kettlebells, starting at 4 kilos (or around 9 pounds) for the women and 12 kilos (around 26 pounds) for the men. I have a heavy kettlebell that resembles a basketball with a handle in my home gym; it weighs in at 48 kilos or 106 pounds.

Technique is important when you swing a kettlebell around, unless hernias are unimportant to you. A beginning exercise is holding a kettlebell by the horns, chest-height, and making proper squats, keeping your weight on your heels. You can make like a Harlem Globetrotter by making under leg passes to yourself. Swing the kettlebell around the front of your right leg and through your legs by passing the kettlebell to your left hand behind your left leg.

Need a Demo?

If you're wondering what a Russian kettlebell workout looks like, you can view a full video session of my FIT kettlebell workout by logging on to www.PerfectWeightCanada.com.

Another resource is Russian kettlebell maestro Pavel Tsatsouline, who has a Web site at www .dragondoor.com, which will also give you ideas on how to exercise with kettlebells.

Sprinting

I realize that sprinting will be outside the realm of possibility for many, but alternating brisk walking with ten or fifteen seconds of running as fast as you can is a great high-intensity exercise you can do. Periods of walking in between will allow you to recover.

After having not sprinted much since my high school days, I was pleased to add wind sprints to my training regimen. I wear a special athletic shoe (one with a raised heel) and complete a half-dozen 40-yard sprints behind my house. That pushes my heart rate into the 85 percent zone—and higher—rather quickly!

Resistance Bands

If you travel a great deal as I do and find it hard to work out, then pack resistance bands in your suitcase. Resistance bands are basically giant surgical-like rubber tubing that stretch to provide resistance. Just about any muscle group can be worked using these bands, but they're great for upper- and lower-body strength training.

When I'm in my hotel room, I wrap them around my door handle, turn around, and perform a series of chest presses. Placing the resistance bands under both feet and bringing my hands just over my shoulders are called overhead presses. I press the arms up over my head and then lower.

All you need is a good imagination or a good exercise guidebook to use resistance bands for an excellent workout.

Jumping Rope or Jumping on a Rebounder

Jumping rope or bouncing up and down on a rebounder (or mini-trampoline) are two of the best lung-bursting exercises out there. A mini-trampoline is typically three feet in diameter and about nine inches off the ground. Jumping up and down is one of the best and most complete anaerobic exercises you can do since jumping strengthens muscles, tendons, and ligaments—and demands great energy. The acceleration, deceleration, and gravity pull positively stress your bones, which results in higher bone density. Rebounding affects the efficiency of the lymphatic system, which helps to shuttle nutrients to the cells and remove waste from the body.

Many people are not aware that the lymphatic system, unlike the body's cardiovascular system that uses the heart to pump blood and oxygen cells through the veins and arteries, has no pump. The lymphatic system relies on body movement to open and close the one-way valves that transport lymphatic cells throughout the body, as well as release toxins. The up and down rhythmic bouncing from jumping rope or jumping on a rebounder promotes increased lymph flow by as much as fifteen times. Instead of toxic by-products like germs, viruses, and bacteria remaining locked within the lymphatic system, jumping around on a rebounder breaks up the inertia and sends the germs and toxins on their way to elimination by the body.

If the last time you jumped rope was back in elementary school, bring your jump rope out of mothballs. You'll be surprised how winded you get, but that's a good thing. The same goes for mini-trampolines, which are available at large merchandise and sporting goods stores. You can find good ones for less than fifty dollars, and many come with videos that you can follow.

Extra Credit

It's a triple FIT day when I can have time to do three of my favourite body therapies:

- A twenty-minute FIT workout in my home gym
- A twenty-minute session in my far infrared sauna
- A twenty-minute FIT swim session in my saltwater pool

You know all about the workout with a stability ball and my medicine balls, but let me tell you more about the sauna. When we constructed our new home, we installed a Sunlight Saunas three-person far infrared sauna in the master bathroom area. After a good workout, I like to relax in the sauna and crank up the heat to 150 degrees. Within a few minutes, I can feel the tension and sweat pour out of my body through my skin.

You may be wondering if you can lose weight sitting in a sauna. Yes, a sauna will gently raise the heart rate and increase the number of calories you burn, but any weight loss is likely to be a form of water loss from perspiration. You'll gain weight right back as soon you replace those lost fluids, but you will rid your body of harmful environmental chemicals, fat-soluble toxins, and heavy metals. I have owned and used a far infrared sauna for over eight years and highly recommend it. (For more information on far infrared sauna technology, visit www.PerfectWeightCanada .com.)

After working out and taking a sauna, I'm pretty wiped, so it's nice to jump into our backyard pool for a refreshing dip. The cool water stimulates the body and boosts oxygen use in the cells.

I understand that few folks have a home gym, sauna, and pool on the premises, but fitness clubs do. If you work out hard for twenty minutes, retreat to the club's sauna to open those skin pores. Finish with a few laps in the pool, and you'll have a triple FIT workout in sixty minutes—and feel like a million bucks.

Let the Sun Shine In

You may not see much correlation between sunning yourself and losing weight, but let me explain. When your face or your arms and legs are exposed to sunlight, the skin synthesizes vitamin D from the ultraviolet rays of sunlight. The body needs vitamin D to produce adequate blood levels of insulin.

I recommend intentionally exposing yourself to at least fifteen minutes of sunlight every other day to increase vitamin D levels in the body. That is often not possible because we're indoors during the day, or it's winter and the sun refuses to break through the grey cloud that seems to blanket the eastern half of Canada from November to April. That's why I recommend taking omega-3 cod liver oil, an important source of vitamin D. A teaspoon or three capsules a day are all you need.

Looking for More to Do?

You can go online to www.PerfectWeightCanada.com and view a video demonstration of me going through a FIT exercise routine. In the meantime, here are some of my favourite exercises you can perform during an exercise session. If possible, perform eight to twelve reps for four times, resting one minute in between reps. Don't overdo it, though, especially at the beginning.

V-leg crunches

Begin by lying down comfortably on the floor, preferably carpeted or with a foam pad. Lie so that your knees are bent and your legs up so that your thighs are perpendicular to your body and your calves parallel to the floor. Open your legs so that they form a V shape. Place your fingertips behind your head with your elbows pointing out to the sides.

Exhale as you slowly raise your head, shoulders, and upper back off the floor in a slow, controlled motion. Keep your abs tight and your lower back pressed to the floor. Hold for a count of two. Inhale as you lower your legs. Rest for a few seconds and then restart.

Diagonal curl-ups

Begin once again by lying comfortably on your back with your feet flat on the floor and your back flat. Place your fingertips behind your head with your elbows out to the sides. Slowly raise your head, shoulders, and upper back, rotating so that your left shoulder comes toward your right knee. Exhale as you lift. Many beginners of this exercise have a tendency to pull their left elbows across their bodies. Instead, you want to keep the left elbow pointing out to the side. Hold for a count of two. Slowly lower and inhale. Repeat the exercise in the opposite direction.

Single-knee lifts

Start in the same position as you did for the diagonal curl-ups. Simultaneously raise your left knee and torso, bringing your forehead and both elbows toward the knee. Don't pull on your neck and head with your arms. Exhale as you lift. Hold for a count of two. As you inhale, slowly lower your upper body and leg. Repeat with the opposite leg.

Bent-knee crossovers

This exercise starts differently. You begin by getting down on all fours, paying attention to keeping your back flat. With your left knee bent and at a 90-degree angle, lift up your left leg and back, then cross it over the calf of your right leg. Keep your buttocks tight at all times. Return to the starting position. Do one set, then repeat with the other leg. For those who want an advanced workout, you can add 1-pound ankle weights to make this exercise more difficult.

Lunges

This is an exercise that looks easy to do but leaves you feeling sore afterward. Start by standing with your feet about six inches apart and your toes pointed straight ahead. For balance, rest your hands on your hips. Step forward as far as possible with your left foot. Bending your knees, slowly lower your right knee toward the floor. Don't let your left knee extend beyond your toes. Hold for a count of two. Pressing off with your left foot, stand back up. Do one set of eight to twelve reps, and then repeat with the right leg. For an even more complete workout, try bending down and touching your foot as you extend it out for the lunge. This will make your lunge a two-part exercise as you will be bending your back after you lunge. You can also do this with a pair dumbbells or a medicine ball. This advanced version of the exercise is called a reaching lunge and provides added functionality to an already great exercise.

The Cobra

Equally important are exercises that strengthen your back. The Cobra is a great exercise. Start by lying flat on your stomach. Rest your elbows on the ground and hold your head up. Stretch the stomach and muscles while contracting the back. To deepen the stretch, you can lift up onto your hands. You will feel a greater stretch in your stomach and greater contractions in your back.

Opposite leg-arm lift

Lying flat on your back, lift your left arm off the ground twelve inches while you lift the right leg twelve inches. This exercise strengthens flabby stomach muscles and can also be done on a stability ball, as previously mentioned.

Gluteal tightener

Lie flat on your back. Lift one leg off the ground, keeping the leg as straight as possible, and hold for five seconds. Rest. Lift the opposite leg off the ground and hold for five seconds. This exercise tightens the *gluteus maximus*—the butt muscles—by contracting the glute muscles and extending the hip flexors. Make sure you keep your hips on the ground so that you can gain the maximized stretch.

Hamstring curl

Get on all fours on your knees. Bend your right leg and then lift until you feel mild tension. Hold for five seconds. Never lift to the point of pain. You can feel the contraction in the hamstring and the stretch in your hip. After doing a half-dozen sets, do the other leg. Be sure to breathe out each time you perform the hamstring curl.

Back flexion

Lie flat on your stomach with arms straight ahead of you. Lift your arms, head, and legs off the ground simultaneously. The only thing on the ground is your chest and your belly. This will strengthen the back muscles while stretching the front of your body. All of us very rarely stretch the front side of our torso since we constantly bend over all day long.

Moving On

Exercising with stability balls, medicine balls, and Russian kettlebells are all great examples of intense, strength-resistance movements that push the body to make great gains in strength, balance, and flexibility. Just like making the choice to eat junk food, going through the rest of your days on earth without intentional exercising is tantamount to choosing a shortened life span and lower quality of living. A Finnish study of nearly eight thousand men and women, for instance, found that those who did not exercise increased their risk of dying by 400 percent compared to individuals in the high-activity group.[10]

Next to an excellent diet, exercise is the second essential for achieving and maintaining optimal physical health. When you exercise, you reduce your risk of developing high blood pressure. You reduce your feelings of depression and anxiety. You build and maintain healthy bones, muscles, and joints. You become stronger and better able to perform tasks.

Exercise is essential to losing body weight and visceral or "killer fat." In fact, regular physical activity is one of the simplest, least expensive, and most rewarding ways to maintain a healthy body. For example, when you lose 10 pounds of body weight, it will feel more like a 30-pound weight loss on your knees—and when you walk upstairs, those 10 pounds will feel like 70 less pounds of weight to your knee joints. Losing an excess 10 pounds can have a dramatic impact.

Your knees are not the only beneficiaries of exercise. You can also live "younger." Men who exercise right live eight years younger, and women who do so live nine years younger.[11] Exercise helps restore the metabolism by increasing insulin sensitivity. Overall, people who exercise look younger and have more vitality and fewer health problems than those who do not exercise.

When you exercise, you are actually helping the body remove toxins through breathing more deeply, which releases toxins from the lungs, and from perspiration and muscle activity. If you do not take advantage of the toxic elimination properties of exercise, these toxins may remain in your body, disrupt immune function, and make you more susceptible to infection and illness.

I think—and this is coming from a former personal trainer—that the toughest thing about exercise is not the exertion it demands but finding time to do it. You will have to set your mind to getting the body moving again. You will have to discipline yourself. The good news is that you don't have to spend a lot of hours exercising with the FIT program. I'm talking about twenty to thirty minutes a day, but it'll take four times a week.

When is the best time to exercise? You're probably expecting me to say in the morning, and the morning is the best time, if for no other reason than you can't cancel a workout that you've already finished. But the best time to exercise is when it works for you.

Now, I know what you're thinking. "But Jordan, I don't have time to exercise. You don't know how hectic my life is."

Although I can't walk a mile in your Nikes, we all manage to find time for the things that are important to us, whether it's volunteering to host the Girl Scout troop, pace the sidelines while your son or daughter runs up and down the soccer field, attend an important civic or charity dinner, or view the latest must-see Hollywood release. We are given 168 hours each week, and from that amount, you must find 4, 5, or 6 half hours to exercise most days of the week.

You don't have to belong to a gym to get your workout done. I understand that fitness club memberships are expensive and that there are a host of reasons why they don't work for you: too far away, no babysitting, no time in the day. If that's the case, you will have to work out at home. All you need is to get a start.

You can do deep knee bends, push-ups, lunges, wall squats, and a number of other exercises with no equipment at all. This can be accomplished while cooking dinner or even during the commercials of your favourite TV show. Even better, spend a few bucks to buy a stability ball. While perched on the exercise ball, you can use a bag of potatoes to provide resistance for various exercises. A 16-ounce can of tomato sauce can be a poor man's Russian kettlebell. A jump rope and rebounder are inexpensive additions.

What about used exercise equipment? You often pay a fraction when buying a used elliptical trainer, for example. Check classified advertisements in your hometown. Another idea is to gather a couple of friends in the neighbourhood and hire a personal trainer to come to your house and put everyone through their paces, making it more affordable for everyone.

Whether you're at home or on the road, in the gym or in your living room, whatever you do, just get started. Use your desire to lose weight to give you a dose of determination to carry out your goals. You can promise yourself that tomorrow is the day you'll *finally* work out, but that's just paving another road with good intentions. You won't get FIT for your perfect weight until you get up and do something *today*.

Are You a Sleepy Head?

Sleep seems to be in short supply these days. A nationwide sleep deficit means that we're packing in as much as we can from the moment we wake up until we crawl into bed sixteen, seventeen, or eighteen exhausting hours later. American adults are down to a little less than seven hours of sleep each night, a good two hours less than our great-great-grandparents slept a hundred years ago.[12]

If you're looking to control your weight, sleep can help out. University of Chicago researchers found a link between the lack of sleep and the risk of weight gain. They were able to identify how a lack of sleep boosts the appetite, especially for high-calorie, high-carbohydrate foods. What happens is that sleep lowers leptin, a hormone that tells the brain that it doesn't need more food, and elevates ghrelin, a different hormone that triggers hunger. When test subjects slept only four hours nightly, leptin levels decreased by 18 percent and ghrelin levels increased 28 percent.[13] Canadians are definitely better than Americans in the sleep department, as your national average is closer to eight hours a night, but too many—15 percent—say they sleep less than 6.5 hours a night.[14]

How many hours of sleep are you getting nightly? The magic number is eight hours, say the sleep experts. That's because when people are allowed to sleep as much as they would like in a controlled setting, like in a sleep laboratory, they naturally sleep eight hours in a twenty-four-hour time period.

Perfect Weight Recap: Get FIT for Your Perfect Weight

- Realize that aerobic exercises—walking the treadmill and enrolling in low-intensity aerobic classes—burns calories but not body fat. Look for ways to exercise that improve your heart and lung capacity by performing FIT exercises that rev up the body's furnace to burn up fat reserves.
- When you exercise, can you pass the "talk test"? In other words, can you exercise and carry on a conversation at the same time? If so, you're not working yourself anaerobically, which are intense, oxygen-depriving exercises.
- Start working out harder for shorter amounts of time. Lift weights, use strength-training equipment like Nautilus, jump rope, or work out with stability balls, medicine balls, and Russian kettlebells.

- When you perform functional interval exercises, you'll witness near-immediate results and burn fat long after you've finished your workout.
- If it's been years since you've lifted a dumbbell or participated in any meaningful exercise, seek out a medical physical with your primary care doctor.
- If you're looking for motivation and/or deeper instruction when you exercise, look into hiring a personal trainer.
- Make a date in your day planner to exercise at least four times a week, although five or six times weekly will be much better for you.
- If you're getting less than seven hours of sleep each night, you're operating with a sleep deficit. The body needs adequate rest, so turn off the TV and go to bed earlier.

Chapter 10

Reduce Toxins for Your Perfect Weight

WITH APOLOGIES TO King David, I now offer you the Dieter's Psalm, based on Psalm 23:

Strict is my diet. I must not want.
It maketh me to lie down at night hungry.
It leadeth me past the confectioners.
It trieth my willpower.
It leadeth me in the paths of alteration for my figure's sake.
Yea, though I walk through the aisles of the pastry department,
I will buy no sweet rolls, for they are fattening.
The cakes and the pies, they tempt me.
Before me is a table set with green beans and lettuce.
I filleth my stomach with liquids,
My day's quota runneth over.
Surely calorie and weight charts will follow me all the days of my life,
And I will dwell in the fear of scales forever.[1]

Humour is often a welcome salve to the emotional pain that comes from being overweight. Perhaps that's why we see cute bumper stickers warning other drivers: "Caution: Hungry Dieter on Board."

I'm one of those fortunate souls who have never had to lose weight. Wait a minute—before you grab the nearest brick and toss it in my direction, hear me out. As President Bill Clinton once famously said, "I feel your pain," and I can commiserate with you because I've put my body through periodic fasts and Perfect Cleanses. I know what it's like to experience light-headedness, dizzy spells, and an inability to concentrate on anything more than my next plate of food.

If you've struggled with your weight, then you've surely experienced the same sense of deprivation. It doesn't matter what diet you've tried, be it Atkins to cabbage soup to grapefruit halves: by mid-afternoon you wish someone would stuff you into a wooden barrel and push you over Niagara Falls.

Physiologically speaking, there's a reason you feel horrible. The more fat cells that take up residence in your torso, the more toxins you've potentially stored in your body. When you lose fat cells, you release toxins into your bloodstream, which is why you feel atrocious and search for the nearest couch on which to lie down.

We have toxins inside our bodies because they are present everywhere in our environment—the air we breathe, the water we drink, the lotions and cosmetics we rub on our skin, the products we use to clean our home, and even the toothpaste we dab on our toothbrushes. If your blood and urine were tested, lab technicians would uncover dozens if not hundreds of chemical toxins in your bloodstream, including PCBs (polychlorinated biphenyls), dioxins, furans, trace metals, phthalates, VOCs (volatile organic compounds), and chlorine.

The main toxic hit comes through the foods we eat and the beverages we drink. Liz Lipski, PhD, author of *Digestive Wellness*, points out that the average American consumes fourteen pounds of additives a year.[2] I'm sure that Canadians are not far behind. Grocery shelves on both sides of the border are crammed with packaged foods containing food colourings, preservatives, flavourings, emulsifiers, humectants, and antimicrobials.

I've already had something to say about what I believe to be some of the worst—and most widely consumed—additives out there, and they are the no-calorie and low-calorie artificial sweeteners such as aspartame, saccharin, and sucralose. Besides the long-alleged health risks, sugar alcohols and polyols such as sorbitol, malitol, isomalt, and a whole lot of other scientific-sounding names found in popular sweeteners can create significant digestive problems. Dr. Prabhakar Swaroop, assistant professor of gastroenterology at Saint Louis University, said, "These sugar alcohols are made up of long chains, and our bodies have a hard time breaking them down." In large amounts, they can cause diarrhea, gas, and bloating—what people refer to as a "laxative effect," he added.[3]

The digestive system has enough work to do without having to deal with an overload of toxins. Fortunately, some toxins are water soluble, meaning they are rapidly passed out of the body and present little harm. Unfortunately, many more toxins are fat soluble, meaning that it can take months or years before they are completely eliminated—if ever—from your system. Some of the more well-known fat-soluble toxins are dioxins, phthalates, DDT, and chlorine, and when they are not eliminated from the body, they become stored in your fatty tissues. "Consider those love handles as a hiding place for stored toxins and poisons," says Don Colbert, MD, and author of *Toxic Relief*. "In other words, fat is usually toxic, too."[4]

The best way to flush fat-soluble toxins out of your bloodstream is to increase your intake of drinking water, which helps eliminate toxins through the kidneys (which I'll get into shortly). Increasing the fibre in your diet eliminates toxins through the bowel, exercise and sweat eliminate toxins through the lymphatic system, and practicing deep breathing eliminates toxins through the lungs.

Another way to reduce your toxin load is to consume organic or grass-fed meat and dairy. Remember: most commercially produced beef, chicken, and pork act as chemical magnets for toxins in the environment, so they will not be as healthy as eating grass-fed, organic meats. In addition, consuming organic produce purchased at health food stores, roadside stands, and farmers' markets (only if produce is grown locally and unsprayed) will expose you to less pesticide residues as compared to conventionally grown fruits and vegetables.

Canned tuna is another food to eat minimally, although many popular diets include tuna and salad as a lunchtime or dinner staple. Heavy metal compounds, like those of mercury, lead, and aluminum, continue to be found in the fatty tissues of tuna, swordfish, and king mackerel. Shrimp and lobster, which are shellfish that scavenge the ocean floor, are loaded with toxins and should be exorcised from your diet. I recommend you limit the consumption of canned tuna to two cans per week (try low-mercury, high-omega-3 tuna) and avoid shellfish completely.

What to Drink

I've already touted the health benefits of drinking pure water in chapter 4, "Drink for Your Perfect Weight," but when it comes to reducing toxins in your environment, water is especially important because of its ability to flush out toxins and other metabolic wastes from the body. Overweight people tend to have larger amounts of stored toxins.

Our bodies are between 60 percent and 70 percent water. Increasing your intake of water will enhance your metabolism—which can lead to weight loss—and allow your body to assimilate nutrients from the foods you eat and the nutritional supplements you take. Since water is the primary resource for carrying nutrients throughout the body, a lack of adequate hydration results in metabolic wastes assaulting your body—a form of self-poisoning. That's why the importance of drinking enough water cannot be overstated: water is a life force involved in nearly every bodily process, from digestion to blood circulation.

Nothing beats plain old water—a liquid totally compatible with your body—especially when you're trying to lose weight. When the body is properly hydrated, the kidneys function optimally, and the liver can convert stored fat into usable energy. In other words, the liver—acting like a traffic cop—will direct the body to tap into its fat reserves when you are eating leaner, healthier foods and consuming fewer calories; and when you are exercising more.

Since bodies with excess weight tend to have sluggish (fattier) livers, the liver's ability to convert stored fat into usable energy can be greatly increased by the consumption of an abundance of clean, healthy water. Cold or lukewarm, it doesn't matter. Water helps you digest your meals more efficiently, reduces fluid retention, and prevents constipation. You will also notice a difference in your skin as water plumps up the skin, thereby reducing the appearance of fine lines and wrinkles while giving the skin a healthy, well-hydrated glow.

Watch out, though, when water soaks your skin during a shower. Standing underneath a nozzle blast of steaming warm or hot water for ten or fifteen minutes is the toxic equivalent of ingesting six to eight glasses of chlorinated water. Since chlorine is a gas, not only does it penetrate the skin, but it is also inhaled during a shower. Municipalities routinely treat public water supplies with chlorine or chloramine, chemical compounds used as disinfectants to kill, destroy, or control bacteria and algae. These potent chemicals are hard on your skin and give your body one more dangerous toxin to deal with.

You can install a whole-house filtration system that removes the chlorine and other impurities out of the water *before* it enters your household pipes, as we did, but a far less expensive option would be installing an inexpensive carbon-block shower filter. Once installed, these shower filters remove toxic chlorine for six months to a year until the filter needs to be changed.

To Microwave or Not to Microwave?

You won't find a microwave in the Rubin household, which puts us into a diminutive minority in my country—and probably yours. Ninety percent of American kitchens come equipped with a microwave oven to heat up leftovers or frozen meals, but I nixed microwave ovens the day Nicki and I set up house after the honeymoon. I told Nicki that I had done my homework: microwave ovens emit radiation in the form of radio frequencies, and when those waves of energy bombarded food, the agitation caused molecular friction to occur, which heated up the food but also destroyed the fragile structure of vitamins, minerals, and enzymes in food.

The U.S. Food and Drug Administration (FDA) regulates microwave ovens and believes they are safe for use, but the jury is still out on the possibility of a link between microwave exposure and diseases such as cancer. My feelings could be summed in three words: *Why risk it?* Nicki, though skeptical at first, went along with the program, and we haven't had a microwave in any home we've lived in.

I realize some readers think that we must live like the Flintstones since we don't have a microwave in the home. What I've noticed about microwaves, though, is that they're never used to heat up "normal" foods—fruits, vegetables, and meats. Instead, I would wager that microwaves in this country are used 90 percent of the time to heat up frozen, heavily processed meals like Hot Pockets sandwiches, Swanson's chicken pot pies, and Lean Cuisine Chicken Florentine Lasagna. These are definitely not meals you should be eating when you follow the Perfect Weight Canada program.

But what about heating up infant formula or baby food? We survived. When Nicki stopped breastfeeding Joshua, it only took a couple of minutes to heat a pot of water and heat up his bottle. We didn't feed him commercial baby food out of a jar anyway, so heating up those jars was never an issue.

What Nicki and I found was that the old-fashioned toaster oven is more than adequate when it comes to heating up something quick. Our favourite toaster oven meal-on-the-go is making homemade pizzas from sprouted English muffins, which not only are a healthy source of fibre and other nutrients, but also they heat up in a jiffy and don't have a soggy aftertaste as some microwaved foods do. On occasion, we've cooked lamb chops, baked potatoes, and just about any leftover in the fridge with our handy toaster oven. Toaster ovens heat up faster than regular ovens, use less energy, and are easier to clean.

Toxins Elsewhere in Your Environment

There are other toxins lurking in our environment that aren't directly related to your perfect weight but are important enough to mention:

Plastics. There's a reason I carry a 64-ounce polycarbonate water bottle with me: the presence of dioxins and phthalates added in the manufacturing process of plastic. Phthalates are used to increase the flexibility and resiliency of plastic. The problem with phthalates is that this petroleum-derived product has been linked to cancer in lab tests.[5]

Polycarbonate water bottles are safer in regards to the leaching problems associated with plastic. It's impossible to get away from plastic in our modern lives, but Nicki and I make it a point to store leftovers in glass containers and not wrap food in plastic wrap, just to be safe. And you won't find Styrofoam cups in our house either.

Household cleaners. Many of today's commercial house cleaners contain potentially harmful chemicals and solvents that expose people to VOCs—volatile organic compounds—which can cause eye, nose, and throat irritation. There's a reason why companies recommend that you keep these household cleaners out of the hands of children.

All-purpose cleaners contain chlorinated phosphates, complex phosphates, dry bleach, kerosene, petroleum-based surfactants, sodium bromide, glycol ether, and naphtha. These compounds are stored in human fat cells, adding to the toxic load on the liver, and they are not absolutely necessary to keep countertops, sinks, and floors clean. Nicki and I have found that natural ingredients like vinegar, lemon juice, citrus oils, and baking soda are excellent substances that make our home spic and span. Natural cleaning products from companies like Seventh Generation and Ecover aren't harsh, abrasive, or potentially dangerous to your family, and they are becoming more and more available in natural food stores and progressive groceries.

Toothpaste. By reading the fine print, you will find that your tube of toothpaste contains a warning: "In case of accidental swallowing, you should contact the local Poison Control Centre." What's that all about? Most commercially available toothpastes contain artificial sweeteners, potassium nitrate, sodium fluoride, and a whole bunch of long, unpronounceable words. Those red, white, and blue swirls in some of the leading brands don't come from fresh strawberries, coconut, and blueberries.

You can search out a healthy, natural, fluoride-free toothpaste in health food stores. On occasion, we've used natural peppermint oil-based tooth drops to clean Joshua's teeth. We think our son has a great shot at going through life cavity-free since he doesn't eat candy or any treat with refined sugar.

Skin care and body care products. Toxic chemicals such as chemical solvents and phthalates are found in lipstick, lip gloss, lip conditioner, hair colouring, hair spray, shampoo, and soap. Ladies, when you rub a tube of lipstick across your lips, your skin readily absorbs these toxins, and that's unhealthy. Lipstick deserves an award for being the most toxic cosmetic. When you spread lipstick across your lips, you're applying a substance that contains several carcinogens, including poly-vinylpyrrolidone plastic (say that three times), saccharin, mineral oil, and artificial colours. It's human nature to lick your lips, but when that happens, you're merely delivering its toxic ingredients sooner into the body's bloodstream. Mascara, eye shadow, powdered blush, and face powder fall into the same category.

Scented products such as perfumes and colognes are a soup of chemicals, solvents, alcohol, and chemical fragrances and a substitute for something that would actually be good for you—natural essential oils. It's a pity that approximately 95 percent of the ingredients in perfumes are derived from petrochemicals.[6] More research needs to be done on the health effects of scented products, but we have all known friends or family who have experienced skin irritation, headaches, and even nausea when they are around certain perfumes and aftershaves. Others are highly allergenic or environmentally sensitive to the overwhelming smell.

It's tough, though, making cosmetic changes. I have this favourite eye shadow… that's a joke, but in our master bathroom, Nicki prefers her tried-and-true, nonorganic mascara, lipstick, and lip liner, along with a certain hairspray that I'm sure contains every carcinogen known to man. She tried an "organic" hairspray one time, but that left her hair feeling like sticky wax. "I don't go for the crunchy look," she said.

Listen, I've learned something in eight years of marriage: women want to look their best, so when Nicki reaches for the hairspray bottle, I excuse myself from the bathroom. At least I don't have to inhale all those toxins.

Organic cosmetics and skin care products are improving as consumer demand escalates, however. A company called Aubrey Organics, also listed in the PWC Resource Guide, is producing superb natural and organic hair and skin care products free of synthetics and petrochemicals. You should find brands like Aubrey Organics in natural food stores and progressive grocery stores, although they are becoming more widely available in drug stores and beauty stores.

Air quality. We spend 90 percent of our time indoors, according to the American Lung Association, usually in well-insulated and energy-efficient homes and offices with central air conditioning in the summer and forced-air heating during the winter.[7] Double-pane windows, when tamped down shut, don't allow any fresh air into the home and trap "used" air filled with harmful particles such as carbon dioxide, nitrogen dioxide, and pet dander.

Perhaps you've noticed all the attention given to mould-related illnesses and how homes have been torn up to rid walls and studs of spores of green and black mould. Those living in mould-infested environments have been diagnosed with impaired thyroid and adrenal problems, chronic fatigue, and memory impairment. It's tough to stick with a lifestyle change—or remember to do so—if poor indoor air quality drains your energy.

I recommend opening your doors and windows periodically to freshen the air you breathe, even if the temperatures are blazing hot or downright freezing. Just a few minutes of fresh air will do wonders, far better for you and the family than spraying the house with synthetic room fresheners and fragranced cleaning products, which provoke skin, eye, and respiratory reactions. In homes where aerosol sprays and air fresheners are used frequently, mothers suffered 25 percent more headaches and 19 percent more depression, and infants under six months of age had 30 percent more ear infections and 22 percent higher incidence of diarrhea, according to a study done at Bristol University in England.[8]

Don't buy air fresheners, deodorizers, and odour removers. Instead, purchase a quality air filter, which will remove and neutralize tiny airborne particles of dust, soot, pollen, mould, and dander. I have set up four high-quality air purifiers in our home that scrub harmful impurities from the air. Indoor houseplants scrub the air as well, but you could also place flower sachets in strategic areas around the house. Health food stores also sell fragrance jars and dried botanicals.

Perfect Weight Recap: Reduce Toxins for Your Perfect Weight

- Drinking plenty of water will give the body the fluids it needs to pull those toxins out of the bloodstream.
- Install shower filters to remove chlorine and toxins from your water.
- Use glass or polycarbonate containers instead of plastic containers whenever possible.
- Improve indoor air quality by opening windows, strategically placing natural houseplants, or buying an air filtration system.
- Use natural cleaning products for your home.
- Try out organic cosmetics and personal care products, which are good for the body and for the environment.

Chapter 11

Think for Your Perfect Weight

IF YOU'RE AMONG those who've watched *Extraordinary Health,* my half-hour TV program that airs on the Trinity Broadcasting Network and other cable networks, then you've probably enjoyed the cooking segments I've done with Carol Green, a bubbly and talented executive chef from South Africa.

Carol has a lilting accent—not quite British, not quite Australian—that's pleasing to American ears. More importantly, she very much enjoys eating to live and teaching others how to cook for their perfect weight. You wouldn't know it by looking at her while she whips up wonderful flans and creamy sauces on our kitchen set, but Carol was an "emotional" eater for many years, someone whose weight yo-yoed whenever black moods or unsettling stress happened in her life. If you have battled emotional ups and downs that have kept you from reaching your perfect weight, then you'll appreciate Carol's story:

> I grew up in a picturesque province called the Eastern Cape on my parent's wheat farm. I have three brothers: Robert is older, and Michael and Gavin are younger. All my brothers were very athletic—Robert was a national rugby star—but their athletic abilities didn't rub off on me. I was really short, and if truth be told, rather chubby as a child. My sporty brothers could eat a ton of food, so I ate big boy portions as well. I guess I never learned what a normal-sized portion of food really was.
>
> Unlike me, my mum is tall, but she is a lovely lady who was always on and off a diet. She was always searching for the next miracle regimen. When she was on a diet, she starved herself and was miserable; when she was off a diet, she ate all the things she had been deprived of. This behaviour impacted me deeply, especially as I grew older. I was a fat kid and teased unmercifully at school. "Carol the Barrel," they called me. I also heard lots of comments like, "How can you possibly be Robert's sister?" Even back then, I didn't measure up.
>
> So I began to go for long runs—and go on crazy diets. I joined the cross-country running squad in high school and became obsessed with running. The weight melted off, down to a point where I weighed 92 pounds. At 5 feet 3 inches tall, I was really skinny, and I liked that.

My final year at high school, though, I got injured and had to stop running, so I concentrated on studies. The pounds came back, not many, mind you, but enough to capture my attention. I really thought I was headed to the fat farm, although when I look back at photos from that time, I was actually thin. That just goes to show you how completely distorted my body image was becoming.

I went into the fashion industry after finishing school, becoming a buyer for one of the leading department stores in South Africa, working in Cape Town. Looks became super important to me; they were paramount since I worked in the fashion industry, where image was everything. So I had to keep any weight from creeping on, which exacerbated the on-a-diet and off-a-diet cycle that had engulfed Mum. I felt great mental anguish and wondered why I kept failing on diets.

I kept putting on the same 20 to 25 pounds two or three times a year. I had fat clothes and thin clothes in my wardrobe, things I could fit into and things I couldn't fit into. At times, I got up to 150 pounds. When the fat clothes came out of the closet, I'd follow the cabbage soup diet for a week (*blech!*) or eat nothing but grapes.

Whenever I came off a diet, I would eat everything in sight—just like Mum. And the weight would come rushing back, which mentally weighed on me again.

I tried on diets like the models tried on clothes before setting off for the runways. If eating grapefruit for a week straight didn't reap results, I followed Weight Watchers for a while. If the latest miracle cure didn't pan out, I tried Jenny Craig. Over a ten-year period I did 'em all: no fat, low fat, low carb, high protein, high carb—I just mixed and matched the regimens, figuring something had to work.

I thought that leaving the fashion industry might help. Ten years ago, out of the blue, I got an opportunity to sail in the Caribbean on a small yacht as the cook, and being the adventurous sort that I am, I took it, even though I had no formal experience as a chef. I had always loved to cook growing up and even thought of going to cooking school, but back in the mid-1980s, there weren't many opportunities for chefs.

I must tell you that I really enjoyed working in the galley as the private yacht glided across the light blue waters of the Caribbean. I found that cooking for others agreed with me. After my first winter in the Caribbean, I found a better job—this time cooking on a beautiful and swift 130-foot yacht owned by an American couple. I didn't do very well being surrounded by all this fancy food; I constantly snacked and overate, gaining 20 to 25 pounds and two clothing sizes. I hated putting on a bikini to take a refreshing dip in the tropical water and trying to "be good" when I was cooking all the time.

During this time I either cooked or followed the latest diet out there, as the rich, thin ladies I cooked for were always obsessing about their weight, too. I became resigned to the idea that I would always be over-weight. "If I'm going to be fat, by golly, I'm going to enjoy it," was my attitude. I was tired of the mental anguish of always being on a diet.

After a couple of years onboard a luxury yacht, I wanted to take my cooking skills to the next level, so I asked for a sabbatical and traveled to Lyon, France, where I enrolled in a four-month intensive cooking school. I learned the basics of traditional French cooking and *boulangerie*. Several things stood out to me. One, I never cooked with so much butter and eggs and cream in my life—but even with all that butter and cream, the French people weren't fat. They cooked and ate real food, a contrast to the directive to prepare low-fat and fat-free dishes and desserts onboard Caribbean yachts.

I noticed several other things about the French. Inside Carrefours—the big supermarket chain in France—potato chips and other snack foods comprised just one-half of one aisle. But in America, where I spent some time during my Caribbean travels, the potato chips and snack chips were stacked up in *two* aisles. (You could also buy a half-dozen different flavoured versions of Doritos.) And what was the story with fat-free sour cream and chive chips?

In addition, French people ate their meals sitting down. They weren't in a hurry to eat, preferring stimulating discussion and a leisurely pace with their knife and fork along with a glass of Bordeaux, even in the middle of the afternoon. No matter what they had pressing on their schedules, the French took their time whenever a meal was served. The Americans I cooked for on the yachts often wolfed down their meals and didn't appreciate the food or the time I took to prepare it. Some would fill up a paper plate from the buffet line and eat standing up.

After receiving my culinary training in France, I returned to the Carib-bean and cooked on private yachts for a couple more years. Waking up in the Grand Cayman Islands one morning or shopping for provisions in Castries, St. Lucia, was a lifestyle very much removed from reality, so I decided to return to land when I accepted a personal chef posi-tion with a prominent Houston family. During this time, I developed a serious heart condition called atrial fibrillation, which meant the heart wasn't beating properly. I was prescribed strong drugs to control the heartbeat, all of which had terrible side effects. Seeking a different path to getting well, I began researching nutritional supplements that could help me. I took various vitamins and minerals by the handful each day, but nothing seemed to help. This all happened in my late thirties.

I found a doctor who put me on a detox program to cleanse my body. "You know, when your body is clean, it can function much better," he said as he wrote me a "prescription" to go purchase some Garden of Life products—Perfect Food and Super Seed—at a health food store. I felt dramatically better within days, which prompted more curiosity on my part. I looked into the rest of the range and found out that Garden of Life is focused on digestive health.

I also found out the person behind Garden of Life was a fellow named Jordan Rubin. He had a new book out called *The Maker's Diet*. I read the book in nearly one sitting; everything made absolute sense to me. When I graduated off the detox program I ate the food in *The Maker's Diet*, focusing on nutritional healing, and the weight loss followed. I realized the damage I had done to my body for years with yo-yo dieting and artificial "fat-free" diet foods. Over a period of three months I lost 23 pounds and attained my perfect weight.

Maintaining your weight and your health is really the same thing. You begin by focusing on eating real food. If I want cake or ice cream, I want to know if they are made from the best quality ingredients I can find without hydrogenated oils and preservatives in them. I love every bite of a cake or ice cream, when it's made the healthy way. I eat calmly, enjoying every last bite.

If you are dealing with emotional issues that are keeping you from your perfect weight, you need to do three things:

1. **You need to understand the real reason why you overeat.** Deal with emotional issues, and you'll understand why you overeat. Stop self-medicating with food. I had to deal with the reasons why I overate and stop blaming it on a diet that didn't work. No diet is ever going to work unless you make it a lifestyle program.
2. **Focus on only eating real food.** When you super-charge your body with nutrition, cravings are way less, and this will help you stay on the program. That's the message in the "Eat for Your Perfect Weight" chapter, but it's amazing how many folks will purchase factory foods and eat pure junk.
3. **Don't eat on the fly.** How you receive your food is important. Make every meal an occasion. Pray over your food. Eat calmly. Eat with joy every bite.

I've been at my perfect weight for two years. Occasionally when I allow myself too many treats, I do gain a half-kilo or so, but I make sure I follow the Perfect Weight program, exercise, and most importantly, don't stress about it. I don't tell myself, "You're going to weigh

150 pounds again." Instead, I get back to basics, and within a week, I'm in good shape again.

For me, cooking is a joy. I have not only turned my health around, but I have also found my life's purpose, which is helping others achieve their perfect weight and achieve God's purpose for their lives. If you are struggling with your weight today, I urge you to give up all the other fad diets you've ever tried and follow the Perfect Weight Eating Plan. Eat whole and natural foods that have been around for thousands of years. You will look and feel better than you ever have, you will age well, and you will enjoy your life as God intended.

Perfect Peace

I love Carol's story, and it's illustrative of how our active minds have a considerable impact on our weight and our health in ways that we never thought imaginable. The mind-body connection has always fascinated me, but I wanted to bring in an expert who's become a dear friend to me. His name is Alex Loyd, PhD, and he and Ben Johnson, MD, are the creators of an emotional health system called "The Healing Codes."

I asked Alex to read Carol's story and then comment on how readers of *Perfect Weight Canada* can "think" for their perfect weight. Alex believes this area of emotional health could be the missing link to reaching your perfect weight. He'll be providing you with a Healing Codes exercise at the end of this chapter that I recommend you perform two to five times per day. But first, here's what Alex had to say:

> My partner, Dr. Ben Johnson, and I have been lecturing around the world talking about the Healing Codes for over five years now, trying to help people heal the source of their problems. It seems that at every event we are inundated with people who tell us they want to lose weight. "Will the Healing Codes help me lose weight?" they ask. "I've been trying for years. Is this going to be the thing that finally does it for me?"
>
> And our answer every single time is this. "No, because your problem is not what you think your problem is."
>
> Many overweight people think something has gone haywire in their bodies, that something's not working the way it is supposed to work, or they are reacting to foods in ways that they shouldn't react. They are looking for the one magical diet that is going to turn everything around, which was Carol Green's story growing up in South Africa.
>
> I greatly identified with what Carol had to say because when I was growing up, the junior high years were the absolute worst time of my life—period, end of discussion. One of the big reasons why is because I

was overweight. I wasn't obese, however, or anything like that. I was just kind of soft and squishy.

I can vividly remember going to David Lipscomb Junior High School in Nashville, Tennessee, and hearing kids yell across the school yard: "Hey, chunky!" And I would laugh. And then I would go home and cry. Of course, while I was crying, I would snack on a whole bag of Lay's potato chips and maybe a couple of white sugary doughnuts. I learned that one of the things that made me feel good after feeling so *bad* was eating something fattening and good tasting.

Some time late in junior high, I made up my mind that my classmates were never going to make fun of me again because of my weight. I started jogging eight or ten miles every day—just like Carol—and knocking off hundreds of sit-ups and push-ups before I went to bed. I laid off high-fat foods, or if I did indulge, I ate them early in the day so I could burn them off.

Sure enough, I lost weight, and people never made fun of me again. I went from being teased all the time to dating cheerleaders and homecoming queens. Wow, I must have lived happily ever after, after that, right? No, absolutely not. Why? Because I solved my weight issues for all the wrong reasons. My single-handed purpose to lose weight was so that people would look at me and think good things instead of thinking how fat I looked. My problem wasn't on the outside; it was what was on the inside, and that's illustrated by the fact that we have one hundred million sensory receptors for things that are outside, but we have ten thousand billion sensory receptors for things that happening inside our bodies.[1] When things happen on the inside, it's always an emotional or spiritual issue.

Let me share with you how this all came together for me. More than three thousand years ago, wise old King Solomon in the Book of Proverbs said this: "Above all else, guard your heart, for it affects everything you do" (Proverbs 4:23, NLT). I'm told that if you read that original passage in Hebrew—which I can't because I don't know Hebrew—then what Solomon is saying is that heart issues are the source of 100 percent of our problems.

This observation makes sense to me. If you ask anybody who has a weight problem, "Is this an issue for you?" every one of them will reply, "Absolutely." A vast majority will confide that it's the *biggest* issue of their lives. Well, according to Solomon, your issue with being overweight does not originate with your body's thyroid or the health of your endocrine system or how fast your body metabolizes fat. They originate with issues of the heart.

A story in the *Dallas Morning News* on September 13, 2004, really drove this point home. The gist of the news article was that researchers at the University of Texas Southwestern Medical Center were finding that cells record their experiences—called cellular memory—all without the benefit of a brain. Scientists believe these cellular memories might mean the difference between a healthy and unhealthy life, even death.[2]

For instance, cancer can be the result of bad cellular memories replacing good ones. Psychological trauma, addiction, and depression may all be furthered by abnormal memories inside cells. Health issues that crop up later in life may be due to errant memories programmed into cells as people age. Dr. Eric Nestler, the University of Texas chairman of the psychiatry department, said that for many ailments, medical treatments aren't much better than Band-Aids since they treat the symptoms, not the source.[3]

That source is from the heart. If you read the more than eleven hundred passages in the Bible that talk about the heart, including what Solomon said about the heart affecting everything you do, and then consider what the Southwestern Medical Center research says about cellular memory—which really is about what lies inside our hearts—it's the same thing! Modern medical science is finally catching up with what Solomon said thirty centuries ago: that the issues of the heart are the source of just about any problem that we can have in our lives. Said another way, if we can fix the issues of the heart, we can fix just about any problem we have.

Now, is this principle applicable to weight loss? You bet your boots it is, and here's why: Whenever we are experiencing—a lot of times this is unconscious and not conscious—anger or fear or anxiety or low self-worth, we are experiencing issues of the heart. They are the spiritual issues that manifest themselves in a thousand different ways: irritation, being overwhelmed by life's circumstances, being afraid of the future, worries about money, relationship difficulties. We can go on for days just naming them. Those are all issues of the heart.

When we have an issue of the heart like one of the things I just mentioned, there is a mechanism in the brain called the hypothalamus. The hypothalamus is responsible for turning the stress switch in the body on or off. When the stress switch is turned on, the first thing it does is suppress the immune system. The second thing it does is start to suppress or shut down normal bodily functioning, such as food digestion, metabolizing of fat, cleansing the blood of toxins, and movement of the bowels.

Dr. Bruce Lipton of the Stanford University Medical School, in his best-selling book *The Biology of Belief*, says that every cell in your body is in one of two modes: it's either in stress mode, or it's in a growth mode.[4] A cell that is in stress mode does not do the job it's supposed to do, so if it's a cell responsible for metabolism, or the proper digestion of food, or pulling nutrients out of food, or dealing with fat so that it's burned or stored appropriately, it's not going to do the job it's supposed to do. Furthermore, the "stressed" cell does not cooperate with other cells around it. It doesn't grow or reproduce but chooses to do its own thing. These cells cannot absorb nutrients the way they're supposed to or release toxins as they need to. Many bodily functions are put on hold or stopped.

Regarding the stress mode, did you know that you're only supposed to go into stress when you're put into a severe, dangerous situation—like being chased by a bear or confronted by an armed intruder in the house? The problem is—and many studies show this—the average person encounters lower levels of stress many, many times a day. We get stressed out by the MasterCard bill, making the house payment, getting into a fender bender, keeping up with the Joneses, wearing the right dress, driving the right car, and a thousand other things. The cumulative effect makes us feel like we are running as fast as we can on a hamster treadmill but getting nowhere quickly.

Dr. Ben and I talk to people all the time, and invariably we ask them to describe their diets to us. "You know, I eat organic, I eat fruits and vegetables, and if I eat meat, it is very lean and in limited amounts. And I still can't lose any weight and keep it off."

Well, OK, tell me about the rest of your life. Are you stressed?

"Oh, man, to the max, over the top. I am under water. I feel like I am going crazy half the time."

When they are in that situation, their immune system is being suppressed, and the physiological systems that control their weight issues are not functioning the way they're supposed to work. Very often, when you heal the underlying issues of the heart, not only do you feel better emotionally, but your physical systems also start to work the way they should. The Healing Codes can help you deal with the issues of the heart, and when that happens, the hypothalamus will turn off the stress switch. The immune system will come back up, the systems of the body will start doing what they were designed to do, and the cells will start functioning properly the way nutrition and metabolism are concerned.

The following Healing Codes exercise will help you work on and improve the issues of the heart. Normally, I recommend that you go through this exercise early in the morning before you start your day, but Jordan believes that performing the Healing Codes exercise before meals will reduce stress and make for better digestion. In fact, if you are upset, nervous, fearful, angry, or stressed out before *any* meal, you won't digest your food as well, and you're more likely to emotionally overeat, so that's when it would be a good time to perform the Healing Codes exercise.

The Healing Codes Exercise

1. Focus on your overall stress level related to your weight, and rate it from 0 to 10, with 10 being the highest. Your first thought should be: "How much does this [the issue in your life] bother me?" When you think about this stressful situation, what feelings, emotions, or thoughts do you feel? Are they anger, frustration, irritation, or a feeling that life is never going to change? When you think about this issue, where do you feel it in your body? What do you feel—pain, heaviness, flutter, or pressure?

2. Place your hands one on top of the other, with your right palm over your belly button and your left palm over the back of your right hand.

3. Focus on the stress you want to leave your body—physical, emotional, or spiritual.

4. Do power breathing for ten seconds. Breathe rapid and powerful "belly breaths" in and out. Forcefully blow out and suck in through your mouth, using your diaphragm so your belly moves out as you breathe in and moves in as you breathe out. If you feel a little light-headed, breathe the same way, but reduce the intensity.

5. Leave your right hand over your belly button and move your left hand over your heart as you relax for fifty seconds. Think or say "stress out" while you focus on the stress leaving your body. If you like, you can also visualize stress leaving your body as you relax and think or say "stress out."

6. Move your left hand back on top of your right hand over your belly button.

7. Focus on physical, emotional, or spiritual peace.

8. Do power breathing for ten seconds. Breathe rapid and powerful "belly breaths" in and out. Forcefully blow out and suck in through your mouth, using your diaphragm so your belly moves out as you breathe in and moves in as you breathe out. If you feel a little light-headed, breathe the same way, but reduce the intensity.

9. Leave your right hand over your belly button and move your left hand over your heart as you relax for fifty seconds. Think or say "peace" while you focus on peace entering your body. If you like, while you say "peace," imagine peace flowing into your body from God or visualize a peaceful scene that calms and strengthens you.

10. Re-rate your overall stress level from 0 to 10, as you did in step 1.

11. Re-rate your overall stress level ten minutes later.

12. Do another Healing Codes exercise if your stress level is still at 4 or above.

Wrap-up From Jordan

This Healing Codes exercise has greatly helped me deal with the stresses in my life—running an international health and wellness organization with more than one hundred employees, writing books, taping TV shows, speaking around the world, being interviewed by the media, and formulating nutritional products for Garden of Life. Then there are my personal responsibilities that—wonderful as they are—can still be stressful: spending quality time with my wife, Nicki, and being a great father to our son, Joshua. At the same time, I understand my stresses are unique to me, and the daily stresses in your life are unique to you as well. We must all cope with the busyness of life.

The Healing Codes exercise can help you deal with any lingering "issues of the heart." One issue that is often overlooked is unforgiveness, which is common for those who grew up being overweight. Perhaps you were teased unmercifully in the schoolyard, like Carol and Alex. When you reached adulthood, the digs were delivered in a more subtle form: "Are you really going to eat that?" or "Have you thought about trying this diet?"

If you are harbouring resentment in your heart, nursing a grudge into overtime, or plotting revenge against those who hurt you, these issues of the heart will produce toxins similar to bingeing on a dozen glazed doughnuts. The efficiency of your immune system decreases noticeably for up to six hours, and staying angry and bitter about those who have teased you in the past can alter the chemistry of your body—and even prompt you to fall off the healthy food wagon again. An old proverb states it well: "What you are eating is not nearly as important as what's eating you."

This is not the time to revert to old habits: consuming a deep-dish large pizza in one sitting, scarfing a package of Oreo cookies, or plying yourself with "comfort" foods filled with fat and sugar as Alex did back in his junior high days. If you're still annoyed by those who teased you about your body shape, made snide comments about your plus-size clothes, or told you that you'll never lose weight, you have to let it go. The Healing Codes exercise will help you do that.

No matter how badly you've been hurt, put your past in the rear-view mirror and move forward. It's still possible to forgive.

Section III
Change Your World

Chapter 12

Take Weight Off the World

DURING ONE OF my seasonal Perfect Cleanses during the writing of *Perfect Weight America* and the Canadian edition, I conceived a lofty goal: eat only locally grown fruit, salad, and vegetables.

I knew I needed some help, so I enlisted the aid of Paul Nison, one of the world's leading experts on eating raw foods and author of a half-dozen books, including *The Raw Life*. Paul lives in West Palm Beach, Florida, and our paths had crossed several times since we're both speakers and health authors.

In addition, Paul also faced a major health crisis when he was twenty years old— the same age I was—when sudden stomach pains grew so intense that he had to be hospitalized. Doctors diagnosed him with Crohn's disease, just like me, and told him to deal with it because they had no cure. His physicians also declared that he would be on medications for the rest of his life.

Such bleak news prompted Paul to chuck his life as a Wall Street trader and move to West Palm Beach, where he settled into an apartment right next door—as fate would have it—to the Hippocrates Health Institute. He had no idea what the institute did, but he soon learned that they taught people how to live with debilitating diseases with a raw-food diet and lifestyle.

Within months Paul's chubby body was transformed, which set him down a new career path to tell others about the health benefits of eating raw foods. Even though I'm not a raw foodist—someone who primarily consumes raw, uncooked, and unprocessed foods—I certainly agree that many health benefits can be derived from eating raw, especially for short periods of time. After all, the Summer Perfect Cleanse means eating raw fruits during the day and a raw salad for dinner, which was my goal when I contacted Paul about my idea of eating local. We made arrangements to meet one morning in the Garden of Life parking lot.

I hadn't seen Paul in a year or two, so I had forgotten that he was a whirling dervish of energy. Mid-thirties, a bushy beard, hair slicked back, and wearing khaki clothes and leather sandals, Paul looked like an extra from Cecil B. DeMille's *The Ten Commandments* movie set. He stands 5 feet 7 inches and weighs 145 pounds.

Paul brandished a pair of perilous tools in his hands—a mean-looking machete that looked to be razor-sharp and an extension pole pruner to pry away coconuts lodged high in the tall palms of South Florida. The plan that morning, as he outlined it, was to visit a nearby organic farm that cultivated exotic fruits not normally found in supermarkets *or* health foods stores, as well as cherry-pick coconuts from coconut trees growing in the midst of suburbia.

Our first stop was Josan Growers, a mom-and-pop fruit farm located in the rural outskirts of West Palm. With Paul as my personal shopper, we filled the back of my car with eggfruit, durian, mangoes, and a 14-pound jackfruit, which, at $3 per pound, cost $42. My total bill was $91. "You'll like that durian," Paul said. "It tastes like vanilla custard with a hint of garlic and onion."

That's an interesting taste combination...

Meanwhile, Paul kept up a steady chatter, telling me about his life as a "minimalist," even though he rued the fact that he was picking up more "stuff" now that he was in his second year of marriage.

"Really?" I said, cocking an eyebrow.

"Yes," he replied. "Except for the furniture in our apartment, everything I own fits in one suitcase."

By now, nothing that Paul could say would surprise me. There was the time he returned to Central Park in New York City and picked leaves off the trees for a snack—and got arrested. Prior to his marriage, he lived out of a van for a year and foraged empty fields for wild food to keep body and soul together. "There are all sorts of wild foods in South Florida that are quite edible," he instructed. I decided I would take his word for it.

After we filled up my trunk with exotic fruit, we drove around Forest Hill—a tidy bedroom community about seven miles southeast of West Palm Beach—hunting for coconuts in front yard trees. Paul guided us to a neighbourhood where he had knocked on doors before to ask the occupants if it would be OK to snag a few of their coconuts.

"Stop here," he directed. I watched as Paul—with a long, flowing beard that threatened to touch his sternum—approached the front door of a well-kept, mustard-hued single-family home with a menacing machete gripped in his right hand. Whoever answered the door would be more likely to call the cops than give him permission to chop down their coconuts.

After several rejections, we found an owner who said it would be OK to prune the coconut tree in her front yard. Up went the extension pole, and with a jerk of the blade, coconuts rained down. We probably packed fifteen or twenty coconuts for the trip home.

I drove Paul back to his car and thanked him for his time. Over the next several days, I split open the fresh coconuts, gulped the mineral-charged coconut water, and feasted on young coconut spoon meat. My "local" salad came from lettuce grown in a hydroponic tower situated in my backyard patio—but more on that later. One crucial ingredient was missing from my salad, though. Florida's famous avocados, so mouth-watering that I call them "butter pears," were out of season, so I had to purchase organic California avocados at my local health food store.

So much for eating 100 percent local, but I came close. In a small and local way, though, I was participating in a burgeoning movement called "sustainable food," which means the establishment of a shorter food chain by consumers and restaurant chefs eager to buy meat, fruits, and vegetables produced locally.

The transportation of lettuce or any type of food—or just about anything we do in life—leaves a "carbon footprint," a term referring to the impact that human activity has on the environment in terms of the amount of greenhouse gases produced. Eating foods shipped from another state or province, driving a car, taking an airline flight, and heating and air conditioning our homes are some of the everyday examples of leaving a "carbon footprint" on the planet.

The leaders of the sustainable food movement urge consumers to leave a smaller carbon footprint by seeking out local organic alternatives to mainstream food from co-ops, natural food stores, farmer's markets, roadside stands, and backyard gardens and fruit-bearing trees. Every time you shop locally for food, your buying decision has ramifications for the health of your body as well as the planet.

Canada is an ideal country for producing organic food because of its large and varied land base and cooler climate, which reduces pest and disease problems. What's interesting to me was learning that most of Canada's organic production is exported primarily to the United States, the European Union, and Japan, and that 70 to 80 percent of Canada's organic consumption is satisfied by imported organic products. This is due to the fact that some of the most popular commodities, such as bananas and citrus fruits, are not grown in Canada. The good news is that the Canadian organic sector is diversifying.[1]

I understand Canadians' necessity to purchase organic strawberries from California's Salinas Valley, organic lettuce from San Diego County, and organic avocadoes from Florida. While the organic food and farming sector is less advanced than it is in the States, more and more Canadian organic farms are being cultivated to meet the rising demand. I know that those in the organic movement in Canada are trying to get the word out that buying more organic food grown in Canada will stimulate the capacity to grow more organic foods in Canada. Your buying choices send an important message to U.S. agribusiness—namely, you're choosing Canadian organic over imported organic and conventionally grown produce. In fact, shopping for organic fruits and vegetables grown locally (or growing your own lettuce, tomatoes, fruit, and vegetables in your backyard) sends an even better message: you're trying to live a more sustainable life that places less environmental demands on the planet. You're attempting to meet the physical needs of the present without compromising the ability of future generations to provide for their own needs.

Living sustainably is an important part of "living green," which is the idea that we should use our natural resources wisely to restore and maintain a balanced world. The choices we make every day regarding the food we eat, how much water and energy we consume, the type of cleaning products we use in the home, and the kind of car (and how often) we drive have a positive or negative impact on the earth.

The term *sustainable* also applies to our fish habitats.

Scientists at Dalhousie University in Halifax, Canada, are worried that stocks of commercial fishing species will collapse by 2048 due to overfishing. They say that 90 percent of the big fish—tuna, cod, and swordfish—are gone from the oceans and that only 6 percent of the global fish catch can be certified as "sustainable," meaning that fish are not being pulled from the ocean any faster than they can reproduce.[2]

We can do our part for the environment—and help ensure that there will be a nutritious protein source for our children and children's children—by looking for the blue-and-white label from the Marine Stewardship Council that the fish are certified as sustainably caught.

It's important to take weight off the world, too.

Taking Weight Off the Planet

Living a sustainable lifestyle is part of my DNA, and I have my Grandpa Joshua Rubin to thank. My father, Herb Rubin, tells me that his family grew up in Floral Park, New York—a suburb of Long Island—without any grass in their backyard. Grandpa ripped out the lawn to cultivate a vegetable garden, using every available square inch to plant cucumbers, tomatoes, and lettuce. Peach and pear trees delivered scrumptious fruit by the bushel. The soil was incredibly fertile because of a compost pile that took up a good corner of the yard. Dad says he can remember approaching his father as a four- or five-year-old boy—this had to be in the mid-1950s—and asking, "Daddy, how do you know the soil is so rich and wonderful to grow plants in?"

Grandpa replied, "Just put your hands in the soil, son, and let it slide over your hands. Don't you feel the richness and life in that soil? It's a feeling! The deep, dark, almost black colour means the soil is rich in nutrients."

Dad was too young to comprehend what nutrients were in those days, but he knew he could kill twenty worms every time he jammed a spade into the black earth. My grandpa was such a conservationist that he had their family of four share the same bathwater! "That was his way to save water," my father remembers. "Disgusting!"

Grandpa couldn't let all that grey water run down the drain, either. No, they got a bucket brigade going and dumped the dirty bathwater on their compost pile. "We had the largest tomatoes in the neighbourhood," my dad said with a tinge of pride.

When Dad was entering high school, Grandpa had him read Rachel Carson's *Silent Spring*, a book widely credited with launching the environmental movement and inspiring widespread public concerns over pesticides and pollution. "He told me that what Rachel Carson wrote would come to pass if we didn't do something and make a difference."

My father, as I mentioned in the introduction, walked to the beat of a different drummer as he came of age and married. He and Mom were among the first of their generation to pursue a hippie-like "natural" lifestyle, as it was called in the

1970s. Unfortunately, even though my grandfather cared about the environment, he lacked discipline in the area of his personal health. Nearly 60 pounds overweight at the age of sixty-three, my grandfather died of a sudden and massive heart attack when I was nine years old. In the eyes of this youngster, he was my favourite person in the whole wide world. I can still remember seeing the cherry-red, plump tomatoes and hefty cucumbers in his backyard garden.

Although I haven't torn up my backyard to plant a garden, I am growing my own cucumbers as well as four varieties of lettuce in a pair of hydroponic towers situated in my backyard patio.

I can hear the question being asked: *What is a hydroponic tower?*

A hydroponic tower is a way of cultivating plants with water and nutrients without soil. I have two towers, each standing around five feet tall. The bottom of the tower holds a water reserve tank with nutrients. A small low-voltage electric water pump transports the water to the top of the tower and descends by gravity, irrigating the plants and returning to the bottom tank. The plants grow out of small holes in the tower. One can plant lettuce, herbs, leek, broccoli, cauliflower, Swiss chard, cucumbers, strawberries, tomatoes, and medicinal herbs—just about anything you want.

A company called Future Growing produced my hydroponic towers. The owner and president of Future Growing is Tim Blank, who worked for Disney's Epcot theme park in Orlando until 2005. At Epcot, which is an acronym for Experimental Prototype Community of Tomorrow, Blank used his training in hydroponic agricultural to manage Epcot's agriculture showcase of food crops from around the world. "I was responsible for Epcot's futuristic, cutting-edge agricultural display, open 365 days a year, utilizing hydroponics and sustainable growing practices from around the world," Blank explained. "I believe one of the greatest futurists who ever lived was a man named Walt Disney."

Walt Disney's pioneering vision of a better tomorrow is one of the reasons why Tim Blank founded Future Growing with the dream that someday every human on the planet would have access to healthy, pesticide-free food right in their own home and local community. (Check out their Web site at www.futuregrowing.com.) The company installs residential glasshouses and glass rooms that attach to homes like sunrooms so that people can grow their own organic fruits and vegetables year round. Those seeking a smaller investment can purchase hydroponic towers, which cost around $500 U.S. apiece, as a way to get into organic and hydroponic gardening.

"With our Future Growing Tower Gardens, people tend to grow a lot of lettuce, herbs, tomatoes, peppers, and cucumbers, but it's the gourmet lettuce that seems to be making the biggest impact," Blank said. "People are used to spending good money in the store for healthy, clean lettuce, but with our tower systems, they can grow lettuce in half the time at very little cost with no pesticide on the leaves."

Nicki, Joshua, and I can barely keep up with the escarole, endive, and lamb's lettuce sprouting from our tower. Tower 2 is our cucumber tower, which fascinates my son Joshua. As I'm writing these words, he's constantly interrupting me with this three-year-old plea: "Daddy, can we go see the cucumbers?" They're huge—in fact, I just ate part of an 18-inch long cucumber in my dinner salad this evening.

"With our growing systems, you have real quality control of the food going into your body," Blank said. "Our company, Future Growing, is introducing this technology to the green and eco-friendly community. What I tell people is that lettuce is one of the easiest crops in the world to grow. Commercial lettuce production, however, is one of those terrible examples of leaving a huge carbon footprint on the world when you consider the environmental costs to grow, harvest, and deliver that one head of lettuce from the fields to a grocery store near you. Think about it: Farmers of conventional lettuce use lots of water and petroleum-based chemicals to maintain it and grow it. After harvesting, the lettuce is packaged and then refrigerated to keep chilled. All that takes gobs of energy, plus the fuel costs to ship the lettuce across the country. Supermarket lettuce sits on a chilled store shelf for several more days, where it has a very short shelf life."

Blank says the new growing technologies make sustainability fun because the food is exploding with flavour and nutrition. "Children want to eat healthy when the food tastes great, and they can actually help and watch it grow," he said. "My wife, Jessica, and I often enjoy having our friends and family over for dinner, and they literally cannot believe the robust flavours in the lettuces, herbs, and vegetables they are eating. No matter how many times someone has enjoyed a meal in our home, we are always asked why the food in the store doesn't taste nearly as good as our home-grown dinner.

"Although Jessica and I are fairly handy in the kitchen, the real secret is Future Growing's proprietary blend of pH-balanced water-soluble nutrients and minerals that provide the plants with great nutrition and abundant growth. We produce such an abundance of almost labour-free food that our friends usually leave our home with a bag of produce."

The technology behind Future Growing recycles 100 percent of the nutrients and water and uses only 5 to 10 percent of the water that conventional or organic farmers use in the field. "Obviously, we have to use a tiny bit of electricity to run a recirculation pump," Blank said, "but you don't have to store your lettuce in the fridge to keep it cool or chilled. Just pick it when you're ready to make a salad. I see this as being a key component to the future sustainability of our planet."

I do, too. Just as I have a burden to help people take weight off their bodies, I have a burden to do my part to take weight off the planet. Everyone has become aware of the environmental challenges lying ahead of us because of global warming. While there's scientific disagreement behind the root causes of global warming—and this book is not taking sides on this contentious issue—the fact remains that climate changes are happening right before our eyes. I haven't forgotten how hot the summer of 2005 was—the hottest year on record—or the buffeting our home took when Hurricane Wilma roared through South Florida. We are all responsible for climate change when we turn on the air conditioning in our homes; drive our cars to work, school, and on errands; take an airline flight; and consume goods and services.

In a few moments, I'll share some ideas that we can all implement at home that will collectively make a big difference, but for now, let me tell you about some of things we're doing at the Garden of Life headquarters in West Palm Beach to be more "green." Our office building is a fairly typical two-story concrete affair situated in a business park. Early in 2006, our team developed the Garden of Life Green Program that would place our company on a path to produce our products in the "greenest" way possible as well as taking steps to consume less energy to run our business.

We've taken some important steps to get there. Garden of Life purchases renewable energy certificates equal to 100 percent of the company's energy expenditures from our offices and distribution centre, and the light switches in our employee restrooms and several of our common areas automatically go off when the motion sensor doesn't detect anyone inside. Our warehouse ships hundreds of boxes each day, but whenever practical and possible, we use recycled or biodegradable packaging in our shipping boxes, marketing materials, product containers, and wrapping. Our catalogues and product boxes are printed with soy-based inks void of toxins. Of course, we like to think that the natural and organic products we produce under the Garden of Life logo are part of lightening the weight of the planet.

What pleases me most is how some of our employees are buying in. Some have traded in their gasoline-powered cars for hybrids. Some started carpooling. The lunchroom recycling is going great guns. Many of our suppliers had the same reaction and have made the move to using organic or recycled products.

We feel, corporately speaking, that Garden of Life has a chance to expand its mission from "Empowering Extraordinary Health" to being part of the solution to improve our air, water, food sources, homes, and workplaces. We have even donated, on behalf of our top 250 retailers, wind power certificates to offset their electricity usage in their stores. You can learn more about our GOL green initiatives at www.golgreen.com.

The Farm of the Future

A couple of years ago, I spoke at a conference in Grantham, Pennsylvania, where I had the opportunity to visit what I call the farm of the future. Their grass-fed raw-milk ice cream was otherworldly. That afternoon I tried scoops of vanilla, maple, strawberry, and peanut butter and couldn't decide which I liked best.

I'm talking about Hendricks Farm and Dairy in Telford, Pennsylvania (their Web site is www .hendricksfarmsanddairy.com). The owner, Trent Hendricks, has a passion to raise food sustainably and locally. In fact, his award-winning raw-milk cheese, eggs from pastured chickens, and meats like lamb sausage aren't available outside of Pennsylvania, which is why health-minded people drive hundreds of miles to buy their superior grass-fed meats and dairy products.

Hendricks Farms and Dairy is licensed to provide Grade A certified humane grass-fed raw, unpasteurized dairy from cow's, goat's, and sheep's milk—over twenty varieties of cheese, cottage cheese, yogurt, cream, ice cream, and, of course, raw milk. On the meat side, they provide organic beef, chicken, eggs, and lamb and beef sausage. If I lived within two hundred miles of Hendricks Farms, I would be there every other week to pick all the necessary protein foods for my family.

I've come to respect Trent as a leader in the sustainable food movement. We had this question-and-answer exchange, and I thought you would be interested in what he had to say.

Jordan: I know that you urge consumers to seek out local, sustainable alternatives to mainstream food. Why is it important to consume local and sustainable meat and dairy products?

Trent Hendricks: This question can be answered on several levels. First, there is an argument that believes food produced in the same environment as the consumer lives in will lead to the greater health of that consumer, based on the foods' ability to survive that environment. Second, there is the aspect of community building, supporting businesses on a local level, and returning dollars to the region in order to build strength and longevity in our communities, maintaining open spaces, and environmental balance. Third, and perhaps most importantly, local agriculture has the potential to reduce our carbon footprints, thereby protecting and healing the environment. As greater demands are placed on our resources, it behooves us to consider the ramifications not only for ourselves but for future generations as well. Earth can most certainly support our growing population and feed us organically, but it will require stewardship and vision.

Jordan: Why do you think customers drive hundreds of miles, across state lines, to buy your meat and dairy products?

Trent Hendricks: We practice what we preach! We are actively researching a complete package for our energy needs, but in the meantime, we have implemented many conservation, sustainable practices, such as heating our water for the dairy and our buildings with wood that would have otherwise ended up in a landfill. Our buildings are located to take advantage of a natural breeze, eliminating the need for fans for the cattle. We compost our animal manure with leaves and ground wood chips from the community and provide an excellent soil enhancer for gardens, lawns, and fields. We recycle our wastewater and use it to irrigate our pastures. We employ animal traction to supply much of our power needs, such as spreading manure, hauling, and trimming pastures.

Also, we absolutely will not sacrifice quality for quantity. The most valuable way to get folks to "eat better" is to make healthy food "taste better," and our farm produces grass-fed, all-natural, humane, and award-winning food. Make it easy for people to eat well, and they will support a viable, sustainable local business.

Jordan: Is it getting easier to find local and sustainable meat and dairy products, or are operations like yours getting scarcer? Is there good news to report?

Trent Hendricks: There is good news, but too many folks entering the industry are looking to make a buck, or simply "live the dream," and are far less focused on the above-mentioned aspects that we feel are very important. This industry is screaming for strong leadership, which is something we hope to assist in providing.

Jordan: Do you consider Hendricks Farm and Dairy a "farm of the future"? If so, why?

Trent Hendricks: Absolutely! We have embraced the best of the old along with the best of the new. We use mules to spread manure to reduce our usage of fossil fuels, yet we have one of the nation's first fully robotic cow milkers, allowing true free-range options to our cows. We are certified humane, certified freedom milk, and we have a fully integrated product line, taking healthy, local, sustainable grass-fed products into universities, hospitals, schools, and outlying communities, educating and feeding folks along the way. Our commitment to social stewardship is unrivaled, and we most definitely have put our money where our mouths are.

A Dozen Ideas for a Greener Home

Simple changes around the house can also make a big difference for the environment. With inspiration from my friend Stephen Hennessey's *In Pink* magazine,[3] here are some suggested changes that we all could afford to do:

1. Change your incandescent light bulbs to compact fluorescent.

Here's an idea that's really caught on, but it's a no-brainer since fluorescent light bulbs burn twelve times as long as regular light bulbs and consume 50 to 80 percent less energy. When we built a new home a year ago, we asked the contractor to install full-spectrum fluorescent light bulbs, which is even better for the environment than compact fluorescent. Full-spectrum lights effectively emit the same kind of light that streams from the sun, as well as ultraviolet rays, which makes this type of lighting extremely healthy since UV light causes the body to produce vitamin D. Full-spectrum lights are more yellowish, which makes reading bedtime books to Joshua easier with less eyestrain.

2. Bring your own shopping bags or reusable canvas bags to the health food or grocery store.

Whenever I travel to Europe, I notice that the supermarkets don't provide plastic bags for their customers. Instead, paper bags can be purchased for around 25 cents each, so the locals bring leather satchels or recycle paper bags from previous trips. What a simple yet effective "green" habit to get behind.

I think supermarket chains on this side of the Atlantic should adopt the same "bring your own bag" policy. One warehouse club already has: Costco stopped providing plastic bags for their customers in the summer of 2007, and I predict other retailers will follow in their footsteps. Plastic bags, made from toxic polyethylene, are not biodegradable and litter the landscape whenever the wind kicks up.

3. Use rechargeable batteries.

Did you know that you're not supposed to throw your old batteries in the trash? In most parts of the United States and Canada, used batteries are considered "e-waste," just like computers and old TV sets. Batteries contain a high concentration of metals that seep into the ground when the casing erodes. The technology behind rechargeable batteries is improving all the time.

4. Recycle your newspapers, junk mail, and plastic bottles.

You want to know what I dislike about my neighbourhood? We don't have separate bins to recycle our newspapers and paper trash. Recycling just the fat Sunday papers alone would save more than a half million trees every week. I can always tell when I have California visitors to my home: they ask where the recycling bin is when they have some paper or plastic trash to throw away.

5. Watch the thermostat.

That's something Nicki and I are constantly doing. Our home is definitely not an icebox during the torrid Florida summers. We keep the thermostat between 76–78 degrees inside the house, which does feel a tad warm, but we're used it. It's still cooler than the inferno outside. When we leave the home, even for a few hours, we turn the AC off.

6. Clean out the bathroom cabinet.

I already touched on this in chapter 10, "Reduce Toxins for Your Perfect Weight," but many personal care products contain parabens, synthetic chemicals used as a preservative. Try out natural products and see if they work for you.

7. Unplug cell phone chargers when not in use.

Most people—including myself—were not aware that electrical devices continue to draw electricity when plugged in. I'm talking about plasma screens, DVD players, and even cell phone chargers. It's not practical to unplug every electronic device in the home—who wants to watch a blinking "12:00" on the DVD player—but we can all be mindful of unplugging our chargers for the iPod, cell phone, BlackBerry, and the like.

8. Think green in the laundry room.

Conventional fabric softeners and static cling products use formaldehyde to make clothes softer. You can substitute a half-cup of vinegar to your wash or dip your favourite essential oil on a cloth and dry with your clothes. Seventh Generation produces some great "green" laundry detergents.

9. Check your cookware.

Pots and pans with nonstick coating are popular with the cook and the person doing the clean up. (Nicki says that person is one and the same in our household.) Yet nonstick pans are coated with perfluorooctanoic acid, or PFOA, which has shown up in trace amounts in blood samples taken from people across the country. The Centers for Disease Control estimates that PFOA is in the blood of 95 percent of Americans, and the Environmental Protection Agency advisory panel has labelled PFOA as a likely carcinogen in humans.[4] Environmentally acceptable cookware is stainless steel, ceramic coated, or stoneware.

10. Choose paper products from recycled ingredients.

It's getting easier and easier to find toilet paper, paper towels, and paper napkins made from recycled paper that are either unbleached or nonchlorine bleached to keep dangerous toxins out of the environment and off your skin and your food.

11. Use air filters.

This is another idea to reduce toxins in your home. Since indoor air is three times more polluted than outdoor air, it behooves you to choose an excellent air filter that removes and neutralizes tiny airborne particles of dust, soot, pollen, mould, and dander. I have set up four high-quality air purifiers in our home that scrub harmful impurities out of the air. We also open up our doors and windows to freshen the air.

12. Start your own compost pile.

All you need is some unwanted space in the backyard, and you can set up a handy compost pile. It sure worked for my grandpa!

Become a Green Patriot by David Steinman

As the author of *Safe Trip to Eden: Ten Steps to Save the Planet From the Global Warming Meltdown*, I make the case that one of the benefits of environmentalism is taking steps to reduce our dependence upon foreign oil, which can strengthen America's national security. That's why I'm trying to field an army of Green Patriots (check out www.greenpatriot.us) who can help spread the message that our individual shopping choices truly have a profound impact on change.

When consumers choose healthy, organic foods and emphasize a more plant-based diet with organic fresh produce and foods that are minimally processed, not only are they improving their personal health, but they are also taking weight off the planet.

That's because organic foods are grown without the use of petrochemical pesticides and fertilizers, which are linked to a myriad of health defects, including cancer, reproductive toxicity, and neurological damage. So one of the best decisions you can make for your personal health just happens to be one of the best decisions you can make for improving our planetary health.

Also, when consumers consume meat from animals that were grass-fed and fish caught sustainably, once again, they are doing something that's both important for their health and for the planet. When you choose grass-fed beef, for example, you're putting a value on grass management, which is synonymous with wildlife habitat. Grass-fed animals spend most of their time in open pastures, where ecology is critical. Mel Coleman, founder of Coleman Purely Natural Products, once told me that all ranchers are really grass managers and that America's private grasslands, when taken in total, are among the key habitat areas for many of America's most vulnerable animal species.

So instead of choosing antibiotic-riddled animals, or those that have been given growth-stimulating hormones, choose meat from grass-fed animals. You are voting not only for better health for yourself but also for a healthier planet.

Perfect Weight Recap: Take Weight Off Your World

- Think green. Our objective should to be to minimize our disruptive lifestyles that threaten the sustainability of nature's cycles.
- Do your best to eat locally, organically, and sustainably.
- Take steps to adopt a green lifestyle in your home. Switch to fluorescent lighting, unplug appliances not in use, and recycle paper and plastic waste.
- Carbon offsets—also called renewable energy certificates and "green tags"—represent the reduction of CO_2 in one location to offset the CO_2 produced in another, like your home or car. Carbonfund.org reduces CO_2 for just $5.50 per ton, if you are interested in offsetting your climate footprint by supporting wind, efficiency, and other climate-friendly projects.

Chapter 13

Holy Toledo! The Results Are In . . .

I ALMOST DIDN'T get there.

A wave of summertime thunderstorms swept through the Southeast, snarling air traffic into and out of Atlanta's Hartsfield Airport, the world's busiest. I was ticketed to fly from West Palm Beach to Toledo—with a change at Delta's Atlanta hub—on the day before Freedom Fest, the culminating event marking the end of the Healthy Toledo campaign. Situated on the expansive lawns surrounding The Church on Strayer, Freedom Fest would be part health fair and part Independence Day celebration that would end with a terrific fireworks display on Saturday night.

After my flights were cancelled on Friday, things looked bleak on Saturday morning. Somehow, I found space on a Continental nonstop from West Palm Beach to Cleveland, arriving after 3:20 p.m. A two-hour drive would get me to Freedom Fest at 5:30 p.m., just about the time I was scheduled to address the large crowd. I wanted to inspire those in attendance by sharing the terrific results of the 126 participants who finished the Healthy Toledo program.

The other thing on my agenda was to hand out prizes to our "winners." These were the individuals who fully completed the Perfect Weight America program by participating in the various weigh-ins, filling out a health questionnaire, and writing their thoughts about the state of their health in "before" and "after" essays. They also faithfully described what foods they ate and what supplements they took *each day* in the *Perfect Weight America* manual. We couldn't call this group "the biggest losers" because the criteria wasn't about measuring weight loss alone but total life transformation, as you'll see.

I made it to The Church on Strayer campus with a few minutes to spare and took in the Freedom Fest scene. Several thousand people—young, old, and in between—were milling about the well-kept grounds. Preschoolers squealed with delight as they tethered themselves in the trampoline jump. Teens scampered up a rock-climbing wall. At the far end of the property, a burgundy helicopter gave thrill-seekers a quick ride into the blue heavens on this pleasantly warm afternoon in the low eighties.

Hundreds swarmed the food booths, where they could order organic chicken off the barbecue with organic stir-fry veggies or grab a healthy berry smoothie. The younger set was drawn to Freedom Fest's main stage, where a succession of Christian rock bands blasted the energetic crowd with bass-heavy thumping music.

I was scheduled to speak in between sets, so I spent a few moments surveying the Healthy Toledo Health Fair in front of the church entrance. Tables had been set up so that area residents could have their blood pressure and cholesterol levels checked by medical personnel from St. Mary's Hospital. Libby Bauman, a holistic health coach, decorated her table with plastic bags filled with various amounts of white sugar, each representing the amount of sugar found in a 44-ounce soft drink, a 16-ounce sports bar, and a breakfast bar. The sugar bag for the soft drink had to be the size of a baseball pitcher's rosin bag.

I was glad to see the local media represented. A *Toledo Blade* photographer aimed his lens at Healthy Toledo participants being interviewed by reporter Ali Seitz. The following morning, a feature story about the Healthy Toledo campaign would be displayed above the fold on page 1 of the Metro section.

I looked over and noticed Stephen Nepa, the project manager whom I had put in charge of directing Healthy Toledo, handing out copies of my previous books—free for the taking—as well as samples of Garden of Life food bars and Rainforest Cacao Chocolate.

"You missed the healthy dessert contest," Stephen teased. The Health Fair sponsored a contest that drew nine entries, ranging from Heavenly Cheesecake to strawberry shortcake. Once the judging was over, several dozen stampeded the table to receive a sweet sample. Since I was in the midst of my ten-day summer Perfect Cleanse, I passed on dessert.

What was even sweeter to me, however, was news that Healthy Toledo was a grand success. Stephen and the team at The Church on Strayer—Melony Bradley, Dr. Tom Baur, and Holly Urbina—had completed the final weigh-ins on Thursday night and immediately began crunching the numbers. We were delighted by the high participation because the eleven-week program was not geared for casual bystanders.

Back in April, after encouraging The Church on Strayer congregation to make a difference in their lives by taking the Healthy Toledo campaign to heart, I also cautioned people not to sign up if they felt any hesitation about seeing this through to the end. (We originally wanted Healthy Toledo to be a twelve-week program, but with Freedom Fest taking place on June 30, 2007, that gave us roughly ten and a half weeks to work with.)

Overall, I was very pleased with Healthy Toledo's weight-loss results and improvement in health markers. The average age of participants was 44.4 years. We had people ranging in age from 18 to 80. When the data came in, we learned that eight participants *gained* weight while participating in Healthy Toledo, which calls for an explanation. Jeff Gertz (whose wife, Melissa, was featured in chapter 5, "Snack for Your Perfect Weight"), added the most poundage: Jeff weighed 190 pounds at the initial weigh in but came in at 203.6 pounds eleven weeks later. He had a normal body weight for his size.

We asked him, "How did that happen?" Jeff replied that he didn't cheat a whole lot, had been gluten intolerant, and had a history of being in the gym. "Maybe my body was remembering what it was like being healthy," he offered as way of explanation. "This is the weight where my body needs to be, and I feel good."

We noticed that of the nine persons who either gained weight or had no weight change, only two started in the "obese" category based on their body mass index. One of the obese individuals attended only one weigh-in during the eleven weeks; the other attended no weigh-ins at all. (We asked Healthy Toledo participants to come to The Church on Strayer every two weeks to be weighed in and receive counseling.)

The other seven participants who gained or maintained their weight started with normal body sizes and their weight in the correct range already, like Jeff Gertz. Situations like Jeff's revealed that Perfect Weight America, for some, is a weight-stabilization program, not a weight-loss program. Either by lack of participation or by being in good shape when they started Healthy Toledo, we removed these nine participants from the weight-loss averages.

Thus, the following results for the Healthy Toledo participants are based on 126 people who lost weight. Eighty of the 126 participants had BMIs putting them in the "obese" or "overweight" category, so we categorized this group as well. Here are some interesting statistics:

Weight loss

- The top 3 each lost an average of 43.7 pounds.
- The top 25 lost an average of 28.7 pounds.
- The top 50 lost an average of 23.0 pounds.
- The 126 participants lost an average of 13.5 pounds.

Body fat

The average body fat loss for the 126 individuals was 4.3 percentage points, or a 14.9 percent improvement. As an example, this means that an individual with 34.3 percent body fat at the initial weigh-in dropped to 30 percent body fat eleven weeks later. We also found that men were more likely than women to see a greater reduction in body fat. Guys won the category hands down because women, on average, have 11 percent more body fat and 8 percent less muscle mass than men.

Inches off the waist

- The 126 individuals in Healthy Toledo lost an average of 3.15 inches.
- The 80 overweight individuals lost an average of 3.6 inches.

Blood pressure

Two numbers are used to describe blood pressure: systolic pressure and diastolic pressure. The systolic pressure, which is always higher and listed first, measures the force that blood exerts on the arterial walls as the heart pumps blood through the body's cardiovascular system. The diastolic pressure, which is always lower and called out second, is the measurement of force as the heart relaxes to allow blood to flow back into the heart. Of the 126 Healthy Toledo participants, 77 percent showed a reduction in systolic, diastolic, or both readings. The average reduction was 9.6 mmHg in systolic and 11.2 mmHg in diastolic readings

A systolic blood pressure reading higher than 120 is viewed as an indicator of heart troubles down the road. A diastolic blood pressure reading higher than 80 is a predictor of heart attacks and strokes in young adults or people of any age suffering from hypertension. Optimal blood pressure is anything below 120/80, and normal blood pressure is between 120/80 and 130/85. Anything above those numbers is considered high blood pressure.

Blood pressure often decreases when weight decreases, and the greater the weight loss, the greater the reduction in blood pressure. In essence, due to weight loss and better food choices, Healthy Toledo participants lost around 10 points in their systolic and diastolic pressure readings, and 25 percent saw their blood pressure fall below 140/90, which signifies hypertension or high blood pressure.

Women power

Since 70 of the 126 participants were women, or 55 percent, we separated their results by gender. These women lost, on the average:

- 10.8 pounds in approximately eleven weeks (1 pound per week)
- 3.2 inches off their waist
- 2.2 inches off their hips

Women also lost, on the average, 4.1 percent of body fat.

My view

A few observations are in order. First, more than ⅓ of the test group lost 23.0 pounds, which is 2 pounds a week. Twenty-three pounds is significant: for men, that usually means two waist sizes (like from a size 38 to 36); for women, 23 pounds usually results in a loss of two or three dress sizes.

Some other comments:

- The average drop in body weight percentile was 9.3 percent, which was a good number after only eleven weeks.
- Twenty-six percent of the participants lost at least 10 percent of their body weight, meaning one-fourth of the Healthy Toledo participants made significant strides toward reaching their perfect weight.
- The average number of inches lost off waists was 3.15 inches, but 28 percent lost at least 5 inches off their waist. When going through the data, we determined that women were more likely than men to see a reduction in their waist measurements.

We also analyzed the answers on the health questionnaire. Not everyone completed the questionnaire, but just over 100 people gave us these observations:

- Sixty-five percent reported an increase in energy.
- Fifty percent reported they were happier.
- Seventy-five percent reported that they were healthier.
- Forty-two percent reported a decrease in occasional heartburn.
- Forty-three percent reported a decrease in symptoms of abdominal distension, such as gas or bloating.
- Forty-three percent reported that it was easier for them to fall asleep.
- Sixty-nine percent reported feeling more refreshed upon waking.

I am extremely pleased with these results, although I will not rest until 100 percent report that they are healthier, happier, and have more energy.

The results of Healthy Toledo, the first stop on our Perfect Weight campaign, are a great example of the remarkable health and life changes that can be achieved by committing to and following the Perfect Weight Eating Plan. If you have been inspired by the results of the Healthy Toledo group and would like to bring the Perfect Weight program to your hometown, log on to www.PerfectWeightCanada .com and shoot us an e-mail. We'd love to help your neighbours reach their perfect weight.

Awards Time

When one of the Christian bands finished their set, I bounded on the Freedom Fest stage and addressed the crowd sitting on lawn chairs and blankets. After expressing appreciation for the effort from everyone connected with Healthy Toledo, I noted, "This is the first time the program was tested, and the results were phenomenal. Now we're ready to take Healthy Toledo to other cities, so I thank you for that."

The crowd offered polite applause. "Now I'd like all the Healthy Toledo participants to come before the stage so that we can honour you," I announced. As many of these men and women filed to the front, I quipped, "Man, what a good-looking bunch," and I meant it. I was just as proud of those who had lost weight and improved their health as they were.

"It's time to hand out some awards, and here are our winners." Before calling the thirteen finalists to the stage, I took a few moments to explain how a team of four—chaired by Stephen Nepa—reviewed the journals, read the essays, and made the tough call of who would receive various prizes. The winner would not necessarily be the person who lost the most weight but the one who impressed the jury with his or her attitude, determination, and personal testimony. I was not part of the decision-making team.

I first announced the ten second-place winners, who each received a four-month supply of fücoTHIN. They were:

- Nancy Beck
- Bell Mae Belle
- Carolyn Bender

- Bernard Flath
- James Huffman
- Terri Huffman
- Judi Mahaney
- Maya Robles
- Tanae Winzeler
- Jim Wrozek

Next came a pair of first-place winners, who each received a year's supply of Garden of Life supplements.

- Pat Cannon, who lost 40.4 pounds. Earlier that morning, he and Pastor Tony Scott got up early and drove to the WTOL-TV studios to be interviewed on the local morning news show. Pat said he was thrilled to lose so much weight, but he still had another 8 pounds to go. (This was an extraordinary result, and results will vary.)
- James Maheny, who lost the most weight of anyone—46.7 pounds. Friends marvelled at his newfound appearance. (Another extraordinary result, and results will vary.)

Then it came time to announce our grand prize winner—the person who would receive a year's supply of Garden of Life supplements as well as an all-expenses-paid trip to one of my Weekend of Wellness seminars held in Delray Beach, Florida; Atlanta, Georgia; and San Diego, California. "Let's congratulate Kari Diepenhorst!" I exclaimed. "Kari has tried every diet program on the planet, but until Healthy Toledo came along, nothing worked. I believe the judges made the right decision due to her determination to reach her perfect weight."

The thirty-three-year-old mother of two held her hands over her face in surprise as others patted her on the back. When I asked her to tell the cheering audience what she had learned in the eleven weeks, Kari said, "I can now put food in the right perspective."

After the success with Healthy Toledo, I became more convinced than ever that Americans and Canadians are ready to reach their perfect weight. I heard participant after participant in Toledo say they didn't go on a diet—they went for an entire lifestyle change. A match was lit in Toledo, and I don't believe the flames can be contained in the Buckeye Basin. What the Healthy Toledo participants accomplished just may be the spark that sets the Perfect Weight campaign on fire.

A New Catchphrase for Toledo

A popular catchphrase when my parents were growing up was "Holy Toledo!" Just as U.S. sportscaster Dick Enberg says "Oh, my!" whenever an exciting play has occurred, "Holy Toledo!" was the trademark exclamation for Bill King, the radio voice for the Oakland Raiders, Oakland A's, and San Francisco Warriors before his death in 2005. The last of the Mohicans is eighty-year-old Milo Hamilton, the long-time Houston Astros radio announcer. A home run by the good guys usually gets this call from Hamilton: "Well hit…back goes Bonds, to the warning track, it's gone! Holy Toledo!"

Since you don't live in Houston, the only other time you can hear "Holy Toledo!" these days is on *MASH* reruns, like when Corporal Klinger catches his dress in the door. So here's my thinking: wouldn't it be cool if "Holy Toledo!" morphed into "Healthy Toledo!" after what happened during the eleven-week Healthy Toledo campaign in the Glass City?

The results were quite a turnaround for this medium-sized city, which has a well-deserved reputation for its unhealthy ways. At The Church on Strayer, a fellow about my age said he worked in the corporate health insurance industry, and he told me that health-care costs per Toledo employee were double the national average ($15,000 versus $7,500), a very unhealthy demographic statistic. This insurance fellow said they studied the actuaries, and right about 1984—the same year that McDonald's started its "supersize" campaign—insurance companies noticed a dramatic leap in health-care costs.

His observation made sense to me because a former McDonald's executive told me that the fast-food behemoth discovered that they could put in *three times* the number of McDonald's restaurants into Toledo than they could elsewhere because the market was that huge for Big Macs, chicken nuggets, and their famous fries.

Then Healthy Toledo came along, and the needle of health budged off "totally unhealthy" by a few degrees. So was Healthy Toledo a mere pebble thrown into a large lake or the start of a ripple effect that touches shorelines far from the city's borders?

That's a great question, and I don't think we'll know the answer for a while. But I do know how Perfect Weight Canada can make a difference in your hometown, and that's because you're holding this book in your hands. You have been given the tools to make a difference in your life, the lives of your loved ones, and the lives of those living in your community. Are you willing to bring Perfect Weight Canada to your community?

If so, we would love to partner with you.

Chapter 14

Success Stories

I ASKED THE Healthy Toledo winners and several other participants to share their stories and their observations about being on the program. Please know that these are the real-life experiences of some of the Healthy Toledo participants. Some results are average (a weight loss of 10.8 pounds in eleven weeks), some less than average, while others are extraordinary. Your results will vary and depend on how much weight you need to lose, coupled with your dedication to the program.

Here's what they had to say:

Kari Diepenhorst
Healthy Toledo Grand Prize Winner
Age: 33
Hometown: Toledo, Ohio
Starting weight: 293 pounds
Ending weight: 248.9 pounds
Weight loss during Healthy Toledo: 44.1 pounds

Healthy Toledo came at a time in my life when I really needed a change. My diet was poor, and so was my health. I would start a diet every Monday, but by the end of the first day, I felt like I was already in a prison and needed to escape. Before Jordan came and spoke at our church, I was really on my last legs. I was done with everything. I didn't know where to turn or what I needed to do, but I knew that I needed to do this for health and for other reasons. I registered for Healthy Toledo on that day, and it's been history ever since.

I would say there has been a big improvement in my weight, but I'm not yet done. I plan on continuing with this program for the rest of my life, as well as exercising more in my daily routine. Healthy Toledo didn't feel like it was a fad thing. It felt like this was going to be the change of my life for the rest of my life.

Learning how to eat better helped me to lose 44 pounds and two dress sizes. I lost 7 inches in my waist and 5 inches in my hips. I can't wait to claim my prize—a Weekend of Wellness with Jordan and his team. Let me tell you: for someone from Toledo, South Florida in January sounds great to me!

Pat Cannon
First Place Winner
Age: 47
Hometown: Perrysburg, Ohio
Starting weight: 234.2 pounds
Ending weight: 193.8 pounds
Weight loss during Healthy Toledo: 40.4 pounds

I've struggled with my weight all my life. It would take six months for me to lose some weight, but then I'd gain it all back in five minutes. That was really frustrating. I used to use food as a reward, and what Healthy Toledo did was help me see food as a source of health. I really want to eat to live and not live to eat. Food is there for fuel. I've changed my thinking on why I eat.

I actually started Jordan's program a month or so before the start of Healthy Toledo, so when you add what I lost before the official start, I've lost 50 pounds in the last fifteen weeks or so. Since I haven't been under 200 pounds for seventeen years, people tell me that I look like a different person! Now I have a very high energy level and sleep great every night, and believe me, I need the rest with four children, including two teenagers in the house.

James Mahaney
First Place Winner
Age: 61
Hometown: Oregon, Ohio
Starting weight: 246.6 pounds
Ending weight: 199.9 pounds
Weight loss during Healthy Toledo: 46.7 pounds

Before Jordan spoke to us about Healthy Toledo, my body had been giving out for a long time. My joints ached, I had lower back pain, and the abdominal pain never went away. My knees and joints would snap, crackle, and pop whenever I moved about.

Like Pat Cannon, I got a head start on Healthy Toledo when I went through Jordan Rubin's 7 Weeks of Wellness program here at The Church on Strayer, so I've really lost 56 pounds in the last four months. Now I can do things I never could do before—like crossing my legs.

One time, while relaxing in the living room, I naturally crossed my legs. Then I realized what I did. I called my wife, Judi, over and said, "Look, I crossed my leg without any help!" Before, I had to grab the bottom of my pants leg and lift my leg, one over the other. Just being able to do simple physical acts like this is such a blessing.

I just got back from four days in Florida with my son's family, including a pair of granddaughters, ages six and two and a half. After a day at Disney World, pushing strollers, carrying the girls around, standing in long lines...I wasn't sore or overtired.

It's great having a new wardrobe. It's great having friends ask me, "What did you do?" It's great telling them how I started eating right, taking supplements, and started exercising again.

Judi Mahaney
Second Place Winner
Age: 59
Hometown: Oregon, Ohio
Starting weight: 136.8 pounds
Ending weight: 114.4 pounds
Weight loss during Healthy Toledo: 22.4 pounds

What a change for me—I now feel great! I love life, myself, and God even more because my outlook has changed.

I dropped four sizes, but I also think I lost more weight percentage-wise than anyone else in the Healthy Toledo program: 16.37 percent of my body weight in just eleven weeks.

Tanae Winzeler
Age: 19
Hometown: Blissfield, Michigan
Starting weight: 150.6 pounds
Ending weight: 146.8 pounds
Weight loss during Healthy Toledo: 3.8 pounds

The past eleven weeks have been both easy and hard. I loved ranch dressing on my salad before this program; now that processed salad dressing almost disgusts me. Even though there were periods when I cheated during Healthy Toledo, I did really well. I am constantly hearing, "Have you lost weight?" "Your hair looks so healthy," or "Where are you? I can barely see you anymore."

This is the first time in my entire life that I can actually say I feel good about how I look. I like it that I don't think I'm ugly or fat anymore, and that is a really nice feeling.

Carolyn Bender
Second Place Winner
Age: 51
Hometown: Fremont, Ohio
Starting weight: 244.4 pounds
Ending weight: 218.6 pounds
Weight loss during Healthy Toledo: 25.8 pounds

Healthy Toledo has been a wonderful experience for me, especially because I lost nearly 9 inches around my waist. I didn't think I'd be able to set aside certain foods, like white potatoes. They were a dinnertime staple when I was a little girl growing up on a dairy farm in Devon, Ohio. After a time, though, I forgot about potatoes and focused on the many foods that are good for my body. I am in the process of learning to "eat to live" rather than "live to eat."

For instance, I didn't eat fruit before, but now I like to eat strawberries, melons, and pineapple. When I make a salad, I use a variety of vegetables. Before, I used to make salads with romaine lettuce, carrots and celery, but now I add broccoli, cauliflower, cucumbers, pumpkin seeds, sesame seeds, walnuts, almonds, and pecans.

My goal is to lose another 50 pounds, and when I do, I have a special reward waiting for me. Four years ago, I signed up for a drawing at the Sandusky County Fair and won a Harley-Davidson Sportster. Because of my excessive weight, the bike has been in the garage all this time. I've ridden just twice in our long driveway; there are only eleven miles on the odometer.

Now that I'm on the road to being healthy, I'm looking forward to going out on the open highway with my Harley. I've taken all the tests; I'm legal to drive it, but I just want to lose a few more pounds before I buy my black leather outfit.

At the rate things are going, I'll be tooling on my Harley in no time.

Dale Bender
Age: 51
Hometown: Fremont, Ohio
Starting weight: 231.5 pounds
Ending weight: 204.6 pounds
Weight loss during Healthy Toledo: 26.9 pounds

It was Carolyn who got me to do Healthy Toledo with her, and she didn't have to yank on my ear. I knew this was the season to get into it. Three years ago I was in pretty good shape: I weighed

200 pounds, but then I steadily gained weight until I tipped the scales at 232 pounds, which means a weight gain of almost a pound a month. I went from a size 34 to a size 36 in my pants. When Healthy Toledo came around, I knew it was time to get back in shape. I also figured it would be fun since I knew a lot of the people doing the program.

After a week or two in, though, I was saying to myself, "What was I thinking?" I wasn't having much fun at all, but I hung in there because Carolyn was doing so well, and we lost weight together. Between us, with my 27 pounds, we lost 52.7 pounds. I thought that was the most for any couple in Healthy Toledo, but then I heard Warren and Donna Heady just beat us out by losing a collective 54.6 pounds.

We've lost an amazing amount of weight, and just as amazing will be seeing my wife in black leather on her Harley-Davidson.

Nancy Beck
Second Place Winner
Age: 42
Hometown: Delta, Ohio
Starting weight: 205.5 pounds
Ending weight: 187.2 pounds
Weight loss: 18.3 pounds

I'm a manager at a busy restaurant, on my feet all day. When I came home, I didn't have energy to cook for my family or myself, so we relied on microwave meals and a lot of processed foods that weren't good for our health.

During Healthy Toledo, though, I got into the habit of exercising. I used to dread working out, but now if I don't exercise every day, I miss it. I can even state that it has become fun to exercise. (Did I just say that?) I am so full of energy. People at work joke and tell me to slow down. I'm trying hard not to be a complainer. People always ask me, "Why do you sing all the time?" and my reply is, "Because I'm happy." That's what losing 10 inches around your waist will do.

I have more regularity. I used to go for days without going to the bathroom; now it's daily. I didn't like feeling bloated and uncomfortable, and now my digestion and elimination are improved.

David Beck
Age: 43
Hometown: Delta, Ohio
Starting weight: 246.8 pounds
Ending weight: 222.8 pounds
Weight loss during Healthy Toledo: 24 pounds

As Nancy's husband, I've sure seen a difference in her disposition. She is a happier person, and that's been great for our marriage. We had never done anything like this for eleven weeks, though. The first few weeks of Healthy Toledo were rough. Once I detoxed, though, the foods on the program tasted better. I love berries and don't miss chocolate, which is a good thing since sweets have always been my downfall.

Another thing is that I used to hate eggs. Couldn't stand them. But I learned real fast that if I didn't want to be hungry in the morning, I better eat eggs. The free-range, omega-3 eggs that Jordan recommended don't have a strong taste like regular supermarket eggs, so now I like these eggs. Nancy cooks us a Mexican omelet in the morning with onions, peppers, salsa on top, and goat cheese. Now I look forward to breakfast.

Nancy even likes the chicken I grill on the barbecue for dinner. She's around chicken all day at her restaurant, but coming home to grilled chicken seasoned with Herbamare works for her.

Beno (Bernard) Flath

Second Place Winner
Age: 55
Hometown: Maumee, Ohio
Starting weight: 161.4 pounds
Ending weight: 143.4 pounds
Weight loss during Healthy Toledo: 18 pounds

I was a cop for fifteen years in Miami Beach, working undercover in violent crimes and investigating armed robbery and home break-ins while working part time as an emergency nurse RN in a level 1 trauma center. Talk about a high-stress lifestyle.

I retired from police work in 2001 and moved back to the Toledo area to be closer to my family. I also took a nursing position in a local ER. I've always been thin and active, and people have complimented my build for years. (I also did some modeling work well into my thirties.) In the last three years, I have run not one but *two* marathons. Staying in shape is important to me, and I remember telling my lovely wife of twenty years—I still think we are on our honeymoon—that I would like to still be waterskiing and snow skiing well past one hundred years of age.

When I heard about Healthy Toledo, I thought this would be a good midlife checkup for me. And was it! I had no idea that I had been abusing my body for so many years.

When I stopped drinking diet sodas and started eating only healthy foods, I lost almost 10 pounds in my first week and felt super. In the final two weeks of Healthy Toledo, I returned to my work as an emergency room nurse full of energy, working twelve-and-a-half-hour shifts. I'm excited to see that even though I lost 18 pounds, I'm actually stronger because I'm eating only good food. I've told dozens of patients and co-workers about Healthy Toledo.

My eating habits are forever changed.

Marty Wcislek

Age: 60
Hometown: Toledo, Michigan
Starting weight: 160.2 pounds
Ending weight: 153.2 pounds
Weight loss during Healthy Toledo: 7 pounds

Healthy Toledo was somewhat difficult for me to do because I had never thought about the state of my health before. I guess I took my health for granted.

I must say that after going on the Healthy Toledo program, I have more energy and just feel better about myself. My neighbors have commented about how much better I look. I think a lot of that was eliminating our visits to fast-food places.

The hardest and most challenging part of Healthy Toledo was going on a weeklong cruise about two weeks into the program. Staying away from pork products, pastries, rolls, and some desserts was hard, but we managed to do relatively well. We now eat turkey bacon for breakfast, and I've really grown to like it. One change I've noticed is that my taste buds have changed. I recently tried eating a fast-food hamburger, and it tasted pretty bad. Overall, I'm very pleased with my lifestyle, and I appreciate all the support in achieving it.

Jim Wrozek

Second Place Winner
Age: 52
Hometown: Blissfield, Michigan
Starting weight: 227 pounds
Ending weight: 191.8 pounds
Weight loss through Healthy Toledo: 35.2 pounds

About two weeks into the program, I began sleeping like a baby again. What a relief! I do get up in the middle of the night, but that's to use the bathroom due to all the water I'm drinking.

I go to bed between 10:00 and 11:00 p.m. and get up at 5:00 a.m. with a lot more energy and spring in my step.

About that spring in my step. People have really noticed a change in me—my appearance at first and then my attitude. I have even been told that I am more humble now.

I find myself looking at people who have the same problems I had and thinking maybe I could help them—if they would only listen to how easy it really is. If Healthy Toledo worked for me, it can work for anyone.

Terri Huffman
Second Place Winner
Age: 49
Hometown: Maumee, Ohio
Starting weight: 199.2 pounds
Ending weight: 186.6 pounds
Weight loss during Healthy Toledo: 12.6 pounds

I started Healthy Toledo about 40 or 50 pounds overweight. I had aches and pains constantly around my ankles, no doubt due to carrying all the extra weight. I've been on diets all my life, and I've never lost weight, always gained, but Healthy Toledo changed that. People have noticed that I lost weight and ask how I did it. Changing my eating habits helped a great deal. Making exercise a daily part of my routine made my energy levels soar.

James Huffman
Second Place Winner
Age: 45
Hometown: Maumee, Ohio
Starting weight: 240 pounds
Ending weight: 210.6 pounds
Weight loss during Healthy Toledo: 29.4 pounds

I've lost nearly 30 pounds, and my energy level has increased tenfold at least. I used to be a sit-around guy all the time, but now I'm constantly doing something. I actually enjoy eating broccoli and asparagus, which is a miracle in itself. I'm not sure how much I lost in waist size, but I sure do feel a lot better.

Debbie Fisher

Age: 52

Hometown: Sandusky, Ohio

Starting weight: 145.8 pounds

Ending weight: 129.7 pounds

Weight loss during Healthy Toledo: 16.1 pounds

When I started Healthy Toledo, I stepped into our local health food store and felt like I was in a foreign country. I ran into a close friend, Sheri Wittmer, and she showed me around. I had never heard of foods like buckwheat, quinoa, and cottonseed oil, but I soon got the hang of it.

I haven't weighed under 130 pounds since I was a teenager. My husband, Jeff, lost 30 pounds, and his 38 pants used to be tight on him, but now he can comfortably fit into 34s. My twenty-six-year-old son, Chad, lost 14.2 pounds. His wife, Katie, was pregnant with their first child, so she couldn't do the program.

Holiday dinners in the future will be interesting. I'm sure we'll have turkey, but it looks like the bird will have to be organic. I don't know if stuffing fits into the picture, but we'll find good things to eat.

Rose Martinez

Age: 65

Hometown: Ottawa Lake, Michigan

Starting weight: 124.2 pounds

Ending weight: 115 pounds

Weight loss during Healthy Toledo: 9.2 pounds

I'm just so glad that my husband, Al, and I stuck through all the phases of Healthy Toledo. We took the supplements on a regular basis and enjoyed that.

Al Martinez

Age: 69

Hometown: Ottawa Lake, Michigan

Starting weight: 182.6 pounds

Ending weight: 177.2 pounds

Weight loss during Healthy Toledo: 5.4 pounds

I had an interesting experience. At first, I gained nearly 5 pounds, but I lost two notches off my belt. "Oh, boy, what's going here?" I thought. Then I realized that's the fat turning into muscle. I went from a tight 36-inch waist to a comfortable 34, and by the end of Healthy Toledo,

I had lost 5.4 pounds, but really, I lost around 10 pounds to get there. My energy level went up, and I feel stronger. I used to toss and turn, toss and turn, in bed, but now I go right back to sleep.

Melissa Gertz
Age: 41
Hometown: Findlay, Ohio
Starting weight: 189.9 pounds
Ending weight: 180 pounds
Weight loss during Healthy Toledo: 9.9 pounds

Much of my story is told at the beginning of chapter 5, "Snack for Your Perfect Weight," but when I was at my worst—snacking and eating out of control—what I was doing was feeding my depression, which made me feel even more depressed.

I asked God, "What can I do?"

I went to a bookstore and prayed for God to show me the right book. I was directed to Jordan's book *The Maker's Diet*. I followed that plan and lost 35 pounds, which changed my life. I was amazed when I heard Jordan was coming to The Church on Strayer to urge us to become part of Healthy Toledo.

I kept right on going with Healthy Toledo, and over a six-month period or so, I went down seven pant sizes and lost over 60 pounds. Now I have control over food; food doesn't have control over me. I don't need ice cream anymore. I don't need Dove chocolate anymore.

During Healthy Toledo, I became a mentor to others. "I've been there. I've done that. This does work," I said. I told people not to give up, and you shouldn't either.

(A note from Jordan: I asked Melissa to join me on my television show, *Extraordinary Health*, a few months after Healthy Toledo, and she was down another 20 pounds to 160!)

Final Thought

I'd now like to give the pulpit, so to speak, to Pastor Tony Scott, who didn't officially participate in the eleven-week program because he's been practicing what he preaches about good health for twenty years. But without him and his incredible energy and dedication to ministering to others, Healthy Toledo never would have happened. Thank you, Pastor Tony, for your leadership.

Our message has always been living a balance, disciplined life between spirit, soul, and body. And I started with myself twenty years ago and turned away from junk foods and started eating right, listening to the right people, reading the right books, listening to the right tapes, reading the Bible, and saying, "What should I be eating?"

As a show of support, I followed Healthy Toledo on my own. Well, I lost 10 pounds and 2½ inches off my waist, which I got very excited about it, but here's the important thing that happened to me: Most of my life, I've been a very light sleeper. I go to bed, sleep for two or three hours, wake up, and repeat this pattern. When I was into about the tenth or twelfth day of this program, I woke up one morning, looked at the clock, and realized I'd been asleep for seven and a half hours! That may have been a first in my adult life, sleeping right through for seven and a half hours with no waking up. That pattern has continued. I go to bed now, sleep six, seven, or seven and a half hours, and then wake up feeling refreshed and energetic.

I would say that Jordan Rubin's message is an inspiration to become everything that God created us to be. God wants you to be everything that you can be spiritually, He wants you to be everything that you can be in your soul, and He wants you to be everything that you can be in your body.

There are so many pastors who aren't healthy, who are overweight, who are on high blood pressure medication, and there's no reason for that. God has put the foods in the earth that heal. I've been praying and believing God will spread this message of good health beyond Toledo, so I'm excited to see what happens with Jordan's Perfect Weight America campaign.

—Pastor Tony Scott

Chapter 15

The Perfect Weight Daily Health Plan

BACK IN CHAPTER 7, I outlined the Perfect Weight Eating Plan that was broken down into a sixteen-week, four-phase program. I also asked you to answer the nutritional type questionnaire in chapter 3, "Eat for Your Perfect Weight," on page 64. If you haven't filled out the questionnaire, you should go back and complete it at this time.

The following plans are divided by gender and whether you're a meat type or a potato type. As a reminder, under the listing for "Get FIT for your perfect weight," I've given you a rigorous regimen that you can follow. If you believe the physical demands are too great, pick and choose the exercises you feel comfortable performing.

Female Meat Type
Phase I (Weeks 1–4)

Day 1

Upon waking

Drink for your perfect weight: 16–24 ounces of water

Think for your perfect weight: Spend some time this morning picturing yourself at your perfect weight. See yourself doing the things you think you can't do now or don't do because you're not at your perfect weight. Picture yourself looking great, free from all of the diseases that people said you're at a high risk for. Next, picture yourself at your perfect weight, inspiring your family and friends, who remark how great you look. Now stand in front of the mirror and repeat:

Today I am going to take another positive step toward achieving my perfect weight.

Then perform the Healing Codes Exercise, which is on page 189. I recommend that you perform the Healing Codes Exercise at least twice a day—once in the morning and once in the evening—but feel free to try this two-minute exercise three, four, or five times a day.

Get FIT for your perfect weight: Perform FIT exercises for twenty minutes, choosing

from physical activities like sprinting, bodyweight exercises, strength training with bands, medicine balls, dumbbells or kettlebells, stationary bike, or the stair stepper. (Video examples of these exercises can be found at www.PerfectWeightCanada.com.)

Breakfast (approximately 7:30 a.m.)

Drink for your perfect weight: 8–12 ounces of water

Make a smoothie in a blender with the following ingredients:

- 1 cup plain whole-milk yogurt or kefir
- 1 tsp. organic flaxseed oil
- 1 tsp. organic extra-virgin coconut oil
- 1 Tbsp. organic raw honey
- 1 cup organic fruit, fresh or frozen (berries, peaches, pineapple, etc.)
- 1 scoop goat's milk protein powder (see the PW Resource Guide on page 322 for recommendations)
- Dash of vanilla extract (optional)

Supplement for your perfect weight: Take two or three whole-food multivitamin caplets and one to four capsules of concentrated fucoxanthin. (See the PWC Resource Guide on page 322 for recommended products.)

Perfect Snack (approximately 10:00 a.m.)

Drink for your perfect weight: 8–12 ounces of water

One Perfect Weight America Peanut Butter fücoProtein whole-food nutrition bar (see the PWC Resource Guide on page 322 for recommended products)

or

One serving of Perfect Meal chocolate-flavoured meal supplement with native whey protein and glucomannan fibre mixed with 12 ounces of water

Lunch (approximately 12:30 p.m.)

Drink for your perfect weight: 12–16 ounces of water

Toss a large green salad with mixed greens, avocado, carrots, cucumbers, celery, tomatoes, red cabbage, red peppers, red onions, sprouts, 2 ounces of canned beans (black, garbanzo, and pinto), and two hard-boiled omega-3 eggs.

For the salad dressing, mix extra-virgin olive oil, apple-cider vinegar or lemon juice, naturally brewed soy sauce, liquid aminos, Celtic Sea Salt, herbs, and spices, or use a healthy store-bought dressing. (See the PWC Resource Guide for recommended brands.)

Supplement for your perfect weight: Take two or three whole-food multivitamin caplets and one to three capsules of concentrated fucoxanthin.

Perfect Snack (approximately 3:30 p.m.)

Drink for your perfect weight: 8–12 ounces of water

One Perfect Weight America Chocolate MacNut Crunch fücoProtein whole-food nutrition bar

or

One serving of Perfect Meal vanilla-flavoured meal supplement with native whey protein and glucomannan fibre mixed with 12 ounces of water

Dinner (approximately 6:15 p.m., but try to finish eating dinner by 7:00 p.m.)

Drink for your perfect weight: 12–16 ounces of water

Baked, poached, or grilled wild-caught salmon

Steamed broccoli

Toss a green salad with mixed greens, avocado, carrots, cucumbers, celery, tomatoes, red cabbage, red peppers, red onions, and sprouts.

For the salad dressing, mix extra-virgin olive oil, apple-cider vinegar or lemon juice, naturally brewed soy sauce, liquid aminos, Celtic Sea Salt, herbs, and spices, or use a healthy store-bought dressing.

Supplement for your perfect weight: Take two or three whole-food multivitamin caplets, one to three capsules of concentrated fucoxanthin, and 1 to 3 teaspoons (or three to nine capsules) of a high omega-3 cod liver oil complex. (See the PWC Resource Guide on page 322 for recommended products.)

Before bed

Think for your perfect weight: Perform the Healing Codes Exercise on page 189.

Drink for your perfect weight: 8–12 ounces of water (optional, of course)

Get FIT for your perfect weight: Perform five minutes of deep-breathing exercises by taking a slow, five-second breath in through your nose (inhale), holding for one second, followed by a forceful quick exhale through your mouth, completely emptying your lungs with each exhalation and completely filling your lungs with each inhalation. Repeat for two to five minutes.

Sleep for your perfect weight: Go to bed by 10:30 p.m.

Day 2

Upon waking

Drink for your perfect weight: 16–24 ounces of water

Think for your perfect weight: Spend some time this morning picturing yourself at your perfect weight. See yourself doing the things you think you can't do now or don't do because you're not at your perfect weight. Picture yourself looking great, free from all of the diseases that people said you're at a high risk for. Next, picture yourself at your perfect weight, inspiring your family and friends, who remark how great you look. Now stand in front of the mirror and repeat:

> *Today I am going to take another positive step toward achieving my perfect weight.*

Then perform the Healing Codes Exercise, which is on page 189. I recommend that you perform the Healing Codes Exercise at least twice a day—once in the morning and once in the evening—but feel free to try this two-minute exercise three, four, or five times a day.

Get FIT for your perfect weight: Perform FIT exercises for twenty minutes, choosing from physical activities like sprinting, bodyweight exercises, strength training with bands, medicine balls, dumbbells or kettlebells, stationary bike, or the stair stepper. (Video examples of these exercises can be found at www.PerfectWeightCanada.com.)

Breakfast (approximately 7:30 a.m.)

Drink for your perfect weight: 8–12 ounces of water

Two eggs any style, cooked in extra-virgin coconut oil (see the PWC Resource Guide on page 322 for recommended products)

Stir-fried onions, mushrooms, and peppers

One grapefruit

Supplement for your perfect weight: Take two or three whole-food multivitamin caplets and one to four capsules of concentrated fucoxanthin.

Perfect Snack (approximately 10:00 a.m.)

Drink for your perfect weight: 8–12 ounces of water

One Perfect Weight America Peanut Butter fücoProtein whole-food nutrition bar (see the PWC Resource Guide on page 322 for recommended products)

or

One serving of Perfect Meal chocolate-flavoured meal supplement with native whey protein and glucomannan fibre mixed with 12 ounces of water

Lunch (approximately 12:30 p.m.)

Drink for your perfect weight: 12–16 ounces of water

Toss a large green salad with mixed greens, avocado, carrots, cucumbers, celery, tomatoes, red cabbage, red peppers, red onions, sprouts, 2 ounces of canned beans (black, garbanzo, and pinto), and 3 ounces of cold, poached, or canned wild salmon.

For the salad dressing, mix extra-virgin olive oil, apple-cider vinegar or lemon juice, naturally brewed soy sauce, liquid aminos, Celtic Sea Salt, herbs, and spices, or mix 1 tablespoon of extra-virgin olive oil with 1 tablespoon of a healthy store-bought dressing.

Supplement for your perfect weight: Take two or three whole-food multivitamin caplets and one to three capsules of concentrated fucoxanthin.

Perfect Snack (approximately 3:30 p.m.)

Drink for your perfect weight: 8–12 ounces of water

One Perfect Weight America Chocolate MacNut Crunch fücoProtein whole-food nutrition bar

or

One serving of Perfect Meal vanilla-flavoured meal supplement with native whey protein and glucomannan fibre mixed with 12 ounces of water

Dinner (approximately 6:15 p.m., but try to finish eating dinner by 7:00 p.m.)

Drink for your perfect weight: 12–16 ounces of water

Roasted organic chicken

Cooked vegetables (carrots, onions, peas, etc.)

Toss a green salad with mixed greens, avocado, carrots, cucumbers, celery, tomatoes, red cabbage, red peppers, red onions, and sprouts.

For the salad dressing, mix extra-virgin olive oil, apple-cider vinegar or lemon juice, naturally brewed soy sauce, liquid aminos, Celtic Sea Salt, herbs, and spices, or mix 1 tablespoon of extra-virgin olive oil with 1 tablespoon of a healthy store-bought dressing.

Supplement for your perfect weight: Take two or three whole-food multivitamin caplets, one to three capsules of concentrated fucoxanthin, and 1 to 3 teaspoons (or three to nine capsules) of a high omega-3 cod liver oil complex.

Before bed

Think for your perfect weight: Perform the Healing Codes Exercise on page 189.

Drink for your perfect weight: 8–12 ounces of water (optional, of course)

Get FIT for your perfect weight: Perform five minutes of deep-breathing exercises by taking a slow, five-second breath in through your nose (inhale), holding for one second, followed by a forceful quick exhale through your mouth, completely emptying your lungs with each exhalation and completely filling your lungs with each inhalation. Repeat for two to five minutes.

Sleep for your perfect weight: Go to bed by 10:30 p.m.

Day 3

Upon waking

Drink for your perfect weight: 16–24 ounces of water

Think for your perfect weight: Spend some time this morning picturing yourself at your perfect weight. See yourself doing the things you think you can't do now or don't do because you're not at your perfect weight. Picture yourself looking great, free from all of the diseases that people said you're at a high risk for. Next, picture yourself at your perfect weight, inspiring your family and friends, who remark how great you look. Now stand in front of the mirror and repeat:

> *Today I am going to take another positive step toward achieving my perfect weight.*

Then perform the Healing Codes Exercise. You can find out what the Healing Codes Exercise is by turning to page 189. I recommend that you perform the Healing Codes Exercise at least twice a day—once in the morning and once in the evening—but feel free to try this two-minute exercise three, four, or five times a day.

Get FIT for your perfect weight: Perform FIT exercises for twenty minutes, choosing from physical activities like sprinting, bodyweight exercises, strength training with bands, medicine balls, dumbbells or kettlebells, stationary bike, or the stair stepper. (Video examples of these exercises can be found at www.PerfectWeightCanada.com.)

Breakfast (approximately 7:30 a.m.)

Drink for your perfect weight: 8–12 ounces of water

6 ounces of organic whole-milk yogurt or cottage cheese with fruit (pineapple, peaches, or berries), honey, and a dash of vanilla extract

Handful of raw almonds

Supplement for your perfect weight: Take two or three whole-food multivitamin caplets and one to four capsules of concentrated fucoxanthin.

Perfect Snack (approximately 10:00 a.m.)

Drink for your perfect weight: 8–12 ounces of water

One Perfect Weight America Peanut Butter fücoProtein whole-food nutrition bar (see the PWC Resource Guide on page 322 for recommended products)

or

One serving of Perfect Meal chocolate-flavoured meal supplement with native whey protein and glucomannan fibre mixed with 12 ounces of water

Lunch (approximately 12:30 p.m.)

Drink for your perfect weight: 12–16 ounces of water

Toss a large green salad with mixed greens, avocado, carrots, cucumbers, celery, tomatoes, red cabbage, red peppers, red onions, sprouts, 2 ounces of canned beans (black, garbanzo, and pinto), and 2 ounces of low-mercury, high-omega-3 canned tuna. (See the PWC Resource Guide on page 322 for recommended products.)

For the salad dressing, mix extra-virgin olive oil, apple-cider vinegar or lemon juice, naturally brewed soy sauce, liquid aminos, Celtic Sea Salt, herbs, and spices, or mix 1 tablespoon of extra-virgin olive oil with 1 tablespoon of a healthy store-bought dressing.

One piece of fruit in season

Supplement for your perfect weight: Take two or three whole-food multivitamin caplets and one to three capsules of concentrated fucoxanthin.

Perfect Snack (approximately 3:30 p.m.)

Drink for your perfect weight: 8–12 ounces of water

One Perfect Weight America Chocolate MacNut Crunch fücoProtein whole-food nutrition bar

or

One serving of Perfect Meal vanilla-flavoured meal supplement with native whey protein and glucomannan fibre mixed with 12 ounces of water

Dinner (approximately 6:15 p.m., but try to finish eating dinner by 7:00 p.m.)

Drink for your perfect weight: 12–16 ounces of water

Red meat steak or ground meat (beef, buffalo, or venison)

Steamed broccoli

Baked winter squash with butter

Toss a green salad with mixed greens, avocado, carrots, cucumbers, celery, tomatoes, red cabbage, red peppers, red onions, and sprouts.

For the salad dressing, mix extra-virgin olive oil, apple-cider vinegar or lemon juice, naturally brewed soy sauce, liquid aminos, Celtic Sea Salt, herbs, and spices, or mix 1 tablespoon of extra-virgin olive oil with 1 tablespoon of a healthy store-bought dressing.

Supplement for your perfect weight: Take two or three whole-food multivitamin caplets, one to three capsules of concentrated fucoxanthin, and 1 to 3 teaspoons (or three to nine capsules) of a high omega-3 cod liver oil complex.

Before bed

Think for your perfect weight: Perform the Healing Codes Exercise on page 189.

Drink for your perfect weight: 8–12 ounces of water (optional, of course)

Get FIT for your perfect weight: Perform five minutes of deep-breathing exercises by taking a slow, five-second breath in through your nose (inhale), holding for one second, followed by a forceful quick exhale through your mouth, completely emptying your lungs with each exhalation and completely filling your lungs with each inhalation. Repeat for two to five minutes.

Sleep for your perfect weight: Go to bed by 10:30 p.m.

Female Meat Type
Phase II (Weeks 5–8)

Day 1

Upon waking

Drink for your perfect weight: 16–24 ounces of water

Think for your perfect weight: Spend some time this morning picturing yourself at your perfect weight. See yourself doing the things you think you can't do now or don't do because you're not at your perfect weight. Picture yourself looking great, free from all of the diseases that people said you're at a high risk for. Next, picture yourself at your perfect weight, inspiring your family and friends, who remark how great you look. Now stand in front of the mirror and repeat:

> *Today I am going to take another positive step toward achieving my perfect weight.*

Then perform the Healing Codes Exercise. You can find out what the Healing Codes Exercise is by turning to page 189. I recommend that you perform the Healing Codes Exercise at least twice a day—once in the morning and once in the evening—but feel free to try this two-minute exercise three, four, or five times a day.

Get FIT for your perfect weight: Perform FIT exercises for twenty minutes, choosing

from physical activities like sprinting, bodyweight exercises, strength training with bands, medicine balls, dumbbells or kettlebells, stationary bike, or the stair stepper. (Video examples of these exercises can be found at www.PerfectWeightCanada.com.)

Breakfast (approximately 7:30 a.m.)

Drink for your perfect weight: 8–12 ounces of water

4–6 ounces of yogurt or cottage cheese with raw honey, berries, sliced almonds, 1 teaspoon of flax oil (optional), and a dash of vanilla extract

Supplement for your perfect weight: Take two or three whole-food multivitamin caplets and one to four capsules of concentrated fucoxanthin. (See the PWC Resource Guide on page 322 for recommended products.)

Perfect Snack (approximately 10:00 a.m.)

Drink for your perfect weight: 8–12 ounces of water

One Perfect Weight America Peanut Butter fücoProtein whole-food nutrition bar (see the PWC Resource Guide on page 322 for recommended products)

or

One serving of Perfect Meal chocolate-flavoured meal supplement with native whey protein and glucomannan fibre mixed with 12 ounces of water

Lunch (approximately 12:30 p.m.)

Drink for your perfect weight: 12–16 ounces of water

Toss a large green salad with mixed greens, avocado, carrots, cucumbers, celery, tomatoes, red cabbage, red peppers, red onions, sprouts, 2 ounces of canned beans (black, garbanzo, and pinto), and two hard-boiled omega-3 eggs.

For the salad dressing, mix extra-virgin olive oil, apple-cider vinegar or lemon juice, naturally brewed soy sauce, liquid aminos, Celtic Sea Salt, herbs, and spices, or use a healthy store-bought dressing. (See the PWC Resource Guide for recommended brands.)

Supplement for your perfect weight: Take two or three whole-food multivitamin caplets and one to three capsules of concentrated fucoxanthin.

Perfect Snack (approximately 3:30 p.m.)

Drink for your perfect weight: 8–12 ounces of water

One Perfect Weight America Chocolate MacNut Crunch fücoProtein whole-food nutrition bar

or

One serving of Perfect Meal vanilla-flavoured meal supplement with native whey protein and glucomannan fibre mixed with 12 ounces of water

Dinner (approximately 6:15 p.m., but try to finish eating dinner by 7:00 p.m.)

Drink for your perfect weight: 12–16 ounces of water

4–6 oz. ground meat burger (beef, buffalo, venison)

Sautéed mushrooms and onions

Toss a green salad with mixed greens, avocado, carrots, cucumbers, celery, tomatoes, red cabbage, red peppers, red onions, and sprouts.

For the salad dressing, mix extra-virgin olive oil, apple-cider vinegar or lemon juice, naturally brewed soy sauce, liquid aminos, Celtic Sea Salt, herbs, and spices, or mix 1 tablespoon of extra-virgin olive oil with 1 tablespoon of a healthy store-bought dressing.

Supplement for your perfect weight: Take two or three whole-food multivitamin caplets, one to three capsules of concentrated fucoxanthin, and 1 to 3 teaspoons (or three to nine capsules) of a high omega-3 cod liver oil complex. (See the PWC Resource Guide on page 322 for recommended products.)

Before bed

Think for your perfect weight: Perform the Healing Codes Exercise on page 189.

Drink for your perfect weight: 8–12 ounces of water (optional, of course)

Get FIT for your perfect weight: Perform five minutes of deep-breathing exercises by taking a slow, five-second breath in through your nose (inhale), holding for one second, followed by a forceful quick exhale through your mouth, completely emptying your lungs with each exhalation and completely filling your lungs with each inhalation. Repeat for two to five minutes.

Sleep for your perfect weight: Go to bed by 10:30 p.m.

Day 2

Upon waking

Drink for your perfect weight: 16–24 ounces of water

Think for your perfect weight: Spend some time this morning picturing yourself at your perfect weight. See yourself doing the things you think you can't do now or don't do because you're not at your perfect weight. Picture yourself looking great, free from all of the diseases that people said you're at a high risk for. Next, picture yourself at your perfect weight, inspiring your family and friends, who remark how great you look. Now stand in front of the mirror and repeat:

> *Today I am going to take another positive step toward achieving my perfect weight.*

Then perform the Healing Codes Exercise. You can find out what the Healing Codes Exercise is by turning to page 189. I recommend that you perform the Healing Codes Exercise at least twice a day—once in the morning and once in the evening—but feel free to try this two-minute exercise three, four, or five times a day.

Get FIT for your perfect weight: Perform FIT exercises for twenty minutes, choosing from physical activities like sprinting, bodyweight exercises, strength training with bands, medicine balls, dumbbells or kettlebells, stationary bike, or the stair stepper. (Video examples of these exercises can be found at www.PerfectWeightCanada.com.)

Breakfast (approximately 7:30 a.m.)

Drink for your perfect weight: 8–12 ounces of water

Two or three eggs any style, cooked in extra-virgin coconut oil (see the PWC Resource Guide on page 322 for recommended products)

One orange

Supplement for your perfect weight: Take two or three whole-food multivitamin caplets and one to four capsules of concentrated fucoxanthin.

Perfect Snack (approximately 10:00 a.m.)

Drink for your perfect weight: 8–12 ounces of water

One Perfect Weight America Peanut Butter fücoProtein whole-food nutrition bar (see the PWC Resource Guide on page 322 for recommended products)

or

One serving of Perfect Meal chocolate-flavoured meal supplement with native whey protein and glucomannan fibre mixed with 12 ounces of water

Lunch (approximately 12:30 p.m.)

Drink for your perfect weight: 12–16 ounces of water

Toss a large green salad with mixed greens, avocado, carrots, cucumbers, celery, tomatoes, red cabbage, red peppers, red onions, sprouts, 2 ounces of canned beans (black, garbanzo, and pinto), and 3 ounces of cold, poached, or canned wild salmon.

For the salad dressing, mix extra-virgin olive oil, apple-cider vinegar or lemon juice, naturally brewed soy sauce, liquid aminos, Celtic Sea Salt, herbs, and spices, or mix 1 tablespoon of extra-virgin olive oil with 1 tablespoon of a healthy store-bought dressing.

Supplement for your perfect weight: Take two or three whole-food multivitamin caplets and one to three capsules of concentrated fucoxanthin.

Perfect Snack (approximately 3:30 p.m.)

Drink for your perfect weight: 8–12 ounces of water

One Perfect Weight America Chocolate MacNut Crunch fücoProtein whole-food nutrition bar

or

One serving of Perfect Meal vanilla-flavoured meal supplement with native whey protein and glucomannan fibre mixed with 12 ounces of water

Dinner (approximately 6:15 p.m., but try to finish eating dinner by 7:00 p.m.)

Drink for your perfect weight: 12–16 ounces of water

Grilled chicken breast

Grilled peppers, onions, and pineapple

Toss a green salad with mixed greens, avocado, carrots, cucumbers, celery, tomatoes, red cabbage, red peppers, red onions, and sprouts.

For the salad dressing, mix extra-virgin olive oil, apple-cider vinegar or lemon juice, naturally brewed soy sauce, liquid aminos, Celtic Sea Salt, herbs, and spices, or mix 1 tablespoon of extra-virgin olive oil with 1 tablespoon of a healthy store-bought dressing.

Supplement for your perfect weight: Take two or three whole-food multivitamin caplets, one to three capsules of concentrated fucoxanthin, and 1 to 3 teaspoons (or three to nine capsules) of a high omega-3 cod liver oil complex.

Before bed

Think for your perfect weight: Perform the Healing Codes Exercise on page 189.

Drink for your perfect weight: 8–12 ounces of water (optional, of course)

Get FIT for your perfect weight: Perform five minutes of deep-breathing exercises by taking a slow, five-second breath in through your nose (inhale), holding for one second, followed by a forceful quick exhale through your mouth, completely emptying your lungs with each exhalation and completely filling your lungs with each inhalation. Repeat for two to five minutes.

Sleep for your perfect weight: Go to bed by 10:30 p.m.

Day 3

Upon waking

Drink for your perfect weight: 16–24 ounces of water

Think for your perfect weight: Spend some time this morning picturing yourself at your perfect weight. See yourself doing the things you think you can't do now or don't do because you're not at your perfect weight. Picture yourself looking great, free from all of the diseases that people said you're at a high risk for. Next, picture yourself at your perfect weight, inspiring your family and friends, who remark how great you look. Now stand in front of the mirror and repeat:

> *Today I am going to take another positive step toward achieving my perfect weight.*

Then perform the Healing Codes Exercise. You can find out what the Healing Codes Exercise is by turning to page 189. I recommend that you perform the Healing Codes Exercise at least twice a day—once in the morning and once in the evening—but feel free to try this two-minute exercise three, four, or five times a day.

Get FIT for your perfect weight: Perform FIT exercises for twenty minutes, choosing from physical activities like sprinting, bodyweight exercises, strength training with bands, medicine balls, dumbbells or kettlebells, stationary bike, or the stair stepper. (Video examples of these exercises can be found at www.PerfectWeightCanada.com.)

Breakfast (approximately 7:30 a.m.)

Drink for your perfect weight: 8–12 ounces of water

6 ounces of organic whole-milk yogurt or cottage cheese with fruit (pineapple, peaches, or berries), honey, and a dash of vanilla extract

Handful of raw almonds

Supplement for your perfect weight: Take two or three whole-food multivitamin caplets and one to four capsules of concentrated fucoxanthin.

Perfect Snack (approximately 10:00 a.m.)

Drink for your perfect weight: 8–12 ounces of water

One Perfect Weight America Peanut Butter fücoProtein whole-food nutrition bar (see the PWC Resource Guide on page 322 for recommended products)

or

One serving of Perfect Meal chocolate-flavoured meal supplement with native whey protein and glucomannan fibre mixed with 12 ounces of water

Lunch (approximately 12:30 p.m.)

Drink for your perfect weight: 12–16 ounces of water

Toss a large green salad with mixed greens, avocado, carrots, cucumbers, celery, tomatoes, red cabbage, red peppers, red onions, sprouts, 2 ounces of canned beans (black, garbanzo, and pinto), and 2 ounces of low-mercury, high-omega-3 canned tuna. (See the PWC Resource Guide on page 322 for recommended products.)

For the salad dressing, mix extra-virgin olive oil, apple-cider vinegar or lemon juice, naturally brewed soy sauce, liquid aminos, Celtic Sea Salt, herbs, and spices, or mix 1 tablespoon of extra-virgin olive oil with 1 tablespoon of a healthy store-bought dressing.

One piece of fruit in season

Supplement for your perfect weight: Take two or three whole-food multivitamin caplets and one to three capsules of concentrated fucoxanthin.

Perfect Snack (approximately 3:30 p.m.)

Drink for your perfect weight: 8-12 ounces of water

One Perfect Weight America Chocolate MacNut Crunch fücoProtein whole-food nutrition bar

or

One serving of Perfect Meal vanilla-flavoured meal supplement with native whey protein and glucomannan fibre mixed with 12 ounces of water

Dinner (approximately 6:15 p.m., but try to finish eating dinner by 7:00 p.m.)

Drink for your perfect weight: 12–16 ounces of water

Red meat steak or ground meat (beef, buffalo, or venison)

Sautéed spinach

Baked sweet potato with butter

Toss a green salad with mixed greens, avocado, carrots, cucumbers, celery, tomatoes, red cabbage, red peppers, red onions, and sprouts.

For the salad dressing, mix extra-virgin olive oil, apple-cider vinegar or lemon juice, naturally brewed soy sauce, liquid aminos, Celtic Sea Salt, herbs, and spices, or mix 1 tablespoon of extra-virgin olive oil with 1 tablespoon of a healthy store-bought dressing.

Supplement for your perfect weight: Take two or three whole-food multivitamin caplets, one to three capsules of concentrated fucoxanthin, and 1 to 3 teaspoons (or three to nine capsules) of a high omega-3 cod liver oil complex.

Before bed

Think for your perfect weight: Perform the Healing Codes Exercise on page 189.

Drink for your perfect weight: 8–12 ounces of water (optional, of course)

Get FIT for your perfect weight: Perform five minutes of deep-breathing exercises by taking a slow, five-second breath in through your nose (inhale), holding for one second, followed by a forceful quick exhale through your mouth, completely emptying your lungs with each exhalation and completely filling your lungs with each inhalation. Repeat for two to five minutes.

Sleep for your perfect weight: Go to bed by 10:30 p.m.

Female Meat Type
Phase III (Weeks 9–12)

Day 1

Upon waking

Drink for your perfect weight: 16–24 ounces of water

Think for your perfect weight: Spend some time this morning picturing yourself at your perfect weight. See yourself doing the things you think you can't do now or don't do because you're not at your perfect weight. Picture yourself looking great, free from all of the diseases that people said you're at a high risk for. Next, picture yourself at your perfect weight, inspiring your family and friends, who remark how great you look. Now stand in front of the mirror and repeat:

> *Today I am going to take another positive step toward achieving my perfect weight.*

Then perform the Healing Codes Exercise. You can find out what the Healing Codes Exercise is by turning to page 189. I recommend that you perform the Healing Codes Exercise at least twice a day—once in the morning and once in the evening—but feel free to try this two-minute exercise three, four, or five times a day.

Get FIT for your perfect weight: Perform FIT exercises for twenty minutes, choosing from physical activities like sprinting, bodyweight exercises, strength training with bands, medicine balls, dumbbells or kettlebells, stationary bike, or the stair stepper. (Video examples of these exercises can be found at www.PerfectWeightCanada.com.)

Breakfast (approximately 7:30 a.m.)

Drink for your perfect weight: 8–12 ounces of water

Make a smoothie in a blender with the following ingredients:

- 1 cup plain whole milk yogurt or kefir
- 1 tsp. organic flaxseed oil
- 1 tsp. organic extra-virgin coconut oil
- 1 Tbsp. organic raw honey
- 1 cup organic fruit, fresh or frozen (berries, banana, peaches, pineapple, etc.)
- 2 scoops goat's milk protein powder (see the PWC Resource Guide on page 322 for recommendations)
- Dash of vanilla extract (optional)

Supplement for your perfect weight: Take two or three whole-food multivitamin caplets and one to four capsules of concentrated fucoxanthin. (See the PWC Resource Guide on page 322 for recommended products.)

Perfect Snack (approximately 10:00 a.m.)

Drink for your perfect weight: 8–12 ounces of water

One Perfect Weight America Peanut Butter fücoProtein whole-food nutrition bar (see the PWC Resource Guide on page 322 for recommended products)

or

One serving of Perfect Meal chocolate-flavoured meal supplement with native whey protein and glucomannan fibre mixed with 12 ounces of water

Lunch (approximately 12:30 p.m.)

Drink for your perfect weight: 12–16 ounces of water

Toss a large green salad with mixed greens, avocado, carrots, cucumbers, celery, tomatoes, red cabbage, red peppers, red onions, sprouts, 2 ounces of canned beans (black, garbanzo, and pinto), and two hard-boiled omega-3 eggs.

For the salad dressing, mix extra-virgin olive oil, apple-cider vinegar or lemon juice, naturally brewed soy sauce, liquid aminos, Celtic Sea Salt, herbs, and spices, or use a healthy store-bought dressing. (See the PWC Resource Guide for recommended brands.)

Supplement for your perfect weight: Take two or three whole-food multivitamin caplets and one to three capsules of concentrated fucoxanthin.

Perfect Snack (approximately 3:30 p.m.)

Drink for your perfect weight: 8–12 ounces of water

One Perfect Weight America Chocolate MacNut Crunch fücoProtein whole-food nutrition bar

or

One serving of Perfect Meal vanilla-flavoured meal supplement with native whey protein and glucomannan fibre mixed with 12 ounces of water

Dinner (approximately 6:15 p.m., but try to finish eating dinner by 7:00 p.m.)

Drink for your perfect weight: 12–16 ounces of water

Meatloaf

Roasted veggies (peas, carrots, and potatoes)

Toss a green salad with mixed greens, avocado, carrots, cucumbers, celery, tomatoes, red cabbage, red peppers, red onions, and sprouts.

For the salad dressing, mix extra-virgin olive oil, apple-cider vinegar or lemon juice, naturally brewed soy sauce, liquid aminos, Celtic Sea Salt, herbs, and spices, or use a healthy store-bought dressing.

Supplement for your perfect weight: Take two or three whole-food multivitamin caplets, one to three capsules of concentrated fucoxanthin, and 1 to 3 teaspoons (or three to nine capsules) of a high omega-3 cod liver oil complex. (See the PWC Resource Guide on page 322 for recommended products.)

Before bed

Think for your perfect weight: Perform the Healing Codes Exercise on page 189.

Drink for your perfect weight: 8–12 ounces of water (optional, of course)

Get FIT for your perfect weight: Perform five minutes of deep-breathing exercises by taking a slow, five-second breath in through your nose (inhale), holding for one second, followed by a forceful quick exhale through your mouth, completely emptying your lungs with each exhalation and completely filling your lungs with each inhalation. Repeat for two to five minutes.

Sleep for your perfect weight: Go to bed by 10:30 p.m.

Day 2

Upon waking

Drink for your perfect weight: 16–24 ounces of water

Think for your perfect weight: Spend some time this morning picturing yourself at your perfect weight. See yourself doing the things you think you can't do now or don't do because you're not at your perfect weight. Picture yourself looking great, free from all of the diseases that people said you're at a high risk for. Next, picture yourself at your perfect weight, inspiring your family and friends, who remark how great you look. Now stand in front of the mirror and repeat:

> *Today I am going to take another positive step toward achieving my perfect weight.*

Then perform the Healing Codes Exercise. You can find out what the Healing Codes Exercise is by turning to page 189. I recommend that you perform the Healing Codes Exercise at least twice a day—once in the morning and once in the evening—but feel free to try this two-minute exercise three, four, or five times a day.

Get FIT for your perfect weight: Perform FIT exercises for twenty minutes, choosing from physical activities like sprinting, bodyweight exercises, strength training with bands, medicine balls, dumbbells or kettlebells, stationary bike, or the stair stepper. (Video examples of these exercises can be found at www.PerfectWeightCanada.com.)

Breakfast (approximately 7:30 a.m.)

Drink for your perfect weight: 8–12 ounces of water

Egg and cheese omelette, cooked in extra-virgin coconut oil

One piece of sprouted or yeast-free toast with butter and 1 ounce of raw cheese

Supplement for your perfect weight: Take two or three whole-food multivitamin caplets and one to four capsules of concentrated fucoxanthin.

Perfect Snack (approximately 10:00 a.m.)

Drink for your perfect weight: 8–12 ounces of water

One Perfect Weight America Peanut Butter fücoProtein whole-food nutrition bar (see the PWC Resource Guide on page 322 for recommended products)

or

One serving of Perfect Meal chocolate-flavoured meal supplement with native whey protein and glucomannan fibre mixed with 12 ounces of water

Lunch (approximately 12:30 p.m.)

Drink for your perfect weight: 12–16 ounces of water

Toss a large green salad with mixed greens, avocado, carrots, cucumbers, celery, tomatoes, red cabbage, red peppers, red onions, sprouts, 2 ounces of canned beans (black, garbanzo, and pinto), and 3 ounces of cold, poached, or canned wild salmon.

For the salad dressing, mix extra-virgin olive oil, apple-cider vinegar or lemon juice, naturally brewed soy sauce, liquid aminos, Celtic Sea Salt, herbs, and spices, or mix 1 tablespoon of extra-virgin olive oil with 1 tablespoon of a healthy store-bought dressing.

Supplement for your perfect weight: Take two or three whole-food multivitamin caplets and one to three capsules of concentrated fucoxanthin.

Perfect Snack (approximately 3:30 p.m.)

Drink for your perfect weight: 8–12 ounces of water

One Perfect Weight America Chocolate MacNut Crunch fücoProtein whole-food nutrition bar

or

One serving of Perfect Meal vanilla-flavoured meal supplement with native whey protein and glucomannan fibre mixed with 12 ounces of water

Dinner (approximately 6:15 p.m., but try to finish eating dinner by 7:00 p.m.)

Drink for your perfect weight: 12–16 ounces of water

Broiled or sautéed white fish

Cooked vegetables (carrots, onions, peas, etc.)

Small serving of whole grain (brown rice, quinoa, millet, amaranth, buckwheat)

Supplement for your perfect weight: Take two or three whole-food multivitamin caplets, one to three capsules of concentrated fucoxanthin, and 1 to 3 teaspoons (or three to nine capsules) of a high omega-3 cod liver oil complex.

Before bed

Think for your perfect weight: Perform the Healing Codes Exercise on page 189.

Drink for your perfect weight: 8–12 ounces of water (optional, of course)

Get FIT for your perfect weight: Perform five minutes of deep-breathing exercises by taking a slow, five-second breath in through your nose (inhale), holding for one second, followed by a forceful quick exhale through your mouth, completely emptying your lungs with each exhalation and completely filling your lungs with each inhalation. Repeat for two to five minutes.

Sleep for your perfect weight: Go to bed by 10:30 p.m.

Day 3

Upon waking

Drink for your perfect weight: 16–24 ounces of water

Think for your perfect weight: Spend some time this morning picturing yourself at your perfect weight. See yourself doing the things you think you can't do now or don't do because you're not at your perfect weight. Picture yourself looking great, free from all of the diseases that people said you're at a high risk for. Next, picture yourself at your perfect weight, inspiring your family and friends, who remark how great you look. Now stand in front of the mirror and repeat:

> *Today I am going to take another positive step toward achieving my perfect weight.*

Then perform the Healing Codes Exercise. You can find out what the Healing Codes Exercise is by turning to page 189. I recommend that you perform the Healing Codes Exercise at least twice a day—once in the morning and once in the evening—but feel free to try this two-minute exercise three, four, or five times a day.

Get FIT for your perfect weight: Perform FIT exercises for twenty minutes, choosing from physical activities like sprinting, bodyweight exercises, strength training with bands, medicine balls, dumbbells or kettlebells, stationary bike, or the stair stepper. (Video examples of these exercises can be found at www.PerfectWeightCanada.com.)

Breakfast (approximately 7:30 a.m.)

Drink for your perfect weight: 8–12 ounces of water

6 ounces of organic whole-milk cottage cheese with fruit (pineapple, peaches, or berries), honey, and a dash of vanilla extract

Supplement for your perfect weight: Take two or three whole-food multivitamin caplets and one to four capsules of concentrated fucoxanthin.

Perfect Snack (approximately 10:00 a.m.)

Drink for your perfect weight: 8–12 ounces of water

One Perfect Weight America Peanut Butter fücoProtein whole-food nutrition bar (see the PWC Resource Guide on page 322 for recommended products)

or

One serving of Perfect Meal chocolate-flavoured meal supplement with native whey protein and glucomannan fibre mixed with 12 ounces of water

Lunch (approximately 12:30 p.m.)

Drink for your perfect weight: 12–16 ounces of water

Toss a large green salad with mixed greens, avocado, carrots, cucumbers, celery, tomatoes, red cabbage, red peppers, red onions, sprouts, 2 ounces of canned beans (black, garbanzo, and pinto), and 2 ounces of low-mercury, high-omega-3 canned tuna. (See the PWC Resource Guide on page 322 for recommended products.)

For the salad dressing, mix extra-virgin olive oil, apple-cider vinegar or lemon juice, naturally brewed soy sauce, liquid aminos, Celtic Sea Salt, herbs, and spices, or mix 1 tablespoon of extra-virgin olive oil with 1 tablespoon of a healthy store-bought dressing.

One piece of fruit in season

Supplement for your perfect weight: Take two or three whole-food multivitamin caplets and one to three capsules of concentrated fucoxanthin.

Perfect Snack (approximately 3:30 p.m.)

Drink for your perfect weight: 8–12 ounces of water

One Perfect Weight America Chocolate MacNut Crunch fücoProtein whole-food nutrition bar

or

One serving of Perfect Meal vanilla-flavoured meal supplement with native whey protein and glucomannan fibre mixed with 12 ounces of water

Dinner (approximately 6:15 p.m., but try to finish eating dinner by 7:00 p.m.)

Drink for your perfect weight: 12–16 ounces of water

Red meat and bean chili

Flax crackers, whole-grain crackers, or baked corn chips

Toss a green salad with mixed greens, avocado, carrots, cucumbers, celery, tomatoes, red cabbage, red peppers, red onions, and sprouts.

For the salad dressing, mix extra-virgin olive oil, apple-cider vinegar or lemon juice, naturally brewed soy sauce, liquid aminos, Celtic Sea Salt, herbs, and spices, or mix 1 tablespoon of extra-virgin olive oil with 1 tablespoon of a healthy store-bought dressing.

Supplement for your perfect weight: Take two or three whole-food multivitamin caplets, one to three capsules of concentrated fucoxanthin, and 1 to 3 teaspoons (or three to nine capsules) of a high omega-3 cod liver oil complex.

Before bed

Think for your perfect weight: Perform the Healing Codes Exercise on page 189.

Drink for your perfect weight: 8–12 ounces of water (optional, of course)

Get FIT for your perfect weight: Perform five minutes of deep-breathing exercises by taking a slow, five-second breath in through your nose (inhale), holding for one second, followed by a forceful quick exhale through your mouth, completely emptying your lungs with each exhalation and completely filling your lungs with each inhalation. Repeat for two to five minutes.

Sleep for your perfect weight: Go to bed by 10:30 p.m.

Female Meat Type
Phase IV (Weeks 13–16)

For Phase IV, you have some options. If you are satisfied with your progress, you should continue on the Phase III plan and finish strong. If you feel that your weight loss has slowed or you liked the way you felt on Phase I or II, you are welcome to repeat one of those phases for the final four weeks.

Female Potato Type
Phase I (Weeks 1–4)

Day 1

Upon waking

Drink for your perfect weight: 16–24 ounces of water

Think for your perfect weight: Spend some time this morning picturing yourself at your perfect weight. See yourself doing the things you think you can't do now or don't do because you're not at your perfect weight. Picture yourself looking great, free from all of the diseases that people said you're at a high risk for. Next, picture yourself at your perfect weight, inspiring your family and friends, who remark how great you look. Now stand in front of the mirror and repeat:

> *Today I am going to take another positive step toward achieving my perfect weight.*

Then perform the Healing Codes Exercise. You can find out what the Healing Codes Exercise is by turning to page 189. I recommend that you perform the Healing Codes Exercise at least twice a day—once in the morning and once in the evening—but feel free to try this two-minute exercise three, four, or five times a day.

Get FIT for your perfect weight: Perform FIT exercises for twenty minutes, choosing from physical activities like sprinting, bodyweight exercises, strength training with bands, medicine balls, dumbbells or kettlebells, stationary bike, or the stair stepper. (Video examples of these exercises can be found at www.PerfectWeightCanada.com.)

Breakfast (approximately 7:30 a.m.)

Drink for your perfect weight: 8–12 ounces of water

Make a smoothie in a blender with the following ingredients:

- 1 cup plain whole-milk yogurt or kefir
- 1 tsp. organic extra-virgin coconut oil
- 2 Tbsp. organic raw honey
- 1 cup organic fruit, fresh or frozen (berries, peaches, pineapple, etc.)
- 1 scoop goat's milk protein powder (see the PWC Resource Guide on page 322 for recommendations)
- Dash of vanilla extract (optional)

Supplement for your perfect weight: Take two or three whole-food multivitamin caplets and one to four capsules of concentrated fucoxanthin. (See the PWC Resource Guide on page 322 for recommended products.)

Perfect Snack (approximately 10:00 a.m.)

Drink for your perfect weight: 8–12 ounces of water

One Garden of Life Fruits of Life organic whole-food nutrition bar (see the PWC Resource Guide on page 322 for recommended products)

or

One serving of Perfect Meal chocolate-flavoured meal supplement with native whey protein and glucomannan fibre mixed with 12 ounces of water

Lunch (approximately 12:30 p.m.)

Drink for your perfect weight: 12–16 ounces of water

Toss a large green salad with mixed greens, avocado, carrots, cucumbers, celery, tomatoes, red cabbage, red peppers, red onions, sprouts, 2 ounces of canned beans (black, garbanzo, and pinto), and two hard-boiled omega-3 eggs.

For the salad dressing, mix extra-virgin olive oil, apple-cider vinegar or lemon juice, naturally brewed soy sauce, liquid aminos, Celtic Sea Salt, herbs, and spices, or use a healthy store-bought dressing.

One apple with skin

Supplement for your perfect weight: Take two or three whole-food multivitamin caplets and one to three capsules of concentrated fucoxanthin.

Perfect Snack (approximately 3:30 p.m.)

Drink for your perfect weight: 8–12 ounces of water

A half-box to one box of Rainforest Cacao Chocolate Macadamia Nuts

or

One serving of Perfect Meal vanilla-flavoured meal supplement with native whey protein and glucomannan fibre mixed with 12 ounces of water

Dinner (approximately 6:15 p.m., but try to finish eating dinner by 7:00 p.m.)

Drink for your perfect weight: 12–16 ounces of water

Baked, poached, or grilled wild-caught salmon

Peas and carrots

Toss a green salad with mixed greens, avocado, carrots, cucumbers, celery, tomatoes, red cabbage, red peppers, red onions, and sprouts.

For the salad dressing, mix extra-virgin olive oil, apple-cider vinegar or lemon juice, naturally brewed soy sauce, liquid aminos, Celtic Sea Salt, herbs, and spices, or use a healthy store-bought dressing.

Supplement for your perfect weight: Take two or three whole-food multivitamin caplets, one to three capsules of concentrated fucoxanthin, and 1 to 3 teaspoons (or three to nine capsules) of a high omega-3 cod liver oil complex.

Before bed

Think for your perfect weight: Perform the Healing Codes Exercise on page 189.

Drink for your perfect weight: 8–12 ounces of water (optional, of course)

Get FIT for your perfect weight: Perform five minutes of deep-breathing exercises by taking a slow, five-second breath in through your nose (inhale), holding for one second, followed by a forceful quick exhale through your mouth, completely emptying your lungs with each exhalation and completely filling your lungs with each inhalation. Repeat for two to five minutes.

Sleep for your perfect weight: Go to bed by 10:30 p.m.

Day 2

Upon waking

Drink for your perfect weight: 16–24 ounces of water

Think for your perfect weight: Spend some time this morning picturing yourself at your perfect weight. See yourself doing the things you think you can't do now or don't do because you're not at your perfect weight. Picture yourself looking great, free from all of the diseases that people said you're at a high risk for. Next, picture yourself at your perfect weight, inspiring your family and friends, who remark how great you look. Now stand in front of the mirror and repeat:

> *Today I am going to take another positive step toward achieving my perfect weight.*

Then perform the Healing Codes Exercise. You can find out what the Healing Codes Exercise is by turning to page 189. I recommend that you perform the Healing Codes Exercise at least twice a day—once in the morning and once in the evening—but feel free to try this two-minute exercise three, four, or five times a day.

Get FIT for your perfect weight: Perform FIT exercises for twenty minutes, choosing from physical activities like sprinting, bodyweight exercises, strength training with bands, medicine balls, dumbbells or kettlebells, stationary bike, or the stair stepper. (Video examples of these exercises can be found at www.PerfectWeightCanada.com.)

Breakfast (approximately 7:30 a.m.)

Drink for your perfect weight: 8–12 ounces of water

Two eggs any style, cooked in extra-virgin coconut oil

Stir-fried onions, mushrooms, and peppers

One serving of grapes

Supplement for your perfect weight: Take two or three whole-food multivitamin caplets and one to four capsules of concentrated fucoxanthin.

Perfect Snack (approximately 10:00 a.m.)

Drink for your perfect weight: 8–12 ounces of water

One Garden of Life Super Seed organic whole-food nutrition bar (see the PWC Resource Guide on page 322 for recommended products)

or

One serving of Perfect Meal chocolate-flavoured meal supplement with native whey protein and glucomannan fibre mixed with 12 ounces of water

Lunch (approximately 12:30 p.m.)

Drink for your perfect weight: 12–16 ounces of water

Toss a large green salad with mixed greens, avocado, carrots, cucumbers, celery, tomatoes, red cabbage, red peppers, red onions, sprouts, 2 ounces of canned beans (black, garbanzo, and pinto), and 2 ounces of cold, poached, or canned wild salmon.

For the salad dressing, mix extra-virgin olive oil, apple-cider vinegar or lemon juice, naturally brewed soy sauce, liquid aminos, Celtic Sea Salt, herbs, and spices, or mix 1 tablespoon of extra-virgin olive oil with 1 tablespoon of a healthy store-bought dressing.

One apple with skin

Supplement for your perfect weight: Take two or three whole-food multivitamin caplets and one to three capsules of concentrated fucoxanthin.

Perfect Snack (approximately 3:30 p.m.)

Drink for your perfect weight: 8–12 ounces of water

A half-box to one box of Rainforest Cacao Chocolate Macadamia Nuts

or

One serving of Perfect Meal vanilla-flavoured meal supplement with native whey protein and glucomannan fibre mixed with 12 ounces of water

Dinner (approximately 6:15 p.m., but try to finish eating dinner by 7:00 p.m.)

Drink for your perfect weight: 12–16 ounces of water

Roasted organic chicken

Cooked vegetable (carrots, onions, peas, etc.)

Toss a green salad with mixed greens, avocado, carrots, cucumbers, celery, tomatoes, red cabbage, red peppers, red onions, and sprouts.

For the salad dressing, mix extra-virgin olive oil, apple-cider vinegar or lemon juice, naturally brewed soy sauce, liquid aminos, Celtic Sea Salt, herbs, and spices, or mix 1 tablespoon of extra-virgin olive oil with 1 tablespoon of a healthy store-bought dressing.

Supplement for your perfect weight: Take two or three whole-food multivitamin caplets and one to three capsules of concentrated fucoxanthin and 1 to 3 teaspoons (or three to nine capsules) of a high omega-3 cod liver oil complex.

Before bed

Think for your perfect weight: Perform the Healing Codes Exercise on page 189.

Drink for your perfect weight: 8–12 ounces of water (optional, of course)

Get FIT for your perfect weight: Perform five minutes of deep-breathing exercises by taking a slow, five-second breath in through your nose (inhale), holding for one second, followed by a forceful quick exhale through your mouth, completely emptying your lungs with each exhalation and completely filling your lungs with each inhalation. Repeat for two to five minutes.

Sleep for your perfect weight: Go to bed by 10:30 p.m.

Day 3

Upon waking

Drink for your perfect weight: 16–24 ounces of water

Think for your perfect weight: Spend some time this morning picturing yourself at your perfect weight. See yourself doing the things you think you can't do now or don't do because you're not at your perfect weight. Picture yourself looking great, free from all of the diseases that people said you're at a high risk for. Next, picture yourself at your perfect weight, inspiring your family and friends, who remark how great you look. Now stand in front of the mirror and repeat:

> *Today I am going to take another positive step toward achieving my perfect weight.*

Then perform the Healing Codes Exercise. You can find out what the Healing Codes Exercise is by turning to page 189. I recommend that you perform the Healing Codes Exercise at least twice a day—once in the morning and once in the evening—but feel free to try this two-minute exercise three, four, or five times a day.

Get FIT for your perfect weight: Perform functional interval training exercises for twenty minutes, choosing from physical activities like sprinting, bodyweight exercises, strength training with bands, medicine balls, dumbbells or kettlebells, stationary bike, or the stair stepper. (Video examples of these exercises can be found at www.PerfectWeightCanada.com.)

Breakfast (approximately 7:30 a.m.)

Drink for your perfect weight: 8–12 ounces of water

4 to 8 ounces of organic whole-milk yogurt with fruit (pineapple, peaches, or berries), honey, and a dash of vanilla extract

Handful of raw almonds

Supplement for your perfect weight: Take two or three whole-food multivitamin caplets and one to four capsules of concentrated fucoxanthin.

Perfect Snack (approximately 10:00 a.m.)

Drink for your perfect weight: 8–12 ounces of water

One Garden of Life Perfect Food Chocolate Greens organic whole-food nutrition bar (see the PWC Resource Guide on page 322 for recommended products)

or

One serving of Perfect Meal chocolate greens-flavoured meal supplement with a green food vegetable blend, native whey protein, and glucomannan fibre mixed with 12 ounces of water

Lunch (approximately 12:30 p.m.)

Drink for your perfect weight: 12–16 ounces of water

Toss a large green salad with mixed greens, avocado, carrots, cucumbers, celery, tomatoes, red cabbage, red peppers, red onions, sprouts, 2 ounces of canned beans (black, garbanzo, and pinto), and 2 ounces of low-mercury, high-omega-3 canned tuna.

For the salad dressing, mix extra-virgin olive oil, apple-cider vinegar or lemon juice, naturally brewed soy sauce, liquid aminos, Celtic Sea Salt, herbs, and spices, or use a healthy store-bought dressing.

One piece of fruit in season

Supplement for your perfect weight: Take two or three whole-food multivitamin caplets and one to three capsules of concentrated fucoxanthin.

Perfect Snack (approximately 3:30 p.m.)

Drink for your perfect weight: 8–12 ounces of water

A half-box to one box of Rainforest Cacao Chocolate Macadamia Nuts

or

One serving of Perfect Meal vanilla-flavoured meal supplement with native whey protein and glucomannan fibre mixed with 12 ounces of water

Dinner (approximately 6:15 p.m., but try to finish eating dinner by 7:00 p.m.)

Drink for your perfect weight: 12–16 ounces of water

Red meat steak (beef, buffalo, or venison)

Steamed broccoli

Toss a green salad with mixed greens, avocado, carrots, cucumbers, celery, tomatoes, red cabbage, red peppers, red onions, and sprouts.

For the salad dressing, mix extra-virgin olive oil, apple-cider vinegar or lemon juice, naturally brewed soy sauce, liquid aminos, Celtic Sea Salt, herbs, and spices, or mix 1 tablespoon of extra-virgin olive oil with 1 tablespoon of a healthy store-bought dressing.

Supplement for your perfect weight: Take two or three whole-food multivitamin caplets, one to three capsules of concentrated fucoxanthin, and 1 to 3 teaspoons (or three to nine capsules) of a high omega-3 cod liver oil complex.

Before bed

Think for your perfect weight: Perform the Healing Codes Exercise on page 189.

Drink for your perfect weight: 8–12 ounces of water (optional, of course)

Get FIT for your perfect weight: Perform five minutes of deep-breathing exercises by taking a slow, five-second breath in through your nose (inhale), holding for one second, followed by a forceful quick exhale through your mouth, completely emptying your lungs with each exhalation and completely filling your lungs with each inhalation. Repeat for two to five minutes.

Sleep for your perfect weight: Go to bed by 10:30 p.m.

Female Potato Type
Phase II (Weeks 5–8)

Day 1

Upon waking

Drink for your perfect weight: 16–24 ounces of water

Think for your perfect weight: Spend some time this morning picturing yourself at your perfect weight. See yourself doing the things you think you can't do now or don't do because you're not at your perfect weight. Picture yourself looking great, free from all of the diseases that people said you're at a high risk for. Next, picture yourself at your perfect weight, inspiring your family and friends, who remark how great you look. Now stand in front of the mirror and repeat:

> *Today I am going to take another positive step toward achieving my perfect weight.*

Then perform the Healing Codes Exercise. You can find out what the Healing Codes Exercise is by turning to page 189. I recommend that you perform the Healing Codes Exercise at least twice a day—once in the morning and once in the evening—but feel free to try this two-minute exercise three, four, or five times a day.

Get FIT for your perfect weight: Perform FIT exercises for twenty minutes, choosing from physical activities like sprinting, bodyweight exercises, strength training with bands, medicine balls, dumbbells or kettlebells, stationary bike, or the stair stepper. (Video examples of these exercises can be found at www.PerfectWeightCanada.com.)

Breakfast (approximately 7:30 a.m.)

Drink for your perfect weight: 8–12 ounces of water

Make a smoothie in a blender with the following ingredients:

- 1 cup plain whole milk yogurt or kefir
- 1 tsp. organic extra-virgin coconut oil
- 2 Tbsp. organic raw honey
- 1 cup organic fruit, fresh or frozen (berries, banana, peaches, pineapple, etc.)

- 1 scoop goat's milk protein powder (see the PWC Resource Guide on page 322 for recommendations)
- Dash of vanilla extract (optional)

Supplement for your perfect weight: Take two or three whole-food multivitamin caplets and one to four capsules of concentrated fucoxanthin. (See the PWC Resource Guide on page 322 for recommended products.)

Perfect Snack (approximately 10:00 a.m.)

Drink for your perfect weight: 8–12 ounces of water

One Garden of Life Fruits of Life organic whole-food nutrition bar (see the PWC Resource Guide on page 322 for recommended products)

or

One serving of Perfect Meal chocolate-flavoured meal supplement with native whey protein and glucomannan fibre mixed with 12 ounces of water

Lunch (approximately 12:30 p.m.)

Drink for your perfect weight: 12–16 ounces of water

Toss a large green salad with mixed greens, avocado, carrots, cucumbers, celery, tomatoes, red cabbage, red peppers, red onions, sprouts, 2 ounces of canned beans (black, garbanzo, and pinto), and two hard-boiled omega-3 eggs.

For the salad dressing, mix extra-virgin olive oil, apple-cider vinegar or lemon juice, naturally brewed soy sauce, liquid aminos, Celtic Sea Salt, herbs, and spices, or use a healthy store-bought dressing.

One piece of fruit

Supplement for your perfect weight: Take two or three whole-food multivitamin caplets and one to three capsules of concentrated fucoxanthin.

Perfect Snack (approximately 3:30 p.m.)

Drink for your perfect weight: 8–12 ounces of water

A half-box to one box of Rainforest Cacao Chocolate Macadamia Nuts

or

One serving of Perfect Meal vanilla-flavoured meal supplement with native whey protein and glucomannan fibre mixed with 12 ounces of water

Dinner (approximately 6:15 p.m., but try to finish eating dinner by 7:00 p.m.)

Drink for your perfect weight: 12–16 ounces of water

Broiled fish

Sautéed spinach

Toss a large green salad with mixed greens, avocado, carrots, cucumbers, celery, tomatoes, red cabbage, red peppers, red onions, and sprouts.

For the salad dressing, mix extra-virgin olive oil, apple-cider vinegar or lemon juice, naturally brewed soy sauce, liquid aminos, Celtic Sea Salt, herbs, and spices, or use a healthy store-bought dressing.

Supplement for your perfect weight: Take two or three whole-food multivitamin

caplets, one to three capsules of concentrated fucoxanthin, and 1 to 3 teaspoons (or three to nine capsules) of a high omega-3 cod liver oil complex. (See the PWC Resource Guide on page 322 for recommended products.)

Before bed

Think for your perfect weight: Perform the Healing Codes Exercise on page 189.

Drink for your perfect weight: 8–12 ounces of water (optional, of course)

Get FIT for your perfect weight: Perform five minutes of deep-breathing exercises by taking a slow, five-second breath in through your nose (inhale), holding for one second, followed by a forceful quick exhale through your mouth, completely emptying your lungs with each exhalation and completely filling your lungs with each inhalation. Repeat for two to five minutes.

Sleep for your perfect weight: Go to bed by 10:30 p.m.

Day 2

Upon waking

Drink for your perfect weight: 16–24 ounces of water

Think for your perfect weight: Spend some time this morning picturing yourself at your perfect weight. See yourself doing the things you think you can't do now or don't do because you're not at your perfect weight. Picture yourself looking great, free from all of the diseases that people said you're at a high risk for. Next, picture yourself at your perfect weight, inspiring your family and friends, who remark how great you look. Now stand in front of the mirror and repeat:

> *Today I am going to take another positive step toward achieving my perfect weight.*

Then perform the Healing Codes Exercise. You can find out what the Healing Codes Exercise is by turning to page 189. I recommend that you perform the Healing Codes Exercise at least twice a day—once in the morning and once in the evening—but feel free to try this two-minute exercise three, four, or five times a day.

Get FIT for your perfect weight: Perform FIT exercises for twenty minutes, choosing from physical activities like sprinting, bodyweight exercises, strength training with bands, medicine balls, dumbbells or kettlebells, stationary bike, or the stair stepper. (Video examples of these exercises can be found at www.PerfectWeightCanada.com.)

Breakfast (approximately 7:30 a.m.)

Drink for your perfect weight: 8–12 ounces of water

2 ounces of raw almonds

One banana

Supplement for your perfect weight: Take two or three whole-food multivitamin caplets and one to four capsules of concentrated fucoxanthin.

Perfect Snack (approximately 10:00 a.m.)

Drink for your perfect weight: 8–12 ounces of water

One Garden of Life Super Seed organic whole-food nutrition bar (see the PWC Resource Guide on page 322 for recommended products)

or

One serving of Perfect Meal chocolate-flavoured meal supplement with native whey protein and glucomannan fibre mixed with 12 ounces of water

Lunch (approximately 12:30 p.m.)

Drink for your perfect weight: 12–16 ounces of water

Toss a large green salad with mixed greens, avocado, carrots, cucumbers, celery, tomatoes, red cabbage, red peppers, red onions, sprouts, 2 ounces of canned beans (black, garbanzo, and pinto), and 2 ounces of cold, poached, or canned wild salmon.

For the salad dressing, mix extra-virgin olive oil, apple-cider vinegar or lemon juice, naturally brewed soy sauce, liquid aminos, Celtic Sea Salt, herbs, and spices, or use a healthy store-bought dressing.

Organic grapes

Supplement for your perfect weight: Take two or three whole-food multivitamin caplets and one to three capsules of concentrated fucoxanthin.

Perfect Snack (approximately 3:30 p.m.)

Drink for your perfect weight: 8–12 ounces of water

A half-box to one box of Rainforest Cacao Chocolate Macadamia Nuts

or

One serving of Perfect Meal vanilla-flavoured meal supplement with native whey protein and glucomannan fibre mixed with 12 ounces of water

Dinner (approximately 6:15 p.m., but try to finish eating dinner by 7:00 p.m.)

Drink for your perfect weight: 12–16 ounces of water

Grilled chicken

Grilled vegetables (onions, peppers, and zucchini)

Baked sweet potato with butter

Supplement for your perfect weight: Take two or three whole-food multivitamin caplets, one to three capsules of concentrated fucoxanthin, and 1 to 3 teaspoons (or three to nine capsules) of a high omega-3 cod liver oil complex.

Before bed

Think for your perfect weight: Perform the Healing Codes Exercise on page 189.

Drink for your perfect weight: 8–12 ounces of water (optional, of course)

Get FIT for your perfect weight: Perform five minutes of deep-breathing exercises by taking a slow, five-second breath in through your nose (inhale), holding for one second, followed by a forceful quick exhale through your mouth, completely emptying your diaphragm with each exhalation and completely filling your diaphragm with each inhalation. Repeat for two to five minutes.

Sleep for your perfect weight: Go to bed by 10:30 p.m.

Day 3

Upon waking

Drink for your perfect weight: 16–24 ounces of water

Think for your perfect weight: Spend some time this morning picturing yourself at your perfect weight. See yourself doing the things you think you can't do now or don't do because you're not at your perfect weight. Picture yourself looking great, free from all of the diseases that people said you're at a high risk for. Next, picture yourself at your perfect weight, inspiring your family and friends, who remark how great you look. Now stand in front of the mirror and repeat:

> *Today I am going to take another positive step toward achieving my perfect weight.*

Then perform the Healing Codes Exercise. You can find out what the Healing Codes Exercise is by turning to page 189. I recommend that you perform the Healing Codes Exercise at least twice a day—once in the morning and once in the evening—but feel free to try this two-minute exercise three, four, or fives times a day.

Get FIT for your perfect weight: Perform FIT exercises for twenty minutes, choosing from physical activities like sprinting, bodyweight exercises, strength training with bands, medicine balls, dumbbells or kettlebells, stationary bike, or the stair stepper. (Video examples of these exercises can be found at www.PerfectWeightCanada.com.)

Breakfast (approximately 7:30 a.m.)

Drink for your perfect weight: 8–12 ounces of water

4 to 8 ounces of organic whole-milk yogurt with fruit (banana, pineapple, peaches, or berries), honey, and a dash of vanilla extract

Handful of raw almonds

Supplement for your perfect weight: Take two or three whole-food multivitamin caplets and one to four capsules of concentrated fucoxanthin.

Perfect Snack (approximately 10:00 a.m.)

Drink for your perfect weight: 8–12 ounces of water

One Garden of Life Perfect Food Chocolate Greens organic whole-food nutrition bar (see the PWC Resource Guide on page 322 for recommended products)

or

One serving of Perfect Meal chocolate-flavoured meal supplement with a green food vegetable blend, native whey protein, and glucomannan fibre mixed with 12 ounces of water

Lunch (approximately 12:30 p.m.)

Drink for your perfect weight: 12–16 ounces of water

Toss a large green salad with mixed greens, avocado, carrots, cucumbers, celery, tomatoes, red cabbage, red peppers, red onions, sprouts, 2 ounces of canned beans (black, garbanzo, and pinto), and 2 ounces of low-mercury, high-omega-3 canned tuna.

For the salad dressing, mix extra-virgin olive oil, apple-cider vinegar or lemon juice, naturally brewed soy sauce, liquid aminos, Celtic Sea Salt, herbs, and spices, or use a healthy store-bought dressing.

One piece of fruit in season

Supplement for your perfect weight: Take two or three whole-food multivitamin caplets and one to three capsules of concentrated fucoxanthin.

Perfect Snack (approximately 3:30 p.m.)

Drink for your perfect weight: 8–12 ounces of water

A half-box to one box of Rainforest Cacao Chocolate Macadamia Nuts

or

One serving of Perfect Meal vanilla-flavoured meal supplement with native whey protein and glucomannan fibre mixed with 12 ounces of water

Dinner (approximately 6:15 p.m., but try to finish eating dinner by 7:00 p.m.)

Drink for your perfect weight: 12–16 ounces of water

Red meat chili

Roasted potatoes

Toss a green salad with mixed greens, avocado, carrots, cucumbers, celery, tomatoes, red cabbage, red peppers, red onions, and sprouts.

For the salad dressing, mix extra-virgin olive oil, apple-cider vinegar or lemon juice, naturally brewed soy sauce, liquid aminos, Celtic Sea Salt, herbs, and spices, or use a healthy store-bought dressing.

Supplement for your perfect weight: Take two or three whole-food multivitamin caplets, one to three capsules of concentrated fucoxanthin, and 1 to 3 teaspoons (or three to nine capsules) of a high omega-3 cod liver oil complex.

Before bed

Think for your perfect weight: Perform the Healing Codes Exercise on page 189.

Drink for your perfect weight: 8–12 ounces of water (optional, of course)

Get FIT for your perfect weight: Perform five minutes of deep-breathing exercises by taking a slow, five-second breath in through your nose (inhale), holding for one second, followed by a forceful quick exhale through your mouth, completely emptying your lungs with each exhalation and completely filling your lungs with each inhalation. Repeat for two to five minutes.

Sleep for your perfect weight: Go to bed by 10:30 p.m.

Female Potato Type
Phase III (Weeks 9–12)

Day 1

Upon waking

Drink for your perfect weight: 16–24 ounces of water

Think for your perfect weight: Spend some time this morning picturing yourself at your perfect weight. See yourself doing the things you think you can't do now or don't do because you're not at your perfect weight. Picture yourself looking great, free from all of the diseases that people said you're at a high risk for. Next, picture yourself at your perfect weight, inspiring your family and friends, who remark how great you look. Now stand in front of the mirror and repeat:

Today I am going to take another positive step toward achieving my perfect weight.

Then perform the Healing Codes Exercise. You can find out what the Healing Codes Exercise is by turning to page 189. I recommend that you perform the Healing Codes Exercise at least twice a day—once in the morning and once in the evening—but feel free to try this two-minute exercise three, four, or five times a day.

Get FIT for your perfect weight: Perform FIT exercises for twenty minutes, choosing from physical activities like sprinting, bodyweight exercises, strength training with bands, medicine balls, dumbbells or kettlebells, stationary bike, or the stair stepper. (Video examples of these exercises can be found at www.PerfectWeightCanada.com.)

Breakfast (approximately 7:30 a.m.)

Drink for your perfect weight: 8–12 ounces of water

Old-fashioned oatmeal with honey, cinnamon, and raisins

2 ounces of cottage cheese and blueberries

Supplement for your perfect weight: Take two or three whole-food multivitamin caplets and one to four capsules of concentrated fucoxanthin.

Perfect Snack (approximately 10:00 a.m.)

Drink for your perfect weight: 8–12 ounces of water

One Garden of Life Fruits of Life organic whole-food nutrition bar (see the PWC Resource Guide on page 322 for recommended products)

or

One serving of Perfect Meal chocolate-flavoured meal supplement with native whey protein and glucomannan fibre mixed with 12 ounces of water

Lunch (approximately 12:30 p.m.)

Drink for your perfect weight: 12–16 ounces of water

Roasted chicken, turkey, or roast beef with lettuce, cheese, tomato, sprouts, and organic mayo (soy oil, not canola) on sprouted or yeast-free whole-grain bread (see the PWC Resource Guide on page 322 for recommended brands)

One apple with skin

Supplement for your perfect weight: Take two or three whole-food multivitamin caplets and one to three capsules of concentrated fucoxanthin.

Perfect Snack (approximately 3:30 p.m.)

Drink for your perfect weight: 8–12 ounces of water

A half-box to one box of Rainforest Cacao Chocolate Macadamia Nuts

or

One serving of Perfect Meal vanilla-flavoured meal supplement with native whey protein and glucomannan fibre mixed with 12 ounces of water

Dinner (approximately 6:15 p.m., but try to finish eating dinner by 7:00 p.m.)

Drink for your perfect weight: 12–16 ounces of water

Baked, poached, or grilled wild-caught salmon

Peas and carrots

Toss a green salad with mixed greens, avocado, carrots, cucumbers, celery, tomatoes, red cabbage, red peppers, red onions, and sprouts.

For the salad dressing, mix extra-virgin olive oil, apple-cider vinegar or lemon juice, naturally brewed soy sauce, liquid aminos, Celtic Sea Salt, herbs, and spices, or use a healthy store-bought dressing.

Supplement for your perfect weight: Take two or three whole-food multivitamin caplets, one to three capsules of concentrated fucoxanthin, and 1 to 3 teaspoons (or three to nine capsules) of a high omega-3 cod liver oil complex.

Before bed

Think for your perfect weight: Perform the Healing Codes Exercise on page 189.

Drink for your perfect weight: 8–12 ounces of water (optional, of course)

Get FIT for your perfect weight: Perform five minutes of deep-breathing exercises by taking a slow, five-second breath in through your nose (inhale), holding for one second, followed by a forceful quick exhale through your mouth, completely emptying your lungs with each exhalation and completely filling your lungs with each inhalation. Repeat for two to five minutes.

Sleep for your perfect weight: Go to bed by 10:30 p.m.

Day 2

Upon waking

Drink for your perfect weight: 16–24 ounces of water

Think for your perfect weight: Spend some time this morning picturing yourself at your perfect weight. See yourself doing the things you think you can't do now or don't do because you're not at your perfect weight. Picture yourself looking great, free from all of the diseases that people said you're at a high risk for. Next, picture yourself at your perfect weight, inspiring your family and friends, who remark how great you look. Now stand in front of the mirror and repeat:

> *Today I am going to take another positive step toward achieving my perfect weight.*

Then perform the Healing Codes Exercise. You can find out what the Healing Codes Exercise is by turning to page 189. I recommend that you perform the Healing Codes Exercise at least twice a day—once in the morning and once in the evening—but feel free to try this two-minute exercise three, four, or five times a day.

Get FIT for your perfect weight: Perform FIT exercises for twenty minutes, choosing from physical activities like sprinting, bodyweight exercises, strength training with bands, medicine balls, dumbbells or kettlebells, stationary bike, or the stair stepper. (Video examples of these exercises can be found at www.PerfectWeightCanada.com.)

Breakfast (approximately 7:30 a.m.)
Drink for your perfect weight: 8–12 ounces of water
Two eggs any style, cooked in 1 tablespoon of extra-virgin coconut oil
One slice of sprouted or yeast-free whole-grain bread with almond butter and honey
Supplement for your perfect weight: Take two or three whole-food multivitamin caplets and one to four capsules of concentrated fucoxanthin.

Perfect Snack (approximately 10:00 a.m.)
Drink for your perfect weight: 8–12 ounces of water
One Garden of Life Fruits of Life organic whole-food nutrition bar (see the PWC Resource Guide on page 322 for recommended products)
or
One serving of Perfect Meal chocolate-flavoured meal supplement with native whey protein and glucomannan fibre mixed with 12 ounces of water

Lunch (approximately 12:30 p.m.)
Drink for your perfect weight: 12–16 ounces of water
Toss a large green salad with mixed greens, avocado, carrots, cucumbers, celery, tomatoes, red cabbage, red peppers, red onions, sprouts, 2 ounces of canned beans (black, garbanzo, and pinto), and 3 ounces of cold, poached, or canned wild salmon.
For the salad dressing, mix extra-virgin olive oil, apple-cider vinegar or lemon juice, naturally brewed soy sauce, liquid aminos, Celtic Sea Salt, herbs, and spices, or use a healthy store-bought dressing.
Organic grapes
Supplement for your perfect weight: Take two or three whole-food multivitamin caplets and one to three capsules of concentrated fucoxanthin.

Perfect Snack (approximately 3:30 p.m.)

Drink for your perfect weight: 8–12 ounces of water

A half-box to one box of Rainforest Cacao Chocolate Macadamia Nuts

or

One serving of Perfect Meal vanilla-flavoured meal supplement with native whey protein and glucomannan fibre mixed with 12 ounces of water

Dinner (approximately 6:15 p.m., but try to finish eating dinner by 7:00 p.m.)

Drink for your perfect weight: 12–16 ounces of water

Grilled chicken kabobs with pineapple, peppers, onions, and zucchini

Toss a green salad with mixed greens, avocado, carrots, cucumbers, celery, tomatoes, red cabbage, red peppers, red onions, and sprouts.

For the salad dressing, mix extra-virgin olive oil, apple-cider vinegar or lemon juice, naturally brewed soy sauce, liquid aminos, Celtic Sea Salt, herbs, and spices, or mix 1 tablespoon of extra-virgin olive oil with 1 tablespoon of a healthy store-bought dressing.

Supplement for your perfect weight: Take two or three whole-food multivitamin caplets, one to three capsules of concentrated fucoxanthin, and 1 to 3 teaspoons (or three to nine capsules) of a high omega-3 cod liver oil complex.

Before bed

Think for your perfect weight: Perform the Healing Codes Exercise on page 189.

Drink for your perfect weight: 8–12 ounces of water (optional, of course)

Get FIT for your perfect weight: Perform five minutes of deep-breathing exercises by taking a slow, five-second breath in through your nose (inhale), holding for one second, followed by a forceful quick exhale through your mouth, completely emptying your lungs with each exhalation and completely filling your lungs with each inhalation. Repeat for two to five minutes.

Sleep for your perfect weight: Go to bed by 10:30 p.m.

Day 3

Upon waking

Drink for your perfect weight: 16–24 ounces of water

Think for your perfect weight: Spend some time this morning picturing yourself at your perfect weight. See yourself doing the things you think you can't do now or don't do because you're not at your perfect weight. Picture yourself looking great, free from all of the diseases that people said you're at a high risk for. Next, picture yourself at your perfect weight, inspiring your family and friends, who remark how great you look. Now stand in front of the mirror and repeat:

> *Today I am going to take another positive step toward achieving my perfect weight.*

Then perform the Healing Codes Exercise. You can find out what the Healing Codes Exercise is by turning to page 189. I recommend that you perform the Healing Codes Exercise at least twice a day—once in the morning and once in the evening—but feel free to try this two-minute exercise three, four, or five times a day.

Get FIT for your perfect weight: Perform FIT exercises for twenty minutes, choosing from physical activities like sprinting, bodyweight exercises, strength training with bands, medicine balls, dumbbells or kettlebells, stationary bike, or the stair stepper. (Video examples of these exercises can be found at www. PerfectWeightCanada.com.)

Breakfast (approximately 7:30 a.m.)

Drink for your perfect weight: 8–12 ounces of water

Organic sprouted dry cereal (see the PWC Resource Guide for recommended brands) or ½ cup of old-fashioned oats, whole corn grits, or seven-grain porridge

4 ounces of organic whole-milk yogurt or cottage cheese with fruit (pineapple, peaches, or berries), honey, and a dash of vanilla extract

Supplement for your perfect weight: Take two or three whole-food multivitamin caplets and one to four capsules of concentrated fucoxanthin.

Perfect Snack (approximately 10:00 a.m.)

Drink for your perfect weight: 8–12 ounces of water

One Garden of Life Super Seed organic whole-food nutrition bar (see the PWC Resource Guide on page 322 for recommended products)

or

One serving of Perfect Meal chocolate-flavoured meal supplement with native whey protein and glucomannan fibre mixed with 12 ounces of water

Lunch (approximately 12:30 p.m.)

Drink for your perfect weight: 12–16 ounces of water

Toss a large green salad with mixed greens, avocado, carrots, cucumbers, celery, tomatoes, red cabbage, red peppers, red onions, sprouts, 2 ounces of canned beans (black, garbanzo, and pinto), and 2 ounces of low-mercury, high-omega-3 canned tuna.

For the salad dressing, mix extra-virgin olive oil, apple-cider vinegar or lemon juice, naturally brewed soy sauce, liquid aminos, Celtic Sea Salt, herbs, and spices, or mix 1 tablespoon of extra-virgin olive oil with 1 tablespoon of a healthy store-bought dressing.

One piece of fruit in season

Supplement for your perfect weight: Take two or three whole-food multivitamin caplets and one to three capsules of concentrated fucoxanthin.

Perfect Snack (approximately 3:30 p.m.)

Drink for your perfect weight: 8–12 ounces of water

A half-box to one box of Rainforest Cacao Chocolate Macadamia Nuts

or

One serving of Perfect Meal vanilla-flavoured meal supplement with native whey protein and glucomannan fibre mixed with 12 ounces of water

Dinner (approximately 6:15 p.m., but try to finish eating dinner by 7:00 p.m.)

Drink for your perfect weight: 12–16 ounces of water

Red meat chili

Steamed quinoa, peas, and carrots

Toss a green salad with mixed greens, avocado, carrots, cucumbers, celery, tomatoes, red cabbage, red peppers, red onions, and sprouts.

For the salad dressing, mix extra-virgin olive oil, apple-cider vinegar or lemon juice, naturally brewed soy sauce, liquid aminos, Celtic Sea Salt, herbs, and spices, or mix 1 tablespoon of extra-virgin olive oil with 1 tablespoon of a healthy store-bought dressing.

Supplement for your perfect weight: Take two or three whole-food multivitamin caplets, one to three capsules of concentrated fucoxanthin, and 1 to 3 teaspoons (or three to nine capsules) of a high omega-3 cod liver oil complex.

Before bed

Think for your perfect weight: Perform the Healing Codes Exercise on page 189.

Drink for your perfect weight: 8–12 ounces of water (optional, of course)

Get FIT for your perfect weight: Perform five minutes of deep-breathing exercises by taking a slow, five-second breath in through your nose (inhale), holding for one second, followed by a forceful quick exhale through your mouth, completely emptying your diaphragm with each exhalation and completely filling your diaphragm with each inhalation. Repeat for two to five minutes.

Sleep for your perfect weight: Go to bed by 10:30 p.m.

Female Potato Type
Phase IV (Weeks 13–16)

For Phase IV, you have some options. If you are satisfied with your progress, you should continue on the Phase III plan and finish strong. If you feel that your weight loss has slowed or you liked the way you felt on Phase I or II, you are welcome to repeat one of those phases for the final four weeks.

Male Meat Type
Phase I (Weeks 1-4)

Day 1

Upon waking

Drink for your perfect weight: 16–24 ounces of water

Think for your perfect weight: Spend some time this morning picturing yourself at your perfect weight. See yourself doing the things you think you can't do now or don't do because you're not at your perfect weight. Picture yourself looking great, free from all of the diseases that people said you're at a high risk for. Next, picture yourself at your perfect weight, inspiring your family and friends, who remark how great you look. Now stand in front of the mirror and repeat:

Today I am going to take another positive step toward achieving my perfect weight.

Then perform the Healing Codes Exercise. You can find out what the Healing Codes Exercise is by turning to page 189. I recommend that you perform the Healing Codes Exercise at least twice a day—once in the morning and once in the evening—but feel free to try this two-minute exercise three, four, or five times a day.

Get FIT for your perfect weight: Perform FIT exercises for twenty minutes, choosing from physical activities like sprinting, bodyweight exercises, strength training with bands, medicine balls, dumbbells or kettlebells, stationary bike, or the stair stepper. (Video examples of these exercises can be found at www.PerfectWeightCanada.com.)

Breakfast (approximately 7:30 a.m.)

Drink for your perfect weight: 8–12 ounces of water
Make a smoothie in a blender with the following ingredients:

- 1 cup plain whole-milk yogurt or kefir
- 1 tsp. organic flaxseed oil
- 1 tsp. organic extra-virgin coconut oil
- 1 Tbsp. organic raw honey
- 1 cup organic fruit, fresh or frozen (berries, banana, peaches, pineapple, etc.)
- One scoop goat's milk protein powder (see the PWC Resource Guide on page 322 for recommendations)
- Dash of vanilla extract (optional)

Supplement for your perfect weight: Take two or three whole-food multivitamin caplets and one to four capsules of concentrated fucoxanthin. (See the PWC Resource Guide on page 322 for recommended products.)

Perfect Snack (approximately 10:00 a.m.)

Drink for your perfect weight: 8–12 ounces of water
One Perfect Weight America Peanut Butter fücoProtein whole-food nutrition bar (see the PWC Resource Guide on page 322 for recommended products)
or
One serving of Perfect Meal chocolate-flavoured meal supplement with native whey protein and glucomannan fibre mixed with 12 ounces of water

Lunch (approximately 12:30 p.m.)

Drink for your perfect weight: 12–16 ounces of water

Toss a large green salad with mixed greens, avocado, carrots, cucumbers, celery, tomatoes, red cabbage, red peppers, red onions, sprouts, 2 ounces of canned beans (black, garbanzo, and pinto), and two hard-boiled omega-3 eggs.

For the salad dressing, mix extra-virgin olive oil, apple-cider vinegar or lemon juice, naturally brewed soy sauce, liquid aminos, Celtic Sea Salt, herbs, and spices, or mix 1 tablespoon of extra-virgin olive oil with 1 tablespoon of a healthy store-bought dressing. (See the PWC Resource Guide for recommended brands.)

Supplement for your perfect weight: Take two or three whole-food multivitamin caplets and one to three capsules of concentrated fucoxanthin.

Perfect Snack (approximately 3:30 p.m.)

Drink for your perfect weight: 8–12 ounces of water

One Perfect Weight America Chocolate MacNut Crunch fücoProtein whole-food nutrition bar

or

One serving of Perfect Meal vanilla-flavoured meal supplement with native whey protein and glucomannan fibre mixed with 12 ounces of water

Dinner (approximately 6:15 p.m., but try to finish eating dinner by 7:00 p.m.)

Drink for your perfect weight: 12–16 ounces of water

Baked, poached, or grilled wild-caught salmon

Steamed broccoli

Toss a green salad with mixed greens, avocado, carrots, cucumbers, celery, tomatoes, red cabbage, red peppers, red onions, and sprouts.

For the salad dressing, mix extra-virgin olive oil, apple-cider vinegar or lemon juice, naturally brewed soy sauce, liquid aminos, Celtic Sea Salt, herbs, and spices, or mix 1 tablespoon of extra-virgin olive oil with 1 tablespoon of a healthy store-bought dressing.

Supplement for your perfect weight: Take two or three whole-food multivitamin caplets, one to three capsules of concentrated fucoxanthin, and 1 to 3 teaspoons (or three to nine capsules) of a high omega-3 cod liver oil complex. (See the PWC Resource Guide on page 322 for recommended products.)

Before bed

Think for your perfect weight: Perform the Healing Codes Exercise on page 189.

Drink for your perfect weight: 8–12 ounces of water (optional, of course)

Get FIT for your perfect weight: Perform five minutes of deep-breathing exercises by taking a slow, five-second breath in through your nose (inhale), holding for one second, followed by a forceful quick exhale through your mouth, completely emptying your diaphragm with each exhalation and completely filling your diaphragm with each inhalation. Repeat for two to five minutes.

Sleep for your perfect weight: Go to bed by 10:30 p.m.

Day 2

Upon waking

Drink for your perfect weight: 16–24 ounces of water

Think for your perfect weight: Spend some time this morning picturing yourself at your perfect weight. See yourself doing the things you think you can't do now or don't do because you're not at your perfect weight. Picture yourself looking great, free from all of the diseases that people said you're at a high risk for. Next, picture yourself at your perfect weight, inspiring your family and friends, who remark how great you look. Now stand in front of the mirror and repeat:

Today I am going to take another positive step toward achieving my perfect weight.

Then perform the Healing Codes Exercise. You can find out what the Healing Codes Exercise is by turning to page 189. I recommend that you perform the Healing Codes Exercise at least twice a day—once in the morning and once in the evening—but feel free to try this two-minute exercise three, four, or five times a day.

Get FIT for your perfect weight: Perform FIT exercises for twenty minutes, choosing from physical activities like sprinting, bodyweight exercises, strength training with bands, medicine balls, dumbbells or kettlebells, stationary bike, or the stair stepper. (Video examples of these exercises can be found at www.PerfectWeightCanada.com.)

Breakfast (approximately 7:30 a.m.)

Drink for your perfect weight: 8–12 ounces of water

Three eggs any style, cooked in 1 tablespoon of extra-virgin coconut oil

Stir-fried onions, mushrooms, and peppers

One grapefruit

Supplement for your perfect weight: Take two or three whole-food multivitamin caplets and one to four capsules of concentrated fucoxanthin.

Perfect Snack (approximately 10:00 a.m.)

Drink for your perfect weight: 8–12 ounces of water

One Perfect Weight America Peanut Butter fücoProtein whole-food nutrition bar (see the PWC Resource Guide on page 322 for recommended products)

or

One serving of Perfect Meal chocolate-flavoured meal supplement with native whey protein and glucomannan fibre mixed with 12 ounces of water

Lunch (approximately 12:30 p.m.)

Drink for your perfect weight: 12–16 ounces of water

Toss a large green salad with mixed greens, avocado, carrots, cucumbers, celery, tomatoes, red cabbage, red peppers, red onions, sprouts, 2 ounces of canned beans (black, garbanzo, and pinto), and 3 ounces of cold, poached, or canned wild salmon.

For the salad dressing, mix extra-virgin olive oil, apple-cider vinegar or lemon juice, naturally brewed soy sauce, liquid aminos, Celtic Sea Salt, herbs, and spices, or mix 1 tablespoon of extra-virgin olive oil with 1 tablespoon of a healthy store-bought dressing.

Supplement for your perfect weight: Take two or three whole-food multivitamin caplets and one to three capsules of concentrated fucoxanthin.

Perfect Snack (approximately 3:30 p.m.)

Drink for your perfect weight: 8–12 ounces of water

One Perfect Weight America Chocolate MacNut Crunch fücoProtein whole-food nutrition bar

or

One serving of Perfect Meal vanilla-flavoured meal supplement with native whey protein and glucomannan fibre mixed with 12 ounces of water

Dinner (approximately 6:15 p.m., but try to finish eating dinner by 7:00 p.m.)

Drink for your perfect weight: 12–16 ounces of water

Roasted organic chicken

Cooked vegetables (carrots, onions, peas, etc.)

Toss a green salad with mixed greens, avocado, carrots, cucumbers, celery, tomatoes, red cabbage, red peppers, red onions, and sprouts.

For the salad dressing, mix extra-virgin olive oil, apple-cider vinegar or lemon juice, naturally brewed soy sauce, liquid aminos, Celtic Sea Salt, herbs, and spices, or mix 1 tablespoon of extra-virgin olive oil with 1 tablespoon of a healthy store-bought dressing.

Supplement for your perfect weight: Take two or three whole-food multivitamin caplets, one to three capsules of concentrated fucoxanthin, and 1 to 3 teaspoons (or three to nine capsules) of a high omega-3 cod liver oil complex.

Before bed

Think for your perfect weight: Perform the Healing Codes Exercise on page 189.

Drink for your perfect weight: 8–12 ounces of water (optional, of course)

Get FIT for your perfect weight: Perform five minutes of deep-breathing exercises by taking a slow, five-second breath in through your nose (inhale), holding for one second, followed by a forceful quick exhale through your mouth, completely emptying your lungs with each exhalation and completely filling your lungs with each inhalation. Repeat for two to five minutes.

Sleep for your perfect weight: Go to bed by 10:30 p.m.

Day 3

Upon waking

Drink for your perfect weight: 16–24 ounces of water

Think for your perfect weight: Spend some time this morning picturing yourself at your perfect weight. See yourself doing the things you think you can't do now or don't do because you're not at your perfect weight. Picture yourself looking great, free from all of the diseases that people said you're at a high risk for. Next, picture yourself at your perfect weight, inspiring your family and friends, who remark how great you look. Now stand in front of the mirror and repeat:

Today I am going to take another positive step toward achieving my perfect weight.

Then perform the Healing Codes Exercise. You can find out what the Healing Codes Exercise is by turning to page 189. I recommend that you perform the Healing Codes Exercise at least twice a day—once in the morning and once in the evening—but feel free to try this two-minute exercise three, four, or five times a day.

Get FIT for your perfect weight: Perform FIT exercises for twenty minutes, choosing from physical activities like sprinting, bodyweight exercises, strength training with bands, medicine balls, dumbbells or kettlebells, stationary bike, or the stair stepper. (Video examples of these exercises can be found at www.PerfectWeightCanada.com.)

Breakfast (approximately 7:30 a.m.)

Drink for your perfect weight: 8–12 ounces of water

8 ounces of organic whole-milk yogurt or cottage cheese with fruit (banana, pineapple, peaches, or berries), honey, and a dash of vanilla extract

Handful of raw almonds

Supplement for your perfect weight: Take two or three whole-food multivitamin caplets and one to four capsules of concentrated fucoxanthin.

Perfect Snack (approximately 10:00 a.m.)

Drink for your perfect weight: 8–12 ounces of water

One Perfect Weight America Peanut Butter fücoProtein whole-food nutrition bar (see the PWC Resource Guide on page 322 for recommended products)

or

One serving of Perfect Meal chocolate-flavoured meal supplement with native whey protein and glucomannan fibre mixed with 12 ounces of water

Lunch (approximately 12:30 p.m.)

Drink for your perfect weight: 12–16 ounces of water

Toss a large green salad with mixed greens, avocado, carrots, cucumbers, celery, tomatoes, red cabbage, red peppers, red onions, sprouts, 2 ounces of canned beans (black, garbanzo, and pinto), and 2 ounces of low-mercury, high-omega-3 canned tuna. (See the PWC Resource Guide on page 322 for recommended products.)

For the salad dressing, mix extra-virgin olive oil, apple-cider vinegar or lemon juice, naturally brewed soy sauce, liquid aminos, Celtic Sea Salt, herbs, and spices, or mix 1 tablespoon of extra-virgin olive oil with 1 tablespoon of a healthy store-bought dressing.

One piece of fruit in season

Supplement for your perfect weight: Take two or three whole-food multivitamin caplets and one to three capsules of concentrated fucoxanthin.

Perfect Snack (approximately 3:30 p.m.)

Drink for your perfect weight: 8–12 ounces of water

One Perfect Weight America Chocolate MacNut Crunch fücoProtein whole-food nutrition bar

or

One serving of Perfect Meal vanilla-flavoured meal supplement with native whey protein and glucomannan fibre mixed with 12 ounces of water

Dinner (approximately 6:15 p.m., but try to finish eating dinner by 7:00 p.m.)

Drink for your perfect weight: 12–16 ounces of water

Red meat steak or ground meat (beef, buffalo, or venison)

Steamed broccoli

Baked winter squash with butter

Toss a green salad with mixed greens, avocado, carrots, cucumbers, celery, tomatoes, red cabbage, red peppers, red onions, and sprouts.

For the salad dressing, mix extra-virgin olive oil, apple-cider vinegar or lemon juice, naturally brewed soy sauce, liquid aminos, Celtic Sea Salt, herbs, and spices, or mix 1 tablespoon of extra-virgin olive oil with 1 tablespoon of a healthy store-bought dressing.

Supplement for your perfect weight: Take two or three whole-food multivitamin caplets, one to three capsules of concentrated fucoxanthin, and 1 to 3 teaspoons (or three to nine capsules) of a high omega-3 cod liver oil complex.

Before bed

Think for your perfect weight: Perform the Healing Codes Exercise on page 189.

Drink for your perfect weight: 8–12 ounces of water (optional, of course)

Get FIT for your perfect weight: Perform five minutes of deep-breathing exercises by taking a slow, five-second breath in through your nose (inhale), holding for one second, followed by a forceful quick exhale through your mouth, completely emptying your lungs with each exhalation and completely filling your lungs with each inhalation. Repeat for two to five minutes.

Sleep for your perfect weight: Go to bed by 10:30 p.m.

Male Meat Type
Phase II (Weeks 5–8)

Day 1

Upon waking

Drink for your perfect weight: 16–24 ounces of water

Think for your perfect weight: Spend some time this morning picturing yourself at your perfect weight. See yourself doing the things you think you can't do now or don't do because you're not at your perfect weight. Picture yourself looking great, free from all of the diseases that people said you're at a high risk for. Next, picture yourself at your perfect weight, inspiring your family and friends, who remark how great you look. Now stand in front of the mirror and repeat:

> *Today I am going to take another positive step toward achieving my perfect weight.*

Then perform the Healing Codes Exercise. You can find out what the Healing Codes Exercise is by turning to page 189. I recommend that you perform the Healing Codes Exercise at least twice a day—once in the morning and once in the evening—but feel free to try this two-minute exercise three, four, or five times a day.

Get FIT for your perfect weight: Perform FIT exercises for twenty minutes, choosing from physical activities like sprinting, bodyweight exercises, strength training with bands, medicine balls, dumbbells or kettlebells, stationary bike, or the stair stepper. (Video examples of these exercises can be found at www.PerfectWeightCanada.com.)

Breakfast (approximately 7:30 a.m.)

Drink for your perfect weight: 8–12 ounces of water

Make a smoothie in a blender with the following ingredients:

- 1 cup plain whole milk yogurt or kefir
- 1 tsp. organic flaxseed oil
- 1 tsp. organic extra-virgin coconut oil
- 1 Tbsp. organic raw honey
- 1 cup organic fruit, fresh or frozen (berries, banana, peaches, pineapple, etc.)
- 1 scoop goat's milk protein powder (see the PWC Resource Guide on page 322 for recommendations)
- Dash of vanilla extract (optional)

Supplement for your perfect weight: Take two or three whole-food multivitamin caplets and one to four capsules of concentrated fucoxanthin. (See the PWC Resource Guide on page 322 for recommended products.)

Perfect Snack (approximately 10:00 a.m.)

Drink for your perfect weight: 8–12 ounces of water

One Perfect Weight America Peanut Butter fücoProtein whole-food nutrition bar (see the PWC Resource Guide on page 322 for recommended products)

or

One serving of Perfect Meal chocolate-flavoured meal supplement with native whey protein and glucomannan fibre mixed with 12 ounces of water

Lunch (approximately 12:30 p.m.)

Drink for your perfect weight: 12–16 ounces of water

Toss a large green salad with mixed greens, avocado, carrots, cucumbers, celery, tomatoes, red cabbage, red peppers, red onions, sprouts, 2 ounces of canned beans (black, garbanzo, and pinto), and two hard-boiled omega-3 eggs.

For the salad dressing, mix extra-virgin olive oil, apple-cider vinegar or lemon juice, naturally brewed soy sauce, liquid aminos, Celtic Sea Salt, herbs, and spices, or mix 1 tablespoon of extra-virgin olive oil with 1 tablespoon of a healthy store-bought dressing. (See the PWC Resource Guide for recommended brands.)

Supplement for your perfect weight: Take two or three whole-food multivitamin caplets and one to three capsules of concentrated fucoxanthin.

Perfect Snack (approximately 3:30 p.m.)

Drink for your perfect weight: 8–12 ounces of water

One Perfect Weight America Chocolate MacNut Crunch fücoProtein whole-food nutrition bar

or

One serving of Perfect Meal vanilla-flavoured meal supplement with native whey protein and glucomannan fibre mixed with 12 ounces of water

Dinner (approximately 6:15 p.m., but try to finish eating dinner by 7:00 p.m.)

Drink for your perfect weight: 12–16 ounces of water

Broiled or steamed fish

Sautéed spinach

Toss a green salad with mixed greens, avocado, carrots, cucumbers, celery, tomatoes, red cabbage, red peppers, red onions, and sprouts.

For the salad dressing, mix extra-virgin olive oil, apple-cider vinegar or lemon juice, naturally brewed soy sauce, liquid aminos, Celtic Sea Salt, herbs, and spices, or mix 1 tablespoon of extra-virgin olive oil with 1 tablespoon of a healthy store-bought dressing.

Supplement for your perfect weight: Take two or three whole-food multivitamin caplets, one to three capsules of concentrated fucoxanthin, and 1 to 3 teaspoons (or three to nine capsules) of a high omega-3 cod liver oil complex. (See the PWC Resource Guide on page 322 for recommended products.)

Before bed

Think for your perfect weight: Perform the Healing Codes Exercise on page 189.

Drink for your perfect weight: 8–12 ounces of water (optional, of course)

Get FIT for your perfect weight: Perform five minutes of deep-breathing exercises by taking a slow, five-second breath in through your nose (inhale), holding for one second, followed by a forceful quick exhale through your mouth, completely emptying your diaphragm with each exhalation and completely filling your diaphragm with each inhalation. Repeat for two to five minutes.

Sleep for your perfect weight: Go to bed by 10:30 p.m.

Day 2

Upon waking

Drink for your perfect weight: 16–24 ounces of water

Think for your perfect weight: Spend some time this morning picturing yourself at your perfect weight. See yourself doing the things you think you can't do now or don't do because you're not at your perfect weight. Picture yourself looking great, free from all of the diseases that people said you're at a high risk for. Next, picture yourself at your perfect weight, inspiring your family and friends, who remark how great you look. Now stand in front of the mirror and repeat:

> *Today I am going to take another positive step toward achieving my perfect weight.*

Then perform the Healing Codes Exercise. You can find out what the Healing Codes Exercise is by turning to page 189. I recommend that you perform the Healing Codes Exercise at least twice a day—once in the morning and once in the evening—but feel free to try this two-minute exercise three, four, or five times a day.

Get FIT for your perfect weight: Perform FIT exercises for twenty minutes, choosing from physical activities like sprinting, bodyweight exercises, strength training with bands, medicine balls, dumbbells or kettlebells, stationary bike, or the stair stepper. (Video examples of these exercises can be found at www.PerfectWeightCanada.com.)

Breakfast (approximately 7:30 a.m.)

Drink for your perfect weight: 8–12 ounces of water

Three eggs any style, cooked in 1 tablespoon of extra-virgin coconut oil

Sautéed tomatoes and onions

One orange

Supplement for your perfect weight: Take two or three whole-food multivitamin caplets and one to four capsules of concentrated fucoxanthin.

Perfect Snack (approximately 10:00 a.m.)

Drink for your perfect weight: 8–12 ounces of water

One Perfect Weight America Peanut Butter fücoProtein whole-food nutrition bar (see the PWC Resource Guide on page 322 for recommended products)

or

One serving of Perfect Meal chocolate-flavoured meal supplement with native whey protein and glucomannan fibre mixed with 12 ounces of water

Lunch (approximately 12:30 p.m.)

Drink for your perfect weight: 12–16 ounces of water

Toss a large green salad with mixed greens, avocado, carrots, cucumbers, celery, tomatoes, red cabbage, red peppers, red onions, sprouts, 2 ounces of canned beans (black, garbanzo, and pinto), and 4 ounces of cold, poached, or canned wild salmon.

For the salad dressing, mix extra-virgin olive oil, apple-cider vinegar or lemon juice, naturally brewed soy sauce, liquid aminos, Celtic Sea Salt, herbs, and spices, or mix 1 tablespoon of extra-virgin olive oil with 1 tablespoon of a healthy store-bought dressing.

One piece of fruit

Supplement for your perfect weight: Take two or three whole-food multivitamin caplets and one to three capsules of concentrated fucoxanthin.

Perfect Snack (approximately 3:30 p.m.)

Drink for your perfect weight: 8–12 ounces of water

One Perfect Weight America Chocolate MacNut Crunch fücoProtein whole-food nutrition bar

or

One serving of Perfect Meal vanilla-flavoured meal supplement with native whey protein and glucomannan fibre mixed with 12 ounces of water

Dinner (approximately 6:15 p.m., but try to finish eating dinner by 7:00 p.m.)

Drink for your perfect weight: 12–16 ounces of water

Meatloaf

Roasted vegetables (potatoes, carrots, onions, peas, etc.)

Toss a green salad with mixed greens, avocado, carrots, cucumbers, celery, tomatoes, red cabbage, red peppers, red onions, and sprouts.

For the salad dressing, mix extra-virgin olive oil, apple-cider vinegar or lemon juice, naturally brewed soy sauce, liquid aminos, Celtic Sea Salt, herbs, and spices, or mix 1 tablespoon of extra-virgin olive oil with 1 tablespoon of a healthy store-bought dressing.

Supplement for your perfect weight: Take two or three whole-food multivitamin caplets, one to three capsules of concentrated fucoxanthin, and 1 to 3 teaspoons (or three to nine capsules) of a high omega-3 cod liver oil complex.

Before bed

Think for your perfect weight: Perform the Healing Codes Exercise on page 189.

Drink for your perfect weight: 8–12 ounces of water (optional, of course)

Get FIT for your perfect weight: Perform five minutes of deep-breathing exercises by taking a slow, five-second breath in through your nose (inhale), holding for one second, followed by a forceful quick exhale through your mouth, completely emptying your diaphragm with each exhalation and completely filling your diaphragm with each inhalation. Repeat for two to five minutes.

Sleep for your perfect weight: Go to bed by 10:30 p.m.

Day 3

Upon waking

Drink for your perfect weight: 16–24 ounces of water

Think for your perfect weight: Spend some time this morning picturing yourself at your perfect weight. See yourself doing the things you think you can't do now or don't do because you're not at your perfect weight. Picture yourself looking great, free from all of the diseases that people said you're at a high risk for. Next, picture yourself at your perfect weight, inspiring your family and friends, who remark how great you look. Now stand in front of the mirror and repeat:

> *Today I am going to take another positive step toward achieving my perfect weight.*

Then perform the Healing Codes Exercise. You can find out what the Healing Codes Exercise is by turning to page 189. I recommend that you perform the Healing Codes Exercise at least twice a day—once in the morning and once in the evening—but feel free to try this two-minute exercise three, four, or five times a day.

Get FIT for your perfect weight: Perform FIT exercises for twenty minutes, choosing from physical activities like sprinting, bodyweight exercises, strength training with bands, medicine balls, dumbbells or kettlebells, stationary bike, or the stair stepper. (Video examples of these exercises can be found at www.PerfectWeightCanada.com.)

Breakfast (approximately 7:30 a.m.)
Drink for your perfect weight: 8–12 ounces of water
6 ounces of organic whole-milk yogurt or cottage cheese with fruit (pineapple, peaches, or berries), honey, and a dash of vanilla extract
Handful of raw almonds
Supplement for your perfect weight: Take two or three whole-food multivitamin caplets and one to four capsules of concentrated fucoxanthin.

Perfect Snack (approximately 10:00 a.m.)
Drink for your perfect weight: 8–12 ounces of water
One Perfect Weight America Peanut Butter fücoProtein whole-food nutrition bar (see the PWC Resource Guide on page 322 for recommended products)
or
One serving of Perfect Meal chocolate-flavoured meal supplement with native whey protein and glucomannan fibre mixed with 12 ounces of water

Lunch (approximately 12:30 p.m.)
Drink for your perfect weight: 12–16 ounces of water
Toss a large green salad with mixed greens, avocado, carrots, cucumbers, celery, tomatoes, red cabbage, red peppers, red onions, sprouts, 2 ounces of canned beans (black, garbanzo, and pinto), and 4 ounces of low-mercury, high-omega-3 canned tuna. (See the PWC Resource Guide on page 322 for recommended products.)
For the salad dressing, mix extra-virgin olive oil, apple-cider vinegar or lemon juice, naturally brewed soy sauce, liquid aminos, Celtic Sea Salt, herbs, and spices, or mix 1 tablespoon of extra-virgin olive oil with 1 tablespoon of a healthy store-bought dressing.

One piece of fruit in season

Supplement for your perfect weight: Take two or three whole-food multivitamin caplets and one to three capsules of concentrated fucoxanthin.

Perfect Snack (approximately 3:30 p.m.)

Drink for your perfect weight: 8–12 ounces of water

One Perfect Weight America Chocolate MacNut Crunch fücoProtein whole-food nutrition bar

or

One serving of Perfect Meal vanilla-flavoured meal supplement with native whey protein and glucomannan fibre mixed with 12 ounces of water

Dinner (approximately 6:15 p.m., but try to finish eating dinner by 7:00 p.m.)

Drink for your perfect weight: 12–16 ounces of water

Red meat steak or ground meat (beef, buffalo, or venison)

Steamed broccoli

Baked sweet potato with butter

Toss a green salad with mixed greens, avocado, carrots, cucumbers, celery, tomatoes, red cabbage, red peppers, red onions, and sprouts.

For the salad dressing, mix extra-virgin olive oil, apple-cider vinegar or lemon juice, naturally brewed soy sauce, liquid aminos, Celtic Sea Salt, herbs, and spices, or mix 1 tablespoon of extra-virgin olive oil with 1 tablespoon of a healthy store-bought dressing.

Supplement for your perfect weight: Take two or three whole-food multivitamin caplets, one to three capsules of concentrated fucoxanthin, and 1 to 3 teaspoons (or three to nine capsules) of a high omega-3 cod liver oil complex.

Before bed

Think for your perfect weight: Perform the Healing Codes Exercise on page 189.

Drink for your perfect weight: 8–12 ounces of water (optional, of course)

Get FIT for your perfect weight: Perform five minutes of deep-breathing exercises by taking a slow, five-second breath in through your nose (inhale), holding for one second, followed by a forceful quick exhale through your mouth, completely emptying your lungs with each exhalation and completely filling your lungs with each inhalation. Repeat for two to five minutes.

Sleep for your perfect weight: Go to bed by 10:30 p.m.

Male Meat Type
Phase III (Weeks 9-12)

Day 1

Upon waking

Drink for your perfect weight: 16–24 ounces of water.

Think for your perfect weight: Spend some time this morning picturing yourself at your perfect weight. See yourself doing the things you think you can't do now or don't do because you're not at your perfect weight. Picture yourself looking great, free from all of the diseases that people said you're at a high risk for. Next, picture yourself at your perfect weight, inspiring your family and friends, who remark how great you look. Now stand in front of the mirror and repeat:

> *Today I am going to take another positive step toward achieving my perfect weight.*

Then perform the Healing Codes Exercise. You can find out what the Healing Codes Exercise is by turning to page 189. I recommend that you perform the Healing Codes Exercise at least twice a day—once in the morning and once in the evening—but feel free to try this two-minute exercise three, four, or fives times a day.

Get FIT for your perfect weight: Perform FIT exercises for twenty minutes, choosing from physical activities like sprinting, bodyweight exercises, strength training with bands, medicine balls, dumbbells or kettlebells, stationary bike, or the stair stepper. (Video examples of these exercises can be found at www.PerfectWeightCanada.com.)

Breakfast (approximately 7:30 a.m.)

Drink for your perfect weight: 8–12 ounces of water

Three-egg tomato and cheese omelette

One piece of sprouted or yeast-free toast with butter

Supplement for your perfect weight: Take two or three whole-food multivitamin caplets and one to four capsules of concentrated fucoxanthin. (See the PWC Resource Guide on page 322 for recommended products.)

Perfect Snack (approximately 10:00 a.m.)

Drink for your perfect weight: 8–12 ounces of water

One Perfect Weight America Peanut Butter fücoProtein whole-food nutrition bar (see the PWC Resource Guide on page 322 for recommended products)

or

One serving of Perfect Meal chocolate-flavoured meal supplement with native whey protein and glucomannan fibre mixed with 12 ounces of water

Lunch (approximately 12:30 p.m.)

Drink for your perfect weight: 12–16 ounces of water

Red meat chili

1 ounce of raw cheese

Whole-grain crackers or baked corn chips

Supplement for your perfect weight: Take two or three whole-food multivitamin caplets and one to three capsules of concentrated fucoxanthin.

Perfect Snack (approximately 3:30 p.m.)

Drink for your perfect weight: 8–12 ounces of water

One Perfect Weight America Chocolate MacNut Crunch fücoProtein whole-food nutrition bar

or

One serving of Perfect Meal vanilla-flavoured meal supplement with native whey protein and glucomannan fibre mixed with 12 ounces of water

Dinner (approximately 6:15 p.m., but try to finish eating dinner by 7:00 p.m.)

Drink for your perfect weight: 12–16 ounces of water

Baked chicken breast

One baked potato with butter

Toss a green salad with mixed greens, avocado, carrots, cucumbers, celery, tomatoes, red cabbage, red peppers, red onions, and sprouts.

For the salad dressing, mix extra-virgin olive oil, apple-cider vinegar or lemon juice, naturally brewed soy sauce, liquid aminos, Celtic Sea Salt, herbs, and spices, or mix 1 tablespoon of extra-virgin olive oil with 1 tablespoon of a healthy store-bought dressing.

Supplement for your perfect weight: Take two or three whole-food multivitamin caplets, one to three capsules of concentrated fucoxanthin, and 1 to 3 teaspoons (or three to nine capsules) of a high omega-3 cod liver oil complex. (See the PWC Resource Guide on page 322 for recommended products.)

Before bed

Think for your perfect weight: Perform the Healing Codes Exercise on page 189.

Drink for your perfect weight: 8–12 ounces of water (optional, of course)

Get FIT for your perfect weight: Perform five minutes of deep-breathing exercises by taking a slow, five-second breath in through your nose (inhale), holding for one second, followed by a forceful quick exhale through your mouth, completely emptying your lungs with each exhalation and completely filling your lungs with each inhalation. Repeat for two to five minutes.

Sleep for your perfect weight: Go to bed by 10:30 p.m.

Day 2

Upon waking

Drink for your perfect weight: 16–24 ounces of water

Think for your perfect weight: Spend some time this morning picturing yourself at your perfect weight. See yourself doing the things you think you can't do now or don't do because you're not at your perfect weight. Picture yourself looking great, free from all of the diseases that people said you're at a high risk for. Next, picture yourself at your perfect weight, inspiring your family and friends, who remark how great you look. Now stand in front of the mirror and repeat:

> *Today I am going to take another positive step toward achieving my perfect weight.*

Then perform the Healing Codes Exercise. You can find out what the Healing Codes Exercise is by turning to page 189. I recommend that you perform the Healing Codes Exercise at least twice a day—once in the morning and once in the evening—but feel free to try this two-minute exercise three, four, or five times a day.

Get FIT for your perfect weight: Perform FIT exercises for twenty minutes, choosing from physical activities like sprinting, bodyweight exercises, strength training with bands, medicine balls, dumbbells or kettlebells, stationary bike, or the stair stepper. (Video examples of these exercises can be found at www.PerfectWeightCanada.com.)

Breakfast (approximately 7:30 a.m.)

Drink for your perfect weight: 8–12 ounces of water
Three eggs any style, cooked in 1 tablespoon of extra-virgin coconut oil
4 ounces cottage cheese, raw honey, and raisins
Supplement for your perfect weight: Take two or three whole-food multivitamin caplets and one to four capsules of concentrated fucoxanthin.

Perfect Snack (approximately 10:00 a.m.)

Drink for your perfect weight: 8–12 ounces of water
One Perfect Weight America Peanut Butter fücoProtein whole-food nutrition bar (see the PWC Resource Guide on page 322 for recommended products)
or
One serving of Perfect Meal chocolate-flavoured meal supplement with native whey protein and glucomannan fibre mixed with 12 ounces of water

Lunch (approximately 12:30 p.m.)

Drink for your perfect weight: 12–16 ounces of water
Toss a large green salad with mixed greens, avocado, carrots, cucumbers, celery, tomatoes, red cabbage, red peppers, red onions, sprouts, 2 ounces of canned beans (black, garbanzo, and pinto), and 4 ounces of cold, poached, or canned wild salmon.

For the salad dressing, mix extra-virgin olive oil, apple-cider vinegar or lemon juice, naturally brewed soy sauce, liquid aminos, Celtic Sea Salt, herbs, and spices, or mix 1 tablespoon of extra-virgin olive oil with 1 tablespoon of a healthy store-bought dressing.

Supplement for your perfect weight: Take two or three whole-food multivitamin caplets and one to three capsules of concentrated fucoxanthin.

Perfect Snack (approximately 3:30 p.m.)

Drink for your perfect weight: 8–12 ounces of water

One Perfect Weight America Chocolate MacNut Crunch fücoProtein whole-food nutrition bar

or

One serving of Perfect Meal vanilla-flavoured meal supplement with native whey protein and glucomannan fibre mixed with 12 ounces of water

Dinner (approximately 6:15 p.m., but try to finish eating dinner by 7:00 p.m.)

Drink for your perfect weight: 12–16 ounces of water

Roasted organic chicken

Roasted vegetables (potatoes, carrots, onions, peas, etc.)

Toss a green salad with mixed greens, avocado, carrots, cucumbers, celery, tomatoes, red cabbage, red peppers, red onions, and sprouts.

For the salad dressing, mix extra-virgin olive oil, apple-cider vinegar or lemon juice, naturally brewed soy sauce, liquid aminos, Celtic Sea Salt, herbs, and spices, or mix 1 tablespoon of extra-virgin olive oil with 1 tablespoon of a healthy store-bought dressing.

Supplement for your perfect weight: Take two or three whole-food multivitamin caplets, one to three capsules of concentrated fucoxanthin, and 1 to 3 teaspoons (or three to nine capsules) of a high omega-3 cod liver oil complex.

Before bed

Think for your perfect weight: Perform the Healing Codes Exercise on page 189.

Drink for your perfect weight: 8–12 ounces of water (optional, of course)

Get FIT for your perfect weight: Perform five minutes of deep-breathing exercises by taking a slow, five-second breath in through your nose (inhale), holding for one second, followed by a forceful quick exhale through your mouth, completely emptying your lung with each exhalation and completely filling your lung with each inhalation. Repeat for two to five minutes.

Sleep for your perfect weight: Go to bed by 10:30 p.m.

Day 3

Upon waking

Drink for your perfect weight: 16–24 ounces of water

Think for your perfect weight: Spend some time this morning picturing yourself at your perfect weight. See yourself doing the things you think you can't do now or don't do because you're not at your perfect weight. Picture yourself looking great, free from all of the diseases that people said you're at a high risk for. Next, picture yourself at your perfect weight, inspiring your family and friends, who remark how great you look. Now stand in front of the mirror and repeat:

Today I am going to take another positive step toward achieving my perfect weight.

Then perform the Healing Codes Exercise. You can find out what the Healing Codes Exercise is by turning to page 189. I recommend that you perform the Healing Codes Exercise at least twice a day—once in the morning and once in the evening—but feel free to try this two-minute exercise three, four, or five times a day.

Get FIT for your perfect weight: Perform FIT exercises for twenty minutes, choosing from physical activities like sprinting, bodyweight exercises, strength training with bands, medicine balls, dumbbells or kettlebells, stationary bike, or the stair stepper. (Video examples of these exercises can be found at www.PerfectWeightCanada.com.)

Breakfast (approximately 7:30 a.m.)

Drink for your perfect weight: 8–12 ounces of water

8 ounces of organic whole-milk yogurt or cottage cheese with fruit (banana, pineapple, peaches, or berries), honey, and a dash of vanilla extract

Handful of raw almonds

Supplement for your perfect weight: Take two or three whole-food multivitamin caplets and one to four capsules of concentrated fucoxanthin.

Perfect Snack (approximately 10:00 a.m.)

Drink for your perfect weight: 8–12 ounces of water

One Perfect Weight America Peanut Butter fücoProtein whole-food nutrition bar (see the PWC Resource Guide on page 322 for recommended products)

or

One serving of Perfect Meal chocolate-flavoured meal supplement with native whey protein and glucomannan fibre mixed with 12 ounces of water

Lunch (approximately 12:30 p.m.)

Drink for your perfect weight: 12–16 ounces of water

Toss a large green salad with mixed greens, avocado, carrots, cucumbers, celery, tomatoes, red cabbage, red peppers, red onions, sprouts, 2 ounces of canned beans (black, garbanzo, and pinto), and 4 ounces of low-mercury, high-omega-3 canned tuna. (See the PWC Resource Guide on page 322 for recommended products.)

For the salad dressing, mix extra-virgin olive oil, apple-cider vinegar or lemon juice, naturally brewed soy sauce, liquid aminos, Celtic Sea Salt, herbs, and spices, or mix 1 tablespoon of extra-virgin olive oil with 1 tablespoon of a healthy store-bought dressing.

One piece of fruit in season

Supplement for your perfect weight: Take two or three whole-food multivitamin caplets and one to three capsules of concentrated fucoxanthin.

Perfect Snack (approximately 3:30 p.m.)

Drink for your perfect weight: 8–12 ounces of water

One Perfect Weight America Chocolate MacNut Crunch fücoProtein whole-food nutrition bar

or

One serving of Perfect Meal vanilla-flavoured meal supplement with native whey protein and glucomannan fibre mixed with 12 ounces of water

Dinner (approximately 6:15 p.m., but try to finish eating dinner by 7:00 p.m.)

Drink for your perfect weight: 12–16 ounces of water

Meatloaf

One baked sweet potato with butter

Steamed broccoli

Toss a green salad with mixed greens, avocado, carrots, cucumbers, celery, tomatoes, red cabbage, red peppers, red onions, and sprouts.

For the salad dressing, mix extra-virgin olive oil, apple-cider vinegar or lemon juice, naturally brewed soy sauce, liquid aminos, Celtic Sea Salt, herbs, and spices, or mix 1 tablespoon of extra-virgin olive oil with 1 tablespoon of a healthy store-bought dressing.

Supplement for your perfect weight: Take two or three whole-food multivitamin caplets, one to three capsules of concentrated fucoxanthin, and 1 to 3 teaspoons (or three to nine capsules) of a high omega-3 cod liver oil complex.

Before bed

Think for your perfect weight: Perform the Healing Codes Exercise on page 189.

Drink for your perfect weight: 8–12 ounces of water (optional, of course)

Get FIT for your perfect weight: Perform five minutes of deep-breathing exercises by taking a slow, five-second breath in through your nose (inhale), holding for one second, followed by a forceful quick exhale through your mouth, completely emptying your lungs with each exhalation and completely filling your lungs with each inhalation. Repeat for two to five minutes.

Sleep for your perfect weight: Go to bed by 10:30 p.m.

Male Meat Type
Phase IV (Weeks 13–16)

For Phase IV, you have some options. If you are satisfied with your progress, you should continue on the Phase III plan and finish strong. If you feel that your weight loss has slowed or you liked the way you felt on Phase I or II, you are welcome to repeat one of those phases for the final four weeks.

Male Potato Type
Phase I (Weeks 1–4)

Day 1

Upon waking

Drink for your perfect weight: 16–24 ounces of water

Think for your perfect weight: Spend some time this morning picturing yourself at your perfect weight, doing the things you think you can't do now or don't do because you're not at your perfect weight. Picture yourself looking great, free from all of the diseases that people said you're at a high risk for. Next, picture yourself at your perfect weight, inspiring your family and friends, who remark how great you look. Now stand in front of the mirror and repeat:

> *Today I am going to take another positive step toward achieving my perfect weight.*

Then perform the Healing Codes Exercise. You can find out what the Healing Codes Exercise is by turning to page 189. I recommend that you perform the Healing Codes Exercise at least twice a day—once in the morning and once in the evening—but feel free to try this two-minute exercise three, four, or five times a day.

Get FIT for your perfect weight: Perform FIT exercises for twenty minutes, choosing from physical activities like sprinting, bodyweight exercises, strength training with bands, medicine balls, dumbbells or kettlebells, stationary bike, or the stair stepper. (Video examples of these exercises can be found at www.PerfectWeightCanada.com.)

Breakfast (approximately 7:30 a.m.)

Drink for your perfect weight: 8–12 ounces of water

Make a smoothie in a blender with the following ingredients:

- 1 cup plain whole-milk yogurt or kefir
- 1 tsp. organic extra-virgin coconut oil
- 2 Tbsp. organic raw honey
- 1 cup of organic fruit, fresh or frozen (berries, banana, peaches, pine-apple, etc.)
- 1 scoop goat's milk protein powder (see the PWC Resource Guide on page 322 for recommendations)
- Dash of vanilla extract (optional)

Supplement for your perfect weight: Take two or three whole-food multivitamin caplets and one to four capsules of concentrated fucoxanthin. (See the PWC Resource Guide on page 322 for recommended products.)

Perfect Snack (approximately 10:00 a.m.)

Drink for your perfect weight: 8–12 ounces of water

One Garden of Life Fruits of Life organic whole-food nutrition bar (see the PWC Resource Guide on page 322 for recommended products)

or

One serving of Perfect Meal chocolate-flavoured meal supplement with native whey protein and glucomannan fibre mixed with 12 ounces of water

Lunch (approximately 12:30 p.m.)

Drink for your perfect weight: 12–16 ounces of water

Toss a large green salad with mixed greens, avocado, carrots, cucumbers, celery, tomatoes, red cabbage, red peppers, red onions, sprouts, 2 ounces of canned beans (black, garbanzo, and pinto), and three hard-boiled omega-3 eggs.

For the salad dressing, mix extra-virgin olive oil, apple-cider vinegar or lemon juice, naturally brewed soy sauce, liquid aminos, Celtic Sea Salt, herbs, and spices, or mix 1 tablespoon of extra-virgin olive oil with 1 tablespoon of a healthy store-bought dressing.

One apple with skin

Supplement for your perfect weight: Take two or three whole-food multivitamin caplets and one to three capsules of concentrated fucoxanthin.

Perfect Snack (approximately 3:30 p.m.)

Drink for your perfect weight: 8–12 ounces of water

A half-box to one box of Rainforest Cacao Chocolate Macadamia Nuts

or

One serving of Perfect Meal vanilla-flavoured meal supplement with native whey protein and glucomannan fibre mixed with 12 ounces of water

Dinner (approximately 6:15 p.m., but try to finish eating dinner by 7:00 p.m.)

Drink for your perfect weight: 12–16 ounces of water

Baked, poached, or grilled wild-caught salmon

Peas and carrots

Toss a green salad with mixed greens, avocado, carrots, cucumbers, celery, tomatoes, red cabbage, red peppers, red onions, and sprouts.

For the salad dressing, mix extra-virgin olive oil, apple-cider vinegar or lemon juice, naturally brewed soy sauce, liquid aminos, Celtic Sea Salt, herbs, and spices, or mix 1 tablespoon of extra-virgin olive oil with 1 tablespoon of a healthy store-bought dressing.

Supplement for your perfect weight: Take two or three whole-food multivitamin caplets, one to three capsules of concentrated fucoxanthin, and 1 to 3 teaspoons (or three to nine capsules) of a high omega-3 cod liver oil complex.

Before bed

Think for your perfect weight: Perform the Healing Codes Exercise on page 189.

Drink for your perfect weight: 8–12 ounces of water (optional, of course)

Get FIT for your perfect weight: Perform five minutes of deep-breathing exercises by taking a slow, five-second breath in through your nose (inhale), holding for one second, followed by a forceful quick exhale through your mouth, completely emptying your lungs with each exhalation and completely filling your lungs with each inhalation. Repeat for two to five minutes.

Sleep for your perfect weight: Go to bed by 10:30 p.m.

Day 2

Upon waking
Drink for your perfect weight: 16–24 ounces of water

Think for your perfect weight: Spend some time this morning picturing yourself at your perfect weight. See yourself doing the things you think you can't do now or don't do because you're not at your perfect weight. Picture yourself looking great, free from all of the diseases that people said you're at a high risk for. Next, picture yourself at your perfect weight, inspiring your family and friends, who remark how great you look. Now stand in front of the mirror and repeat:

> *Today I am going to take another positive step toward achieving my perfect weight.*

Then perform the Healing Codes Exercise. You can find out what the Healing Codes Exercise is by turning to page 189. I recommend that you perform the Healing Codes Exercise at least twice a day—once in the morning and once in the evening—but feel free to try this two-minute exercise three, four, or five times a day.

Get FIT for your perfect weight: Perform FIT exercises for twenty minutes, choosing from physical activities like sprinting, bodyweight exercises, strength training with bands, medicine balls, dumbbells or kettlebells, stationary bike, or the stair stepper. (Video examples of these exercises can be found at www.PerfectWeightCanada.com.)

Breakfast (approximately 7:30 a.m.)
Drink for your perfect weight: 8–12 ounces of water
Three eggs any style, cooked in 1 tablespoon of extra-virgin coconut oil
Stir-fried onions, mushrooms, and peppers
One serving of grapes
Supplement for your perfect weight: Take two or three whole-food multivitamin caplets and one to four capsules of concentrated fucoxanthin.

Perfect Snack (approximately 10:00 a.m.)
Drink for your perfect weight: 8–12 ounces of water
One Garden of Life Super Seed organic whole-food nutrition bar (see the PWC Resource Guide on page 322 for recommended products)
or
One serving of Perfect Meal chocolate-flavoured meal supplement with native whey protein and glucomannan fibre mixed with 12 ounces of water

Lunch (approximately 12:30 p.m.)

Drink for your perfect weight: 12–16 ounces of water

Toss a large green salad with mixed greens, avocado, carrots, cucumbers, celery, tomatoes, red cabbage, red peppers, red onions, sprouts, 2 ounces of canned beans (black, garbanzo, and pinto), and 2 ounces of cold, poached, or canned wild salmon.

For the salad dressing, mix extra-virgin olive oil, apple-cider vinegar or lemon juice, naturally brewed soy sauce, liquid aminos, Celtic Sea Salt, herbs, and spices, or mix 1 tablespoon of extra-virgin olive oil with 1 tablespoon of a healthy store-bought dressing.

One apple with skin

Supplement for your perfect weight: Take two or three whole-food multivitamin caplets and one to three capsules of concentrated fucoxanthin.

Perfect Snack (approximately 3:30 p.m.)

Drink for your perfect weight: 8–12 ounces of water

A half-box to one box of Rainforest Cacao Chocolate Macadamia Nuts

or

One serving of Perfect Meal vanilla-flavoured meal supplement with native whey protein and glucomannan fibre mixed with 12 ounces of water

Dinner (approximately 6:15 p.m., but try to finish eating dinner by 7:00 p.m.)

Drink for your perfect weight: 12–16 ounces of water

Roasted organic chicken

Cooked vegetables (carrots, onions, peas, etc.)

Toss a green salad with mixed greens, avocado, carrots, cucumbers, celery, tomatoes, red cabbage, red peppers, red onions, and sprouts.

For the salad dressing, mix extra-virgin olive oil, apple-cider vinegar or lemon juice, naturally brewed soy sauce, liquid aminos, Celtic Sea Salt, herbs, and spices, or mix 1 tablespoon of extra-virgin olive oil with 1 tablespoon of a healthy store-bought dressing.

Supplement for your perfect weight: Take two or three whole-food multivitamin caplets, one to three capsules of concentrated fucoxanthin, and 1 to 3 teaspoons (or three to nine capsules) of a high omega-3 cod liver oil complex.

Before bed

Think for your perfect weight: Perform the Healing Codes Exercise on page 189.

Drink for your perfect weight: 8–12 ounces of water (optional, of course)

Get FIT for your perfect weight: Perform five minutes of deep-breathing exercises by taking a slow, five-second breath in through your nose (inhale), holding for one second, followed by a forceful quick exhale through your mouth, completely emptying your diaphragm with each exhalation and completely filling your diaphragm with each inhalation. Repeat for two to five minutes.

Sleep for your perfect weight: Go to bed by 10:30 p.m.

Day 3

Upon waking

Drink for your perfect weight: 16–24 ounces of water

Think for your perfect weight: Spend some time this morning picturing yourself at your perfect weight. See yourself doing the things you think you can't do now or don't do because you're not at your perfect weight. Picture yourself looking great, free from all of the diseases that people said you're at a high risk for. Next, picture yourself at your perfect weight, inspiring your family and friends, who remark how great you look. Now stand in front of the mirror and repeat:

> *Today I am going to take another positive step toward achieving my perfect weight.*

Then perform the Healing Codes Exercise. You can find out what the Healing Codes Exercise is by turning to page 189. I recommend that you perform the Healing Codes Exercise at least twice a day—once in the morning and once in the evening—but feel free to try this two-minute exercise three, four, or five times a day.

Get FIT for your perfect weight: Perform FIT exercises for twenty minutes, choosing from physical activities like sprinting, bodyweight exercises, strength training with bands, medicine balls, dumbbells or kettlebells, stationary bike, or the stair stepper. (Video examples of these exercises can be found at www.PerfectWeightCanada.com.)

Breakfast (approximately 7:30 a.m.)

Drink for your perfect weight: 8–12 ounces of water

4 to 8 ounces of organic whole-milk yogurt with fruit (pineapple, peaches, or berries), honey, and a dash of vanilla extract

Handful of raw almonds

Supplement for your perfect weight: Take two or three whole-food multivitamin caplets and one to four capsules of concentrated fucoxanthin.

Perfect Snack (approximately 10:00 a.m.)

Drink for your perfect weight: 8–12 ounces of water

One Garden of Life Perfect Food Chocolate Greens organic whole-food nutrition bar (see the PWC Resource Guide on page 322 for recommended products)

or

One serving of Perfect Meal chocolate-flavoured meal supplement with a green food vegetable blend, native whey protein, and glucomannan fibre mixed with 12 ounces of water

Lunch (approximately 12:30 p.m.)

Drink for your perfect weight: 12–16 ounces of water

Toss a large green salad with mixed greens, avocado, carrots, cucumbers, celery, tomatoes, red cabbage, red peppers, red onions, sprouts, 2 ounces of canned beans (black, garbanzo, and pinto), and 4 ounces of low-mercury, high-omega-3 canned tuna.

For the salad dressing, mix extra-virgin olive oil, apple-cider vinegar or lemon juice, naturally brewed soy sauce, liquid aminos, Celtic Sea Salt, herbs, and spices, or mix 1 tablespoon of extra-virgin olive oil with 1 tablespoon of a healthy store-bought dressing.

One piece of fruit in season

Supplement for your perfect weight: Take two or three whole-food multivitamin caplets and one to three capsules of concentrated fucoxanthin.

Perfect Snack (approximately 3:30 p.m.)

Drink for your perfect weight: 8–12 ounces of water

A half-box to one box of Rainforest Cacao Chocolate Macadamia Nuts

or

One serving of Perfect Meal vanilla-flavoured meal supplement with native whey protein and glucomannan fibre mixed with 12 ounces of water

Dinner (approximately 6:15 p.m., but try to finish eating dinner by 7:00 p.m.)

Drink for your perfect weight: 12–16 ounces of water

Red meat steak (beef, buffalo, or venison)

Steamed broccoli

Toss a green salad with mixed greens, avocado, carrots, cucumbers, celery, tomatoes, red cabbage, red peppers, red onions, and sprouts.

For the salad dressing, mix extra-virgin olive oil, apple-cider vinegar or lemon juice, naturally brewed soy sauce, liquid aminos, Celtic Sea Salt, herbs, and spices, or mix 1 tablespoon of extra-virgin olive oil with 1 tablespoon of a healthy store-bought dressing.

Supplement for your perfect weight: Take two or three whole-food multivitamin caplets, one to three capsules of concentrated fucoxanthin, and 1 to 3 teaspoons (or three to nine capsules) of a high omega-3 cod liver oil complex.

Before bed

Think for your perfect weight: Perform the Healing Codes Exercise on page 189.

Drink for your perfect weight: 8–12 ounces of water (optional, of course)

Get FIT for your perfect weight: Perform five minutes of deep-breathing exercises by taking a slow, five-second breath in through your nose (inhale), holding for one second, followed by a forceful quick exhale through your mouth, completely emptying your lungs with each exhalation and completely filling your lungs with each inhalation. Repeat for two to five minutes.

Sleep for your perfect weight: Go to bed by 10:30 p.m.

Male Potato Type
Phase II (Weeks 5–8)

Day 1

Upon waking

Drink for your perfect weight: 16–24 ounces of water

Think for your perfect weight: Spend some time this morning picturing yourself at your perfect weight. See yourself doing the things you think you can't do now or don't do because you're not at your perfect weight. Picture yourself looking great, free from all of the diseases that people said you're at a high risk for. Next, picture yourself at your perfect weight, inspiring your family and friends, who remark how great you look. Now stand in front of the mirror and repeat:

> *Today I am going to take another positive step toward achieving my perfect weight.*

Then perform the Healing Codes Exercise. You can find out what the Healing Codes Exercise is by turning to page 189. I recommend that you perform the Healing Codes Exercise at least twice a day—once in the morning and once in the evening—but feel free to try this two-minute exercise three, four, or five times a day.

Get FIT for your perfect weight: Perform FIT exercises for twenty minutes, choosing from physical activities like sprinting, bodyweight exercises, strength training with bands, medicine balls, dumbbells or kettlebells, stationary bike, or the stair stepper. (Video examples of these exercises can be found at www.PerfectWeightCanada.com.)

Breakfast (approximately 7:30 a.m.)

Drink for your perfect weight: 8–12 ounces of water

8 ounces of cottage cheese with raw honey and banana

Supplement for your perfect weight: Take two or three whole-food multivitamin caplets and one to four capsules of concentrated fucoxanthin. (See the PWC Resource Guide on page 322 for recommended products.)

Perfect Snack (approximately 10:00 a.m.)

Drink for your perfect weight: 8–12 ounces of water

One Garden of Life Fruits of Life organic whole-food nutrition bar (see the PWC Resource Guide on page 322 for recommended products)

or

One serving of Perfect Meal chocolate-flavoured meal supplement with native whey protein and glucomannan fibre mixed with 12 ounces of water

Lunch (approximately 12:30 p.m.)

Drink for your perfect weight: 12–16 ounces of water

Toss a large green salad with mixed greens, avocado, carrots, cucumbers, celery, tomatoes, red cabbage, red peppers, red onions, sprouts, 2 ounces of canned beans (black, garbanzo, and pinto), and three hard-boiled omega-3 eggs.

For the salad dressing, mix extra-virgin olive oil, apple-cider vinegar or lemon juice, naturally brewed soy sauce, liquid aminos, Celtic Sea Salt, herbs, and spices, or mix 1 tablespoon of extra-virgin olive oil with 1 tablespoon of a healthy store-bought dressing.

One apple with skin

Supplement for your perfect weight: Take two or three whole-food multivitamin caplets and one to three capsules of concentrated fucoxanthin.

Perfect Snack (approximately 3:30 p.m.)

Drink for your perfect weight: 8–12 ounces of water

A half-box to one box of Rainforest Cacao Chocolate Macadamia Nuts

or

One serving of Perfect Meal vanilla-flavoured meal supplement with native whey protein and glucomannan fibre mixed with 12 ounces of water

Dinner (approximately 6:15 p.m., but try to finish eating dinner by 7:00 p.m.)

Drink for your perfect weight: 12–16 ounces of water

Meatloaf

Mashed potato with butter

Steamed broccoli

Supplement for your perfect weight: Take two or three whole-food multivitamin caplets, one to three capsules of concentrated fucoxanthin, and 1 to 3 teaspoons (or three to nine capsules) of a high omega-3 cod liver oil complex. (See the PWC Resource Guide on page 322 for recommended products.)

Before bed

Think for your perfect weight: Perform the Healing Codes Exercise on page 189.

Drink for your perfect weight: 8–12 ounces of water (optional, of course)

Get FIT for your perfect weight: Perform five minutes of deep-breathing exercises by taking a slow, five-second breath in through your nose (inhale), holding for one second, followed by a forceful quick exhale through your mouth, completely emptying your lungs with each exhalation and completely filling your lungs with each inhalation. Repeat for two to five minutes.

Sleep for your perfect weight: Go to bed by 10:30 p.m.

Day 2

Upon waking

Drink for your perfect weight: 16–24 ounces of water

Think for your perfect weight: Spend some time this morning picturing yourself at your perfect weight. See yourself doing the things you think you can't do now or don't do because you're not at your perfect weight. Picture yourself looking great, free from all of the diseases that people said you're at a high risk for. Next, picture yourself at your perfect weight, inspiring your family and friends, who remark how great you look. Now stand in front of the mirror and repeat:

Today I am going to take another positive step toward achieving my perfect weight.

Then perform the Healing Codes Exercise. You can find out what the Healing Codes Exercise is by turning to page 189. I recommend that you perform the Healing Codes Exercise at least twice a day—once in the morning and once in the evening—but feel free to try this two-minute exercise three, four, or five times a day.

Get FIT for your perfect weight: Perform FIT exercises for twenty minutes, choosing from physical activities like sprinting, bodyweight exercises, strength training with bands, medicine balls, dumbbells or kettlebells, stationary bike, or the stair stepper. (Video examples of these exercises can be found at www.PerfectWeightCanada.com.)

Breakfast (approximately 7:30 a.m.)

Drink for your perfect weight: 8–12 ounces of water

Three eggs any style, cooked in 1 tablespoon of extra-virgin coconut oil

4 ounces of old-fashioned oatmeal with butter, honey, raisins, and cinnamon

Supplement for your perfect weight: Take two or three whole-food multivitamin caplets and one to four capsules of concentrated fucoxanthin.

Perfect Snack (approximately 10:00 a.m.)

Drink for your perfect weight: 8–12 ounces of water

One Garden of Life Super Seed organic whole-food nutrition bar (see the PWC Resource Guide on page 322 for recommended products)

or

One serving of Perfect Meal chocolate-flavoured meal supplement with native whey protein and glucomannan fibre mixed with 12 ounces of water

Lunch (approximately 12:30 p.m.)

Drink for your perfect weight: 12–16 ounces of water

Toss a large green salad with mixed greens, avocado, carrots, cucumbers, celery, tomatoes, red cabbage, red peppers, red onions, sprouts, 2 ounces of canned beans (black, garbanzo, and pinto), and 4 ounces of cold, poached, or canned wild salmon.

For the salad dressing, mix extra-virgin olive oil, apple-cider vinegar or lemon juice, naturally brewed soy sauce, liquid aminos, Celtic Sea Salt, herbs, and spices, or mix 1 tablespoon of extra-virgin olive oil with 1 tablespoon of a healthy store-bought dressing.

Organic grapes

Supplement for your perfect weight: Take two or three whole-food multivitamin caplets and one to three capsules of concentrated fucoxanthin.

Perfect Snack (approximately 3:30 p.m.)

Drink for your perfect weight: 8–12 ounces of water

A half-box to one box of Rainforest Cacao Chocolate Macadamia Nuts

or

One serving of Perfect Meal vanilla-flavoured meal supplement with native whey protein and glucomannan fibre mixed with 12 ounces of water

Dinner (approximately 6:15 p.m., but try to finish eating dinner by 7:00 p.m.)

Drink for your perfect weight: 12–16 ounces of water

Grilled chicken

Brown rice

Stir-fried vegetables (peppers, onions, mushrooms, etc.)

Supplement for your perfect weight: Take two or three whole-food multivitamin caplets, one to three capsules of concentrated fucoxanthin, and 1 to 3 teaspoons (or three to nine capsules) of a high omega-3 cod liver oil complex.

Before bed

Think for your perfect weight: Perform the Healing Codes Exercise on page 189.

Drink for your perfect weight: 8–12 ounces of water (optional, of course)

Get FIT for your perfect weight: Perform five minutes of deep-breathing exercises by taking a slow, five-second breath in through your nose (inhale), holding for one second, followed by a forceful quick exhale through your mouth, completely emptying your lungs with each exhalation and completely filling your lungs with each inhalation. Repeat for two to five minutes.

Sleep for your perfect weight: Go to bed by 10:30 p.m.

Day 3

Upon waking

Drink for your perfect weight: 16–24 ounces of water

Think for your perfect weight: Spend some time this morning picturing yourself at your perfect weight. See yourself doing the things you think you can't do now or don't do because you're not at your perfect weight. Picture yourself looking great, free from all of the diseases that people said you're at a high risk for. Next, picture yourself at your perfect weight, inspiring your family and friends, who remark how great you look. Now stand in front of the mirror and repeat:

> *Today I am going to take another positive step toward achieving my perfect weight.*

Then perform the Healing Codes Exercise. You can find out what the Healing Codes Exercise is by turning to page 189. I recommend that you perform the Healing Codes Exercise at least twice a day—once in the morning and once in the evening—but feel free to try this two-minute exercise three, four, or five times a day.

Get FIT for your perfect weight: Perform FIT exercises for twenty minutes, choosing from physical activities like sprinting, bodyweight exercises, strength training with bands, medicine balls, dumbbells or kettlebells, stationary bike, or the stair stepper. (Video examples of these exercises can be found at www.PerfectWeightCanada.com.)

Breakfast (approximately 7:30 a.m.)

Drink for your perfect weight: 8–12 ounces of water

4 to 8 ounces of organic whole-milk yogurt with fruit (pineapple, peaches, or berries), honey, and a dash of vanilla extract

Handful of raw almonds and raisins

Supplement for your perfect weight: Take two or three whole-food multivitamin caplets and one to four capsules of concentrated fucoxanthin.

Perfect Snack (approximately 10:00 a.m.)

Drink for your perfect weight: 8–12 ounces of water

One Garden of Life Perfect Food Chocolate Greens organic whole-food nutrition bar (see the PWC Resource Guide on page 322 for recommended products)

or

One serving of Perfect Meal chocolate-flavoured meal supplement with a green food vegetable blend, native whey protein, and glucomannan fibre mixed with 12 ounces of water

Lunch (approximately 12:30 p.m.)

Drink for your perfect weight: 12–16 ounces of water

Toss a large green salad with mixed greens, avocado, carrots, cucumbers, celery, tomatoes, red cabbage, red peppers, red onions, sprouts, 2 ounces of canned beans (black, garbanzo, and pinto), and 4 ounces of cold, poached, or canned wild salmon.

For the salad dressing, mix extra-virgin olive oil, apple-cider vinegar or lemon juice, naturally brewed soy sauce, liquid aminos, Celtic Sea Salt, herbs, and spices, or mix 1 tablespoon of extra-virgin olive oil with 1 tablespoon of a healthy store-bought dressing.

One piece of fruit in season

Supplement for your perfect weight: Take two or three whole-food multivitamin caplets and one to three capsules of concentrated fucoxanthin.

Perfect Snack (approximately 3:30 p.m.)

Drink for your perfect weight: 8–12 ounces of water

A half-box to one box of Rainforest Cacao Chocolate Macadamia Nuts

or

One serving of Perfect Meal vanilla-flavoured meal supplement with native whey protein and glucomannan fibre mixed with 12 ounces of water

Dinner (approximately 6:15 p.m., but try to finish eating dinner by 7:00 p.m.)

Drink for your perfect weight: 12–16 ounces of water

Red meat chili

Raw cheese

Whole-grain crackers or baked corn chips

Toss a green salad with mixed greens, avocado, carrots, cucumbers, celery, tomatoes, red cabbage, red peppers, red onions, and sprouts.

For the salad dressing, mix extra-virgin olive oil, apple-cider vinegar or lemon juice, naturally brewed soy sauce, liquid aminos, Celtic Sea Salt, herbs, and spices, or mix 1 tablespoon of extra-virgin olive oil with 1 tablespoon of a healthy store-bought dressing.

Supplement for your perfect weight: Take two or three whole-food multivitamin caplets, one to three capsules of concentrated fucoxanthin, and 1 to 3 teaspoons (or three to nine capsules) of a high omega-3 cod liver oil complex.

Before bed

Think for your perfect weight: Perform the Healing Codes Exercise on page 189.

Drink for your perfect weight: 8–12 ounces of water (optional, of course)

Get FIT for your perfect weight: Perform five minutes of deep-breathing exercises by taking a slow, five-second breath in through your nose (inhale), holding for one second, followed by a forceful quick exhale through your mouth, completely emptying your lungs with each exhalation and completely filling your lungs with each inhalation. Repeat for two to five minutes.

Sleep for your perfect weight: Go to bed by 10:30 p.m.

Male Potato Type
Phase III (Weeks 9–12)

Day 1

Upon waking

Drink for your perfect weight: 16–24 ounces of water

Think for your perfect weight: Spend some time this morning picturing yourself at your perfect weight. See yourself doing the things you think you can't do now or don't do because you're not at your perfect weight. Picture yourself looking great, free from all of the diseases that people said you're at a high risk for. Next, picture yourself at your perfect weight, inspiring your family and friends, who remark how great you look. Now stand in front of the mirror and repeat:

> *Today I am going to take another positive step toward achieving my perfect weight.*

Then perform the Healing Codes Exercise. You can find out what the Healing Codes Exercise is by turning to page 189. I recommend that you perform the Healing Codes Exercise at least twice a day—once in the morning and once in the evening—but feel free to try this two-minute exercise three, four, or five times a day.

Get FIT for your perfect weight: Perform FIT exercises for twenty minutes, choosing from physical activities like sprinting, bodyweight exercises, strength training with bands, medicine balls, dumbbells or kettlebells, stationary bike, or the stair stepper. (Video examples of these exercises can be found at www.PerfectWeightCanada.com.)

Breakfast (approximately 7:30 a.m.)

Drink for your perfect weight: 8–12 ounces of water

Make a smoothie in a blender with the following ingredients:

- 1 cup plain whole-milk yogurt or kefir
- 1 tsp. organic extra-virgin coconut oil
- 2 Tbsp. organic raw honey
- 1 cup organic fruit, fresh or frozen (berries, banana, peaches, pineapple, etc.)
- 1 scoop goat's milk protein powder (see the PWC Resource Guide on page 322 for recommendations)
- Dash of vanilla extract (optional)

Supplement for your perfect weight: Take two or three whole-food multivitamin caplets and one to four capsules of concentrated fucoxanthin.

Perfect Snack (approximately 10:00 a.m.)

Drink for your perfect weight: 8–12 ounces of water

One Garden of Life Fruits of Life organic whole-food nutrition bar (see the PWC Resource Guide on page 322 for recommended products)

or

One serving of Perfect Meal chocolate-flavoured meal supplement with native whey protein and glucomannan fibre mixed with 12 ounces of water

Lunch (approximately 12:30 p.m.)

Drink for your perfect weight: 12–16 ounces of water

Roasted chicken, turkey, or roast beef with lettuce, cheese, tomato, sprouts, and organic mayo (soy oil, not canola) on sprouted or yeast-free whole-grain bread (see the PWC Resource Guide page 322 for recommended brands)

One apple with skin

Supplement for your perfect weight: Take two or three whole-food multivitamin caplets and one to three capsules of concentrated fucoxanthin.

Perfect Snack (approximately 3:30 p.m.)

Drink for your perfect weight: 8–12 ounces of water

A half-box to one box of Rainforest Cacao Chocolate Macadamia Nuts

or

One serving of Perfect Meal vanilla-flavoured meal supplement with native whey protein and glucomannan fibre mixed with 12 ounces of water

Dinner (approximately 6:15 p.m., but try to finish eating dinner by 7:00 p.m.)

Drink for your perfect weight: 12–16 ounces of water

Baked, poached, or grilled wild-caught salmon

Peas and carrots

Toss a green salad with mixed greens, avocado, carrots, cucumbers, celery, tomatoes, red cabbage, red peppers, red onions, and sprouts.

For the salad dressing, mix extra-virgin olive oil, apple-cider vinegar or lemon juice, naturally brewed soy sauce, liquid aminos, Celtic Sea Salt, herbs, and spices, or mix 1 tablespoon of extra-virgin olive oil with 1 tablespoon of a healthy store-bought dressing.

Supplement for your perfect weight: Take two or three whole-food multivitamin caplets, one to three capsules of concentrated fucoxanthin, and 1 to 3 teaspoons (or three to nine capsules) of a high omega-3 cod liver oil complex.

Before bed

Think for your perfect weight: Perform the Healing Codes Exercise on page 189.

Drink for your perfect weight: 8–12 ounces of water (optional, of course)

Get FIT for your perfect weight: Perform five minutes of deep-breathing exercises by taking a slow, five-second breath in through your nose (inhale), holding for one second, followed by a forceful quick exhale through your mouth, completely emptying your diaphragm with each exhalation and completely filling your diaphragm with each inhalation. Repeat for two to five minutes.

Sleep for your perfect weight: Go to bed by 10:30 p.m.

Day 2

Upon waking

Drink for your perfect weight: 16–24 ounces of water

Think for your perfect weight: Spend some time this morning picturing yourself at your perfect weight. See yourself doing the things you think you can't do now or don't do because you're not at your perfect weight. Picture yourself looking great, free from all of the diseases that people said you're at a high risk for. Next, picture yourself at your perfect weight, inspiring your family and friends, who remark how great you look. Now stand in front of the mirror and repeat:

> *Today I am going to take another positive step toward achieving my perfect weight.*

Then perform the Healing Codes Exercise. You can find out what the Healing Codes Exercise is by turning to page 189. I recommend that you perform the Healing Codes Exercise at least twice a day—once in the morning and once in the evening—but feel free to try this two-minute exercise three, four, or five times a day.

Get FIT for your perfect weight: Perform FIT exercises for twenty minutes, choosing

from physical activities like sprinting, bodyweight exercises, strength training with bands, medicine balls, dumbbells or kettlebells, stationary bike, or the stair stepper. (Video examples of these exercises can be found at www.PerfectWeightCanada.com.)

Breakfast (approximately 7:30 a.m.)

Drink for your perfect weight: 8–12 ounces of water

Two or three eggs any style, cooked in 1 tablespoon of extra-virgin coconut oil (see the PWC Resource Guide on page 322 for recommended products)

Stir-fried onions, mushrooms, and peppers

One slice of sprouted or yeast-free whole-grain bread with almond butter and honey

Supplement for your perfect weight: Take two or three whole-food multivitamin caplets and one to four capsules of concentrated fucoxanthin.

Perfect Snack (approximately 10:00 a.m.)

Drink for your perfect weight: 8–12 ounces of water

One Garden of Life Fruits of Life organic whole-food nutrition bar (see the PWC Resource Guide on page 322 for recommended products)

or

One serving of Perfect Meal chocolate-flavoured meal supplement with native whey protein and glucomannan fibre mixed with 12 ounces of water

Lunch (approximately 12:30 p.m.)

Drink for your perfect weight: 12–16 ounces of water

Toss a large green salad with mixed greens, avocado, carrots, cucumbers, celery, tomatoes, red cabbage, red peppers, red onions, sprouts, 2 ounces of canned beans (black, garbanzo, and pinto), and 4 ounces of cold, poached, or canned wild salmon.

For the salad dressing, mix extra-virgin olive oil, apple-cider vinegar or lemon juice, naturally brewed soy sauce, liquid aminos, Celtic Sea Salt, herbs, and spices, or mix 1 tablespoon of extra-virgin olive oil with 1 tablespoon of a healthy store-bought dressing.

Organic grapes

Supplement for your perfect weight: Take two or three whole-food multivitamin caplets and one to three capsules of concentrated fucoxanthin.

Perfect Snack (approximately 3:30 p.m.)

Drink for your perfect weight: 8–12 ounces of water

A half-box to one box of Rainforest Cacao Chocolate Macadamia Nuts

or

One serving of Perfect Meal vanilla-flavoured meal supplement with native whey protein and glucomannan fibre mixed with 12 ounces of water

Dinner (approximately 6:15 p.m., but try to finish eating dinner by 7:00 p.m.)

Drink for your perfect weight: 12–16 ounces of water

Roasted organic chicken

Cooked vegetable (carrots, onions, peas, etc.)

Toss a green salad with mixed greens, avocado, carrots, cucumbers, celery, tomatoes, red cabbage, red peppers, red onions, and sprouts.

For the salad dressing, mix extra-virgin olive oil, apple-cider vinegar or lemon juice, naturally brewed soy sauce, liquid aminos, Celtic Sea Salt, herbs, and spices, or mix 1 tablespoon of extra-virgin olive oil with 1 tablespoon of a healthy store-bought dressing.

Supplement for your perfect weight: Take two or three whole-food multivitamin caplets, one to three capsules of concentrated fucoxanthin, and 1 to 3 teaspoons (or three to nine capsules) of a high omega-3 cod liver oil complex.

Before bed

Think for your perfect weight: Perform the Healing Codes Exercise on page 189.

Drink for your perfect weight: 8–12 ounces of water (optional, of course)

Get FIT for your perfect weight: Perform five minutes of deep-breathing exercises by taking a slow, five-second breath in through your nose (inhale), holding for one second, followed by a forceful quick exhale through your mouth, completely emptying your diaphragm with each exhalation and completely filling your diaphragm with each inhalation. Repeat for two to five minutes.

Sleep for your perfect weight: Go to bed by 10:30 p.m.

Day 3

Upon waking

Drink for your perfect weight: 16–24 ounces of water

Think for your perfect weight: Spend some time this morning picturing yourself at your perfect weight. See yourself doing the things you think you can't do now or don't do because you're not at your perfect weight. Picture yourself looking great, free from all of the diseases that people said you're at a high risk for. Next, picture yourself at your perfect weight, inspiring your family and friends, who remark how great you look. Now stand in front of the mirror and repeat:

> *Today I am going to take another positive step toward achieving my perfect weight.*

Then perform the Healing Codes Exercise. You can find out what the Healing Codes Exercise is by turning to page 189. I recommend that you perform the Healing Codes Exercise at least twice a day—once in the morning and once in the evening—but feel free to try this two-minute exercise three, four, or fives times a day.

Get FIT for your perfect weight: Perform FIT exercises for twenty minutes, choosing from physical activities like sprinting, bodyweight exercises, strength training with bands, medicine balls, dumbbells or kettlebells, stationary bike, or the stair stepper. (Video examples of these exercises can be found at www.PerfectWeightCanada.com.)

Breakfast (approximately 7:30 a.m.)
Drink for your perfect weight: 8–12 ounces of water

Organic sprouted dry cereal (see the PWC Resource Guide for recommended brands) or ½ cup of old-fashioned oats, whole corn grits, or seven-grain porridge

4 ounces of organic whole-milk yogurt or cottage cheese with fruit (pineapple, peaches, or berries), honey, and a dash of vanilla extract

Supplement for your perfect weight: Take two or three whole-food multivitamin caplets and one to four capsules of concentrated fucoxanthin.

Perfect Snack (approximately 10:00 a.m.)
Drink for your perfect weight: 8–12 ounces of water

One Garden of Life Super Seed organic whole-food nutrition bar (see the PWC Resource Guide on page 322 for recommended products)

or

One serving of Perfect Meal chocolate-flavoured meal supplement with native whey protein and glucomannan fibre mixed with 12 ounces of water

Lunch (approximately 12:30 p.m.)
Drink for your perfect weight: 12–16 ounces of water

Toss a large green salad with mixed greens, avocado, carrots, cucumbers, celery, tomatoes, red cabbage, red peppers, red onions, sprouts, 2 ounces of canned beans (black, garbanzo, and pinto), and 4 ounces of low-mercury, high-omega-3 canned tuna.

For the salad dressing, mix extra-virgin olive oil, apple-cider vinegar or lemon juice, naturally brewed soy sauce, liquid aminos, Celtic Sea Salt, herbs, and spices, or mix 1 tablespoon of extra-virgin olive oil with 1 tablespoon of a healthy store-bought dressing.

One piece of fruit in season

Supplement for your perfect weight: Take two or three whole-food multivitamin caplets and one to three capsules of concentrated fucoxanthin.

Perfect Snack (approximately 3:30 p.m.)
Drink for your perfect weight: 8–12 ounces of water

A half-box to one box of Rainforest Cacao Chocolate Macadamia Nuts

or

One serving of Perfect Meal vanilla-flavoured meal supplement with native whey protein and glucomannan fibre mixed with 12 ounces of water

Dinner (approximately 6:15 p.m., but try to finish eating dinner by 7:00 p.m.)
Drink for your perfect weight: 12–16 ounces of water

Red meat steak (beef, buffalo, or venison)

Sautéed spinach

Mashed potatoes with butter

Toss a green salad with mixed greens, avocado, carrots, cucumbers, celery, tomatoes, red cabbage, red peppers, red onions, and sprouts.

For the salad dressing, mix extra-virgin olive oil, apple-cider vinegar or lemon juice, naturally brewed soy sauce, liquid aminos, Celtic Sea Salt, herbs, and spices, or mix 1 tablespoon of extra-virgin olive oil with 1 tablespoon of a healthy store-bought dressing.

Supplement for your perfect weight: Take two or three whole-food multivitamin caplets, one to three capsules of concentrated fucoxanthin, and 1 to 3 teaspoons (or three to nine capsules) of a high omega-3 cod liver oil complex.

Before bed

Think for your perfect weight: Perform the Healing Codes Exercise on page 189.

Drink for your perfect weight: 8–12 ounces of water (optional, of course)

Get FIT for your perfect weight: Perform five minutes of deep-breathing exercises by taking a slow, five-second breath in through your nose (inhale), holding for one second, followed by a forceful quick exhale through your mouth, completely emptying your lungs with each exhalation and completely filling your lungs with each inhalation. Repeat for two to five minutes.

Sleep for your perfect weight: Go to bed by 10:30 p.m.

Male Potato Type
Phase IV (Weeks 13–16)

For Phase IV, you have some options. If you are satisfied with your progress, you should continue on the Phase III plan and finish strong. If you feel that your weight loss has slowed or you liked the way you felt on Phase I or II, you are welcome to repeat one of those phases for the final four weeks.

Appendix A

Perfect Recipes From Chef Carol

YOU READ MUCH of Chef Carol Green's compelling story in chapter 11, "Think for Your Perfect Weight." She was raised on a farm in rural South Africa, surrounded by the rhythms of the seasons. Her budding culinary skills were first professionally put to the test when she followed her spirit of adventure and began cooking onboard mega-yachts in the Caribbean.

To truly understand the foundation of good food, she took a hiatus and studied the art of French cuisine and *patisserie* at the *Ecole des Arts Culinaires* in Lyon, France. I first met Carol when I was invited to speak in South Africa in 2006 and was told of her great talent in the kitchen. I asked Carol if she would come to United States and appear on my television show, *Extraordinary Health*, seen weekly on the Trinity Broadcast Network and other cable outlets. Carol and I do these wonderful cooking segments, but the best part is when the cameras are turned off and I get to dig in to the appetizing entrees and dishes that she's prepared.

Below are just sixteen examples of delicious and nutritious recipes created by Chef Carol. For many more of Carol's mouth-watering recipes, visit www.PerfectWeightCanada.com.

Baked Eggs in Tomato Cups With Sautéed Spinach	
4 tomatoes	4 eggs
8 Tbsp. parmesan cheese (raw pecorino)	8 oz. spinach
2 cloves garlic, minced	1 tbsp. Garden of Life Coconut Oil
Herbamare seasoning, as needed	

SPECIAL EQUIPMENT: Muffin tins

Preheat oven to 400°F. Cut off tops of tomatoes, and scoop out all the flesh with a spoon. Place tomatoes in muffin tins and gently break an egg in each one. Sprinkle with Herbamare seasoning; then sprinkle 2 tablespoons of cheese over each tomato. Tent the muffin tin with foil and bake for 20 minutes, or until just set.

While eggs are baking, heat a sauté pan over medium heat, and melt the coconut oil. Add the garlic and sauté for a few minutes; then add the spinach and cook, stirring until just wilted. Season with Herbamare and serve as a side to the eggs.

Serves 4.

Chef Carol's comment: "These individual tomato cups look as good as they taste and are easy and quick to prepare. Serve with a side of sautéed spinach or mushrooms."

Nutritional facts per serving: 116 calories; 6 g fat (47.6 percent calories from fat); 9 g protein; 7 g carbohydrate; 1 g dietary fiber; 191 mg cholesterol; 160 mg sodium.

Perfect Blueberry Clouds

¼ cup hot water

1 cup blueberry juice

1 cup frozen blueberries

4 Tbsp. fresh blueberries, for garnish

1 envelope unflavored beef gelatin

1 cup ice water

2 scoops Garden of Life Perfect Meal Vanilla

Pour hot water into cup, and sprinkle the gelatin over; stir to dissolve. Add blueberry juice and refrigerate until "wobbly," about 1 hour. Then place the jelly in blender and blend on high; add ice water and frozen blueberries. Then add Garden of Life Perfect Meal Vanilla, and blend until fluffy. Serve immediately or pour into individual ramekins and allow to set. Top with reserved fresh blueberries.

Serves 6.

Chef Carol's comment: "The first phase of the Perfect Weight America program is the most challenging. Here is a fluffy and light delicious treat to reward the effort."

Nutritional facts per serving: 114 calories; trace fat (2.8 percent calories from fat); 4 g protein; 24 g carbohydrate; 3 g dietary fiber; 0 mg cholesterol; 53 mg sodium.

Cucumber and Tomato Tzatziki

3 cups Greek yogurt

3 Tbsp. dill, fresh chopped

1 large tomato, chopped fine

1 cucumber

1 clove garlic, minced

Sea salt and pepper as needed

SPECIAL EQUIPMENT: 2 strainers, cheesecloth

Place a strainer over a medium bowl and line with cheesecloth. Spoon yogurt into the lined strainer, and allow to stand at room temperature to drain, about 3 hours. Coarsely grate cucumber, place in another strainer, and let stand at room temperature until most of the liquid drains out, about 3 hours. Discard extra liquids. Mix yogurt and cucumber with dill, garlic, and tomato. Season with salt and pepper.

Serves 6.

Chef Carol's comment: "Diced tomatoes make a colorful addition to this classic Greek yogurt sauce, wonderful when served with fish."

Nutritional facts per serving: 91 calories; 4 g fat (39.9 percent calories from fat); 5 g protein; 9 g carbohydrate; 1 g dietary fiber; 16 mg cholesterol; 63 mg sodium.

Fragrant Chicken and Pineapple Broth Bowl

1 small pineapple

2 Tbsp. Garden of Life Extra-Virgin Coconut Oil

4 cups filtered water

½ pounds of shiitake mushroom, sliced ½-inch thick

2 cloves garlic, minced	2 Tbsp. roasted red chili paste
2 inches fresh ginger, finely grated	3 spring onions, cut on bias
1 stalk lemongrass, crushed	2 skinless boneless chicken breasts, cubed
¼ cup tamari soy sauce	2 limes, zested and juiced
½ tsp. stevia	1 cup bean sprouts
½ cup cilantro, rough chopped	½ cup basil, julienned

Peel and core pineapple; set aside the core and chop the flesh into ¼-inch pieces. Rough chop the core; then place in a blender with 4 cups of water and blend well. Strain through a fine sieve and discard the solids.

Place a stockpot over medium high heat, add the coconut oil. Sauté mushrooms and garlic until softened. Add chili paste, ginger, and spring onions; sauté 1 minute more. Add pineapple broth and lemongrass. Bring to a slow simmer, and cook 10 minutes. Add chicken cubes, and cook until just done, about 3 minutes. Add tamari sauce, lime juice, and a touch of zest. Sweeten with the herbal supplement stevia and salt to taste. Discard lemongrass stalk. Divide into large, deep soup bowls and heap bean sprouts, cilantro, and basil on top.

Serves 4.

Chef Carol's comment: "Light and satisfying, broths are a great way to assist weight loss. Don't let the long list of ingredients deter you from making this wonderful dish. It takes minutes to assemble and can be made with fewer ingredients."

Nutritional facts per serving: 438 calories; 5 g fat (9.7 percent calories from fat); 46 g protein; 80 g carbohydrate; 13 g dietary fiber; 71 mg cholesterol; 2376 mg sodium.

Herbed Pesto

1 cup fresh basil leaves, packed	½ cup parsley leaves, packed
1 Tbsp. fresh thyme leaves	1 Tbsp. fresh oregano leaves
¼ cup fresh mint leaves	½ cup grated Parmesan cheese
1 head garlic, chopped	½ cup pine nuts
½ cup olive oil	

SPECIAL EQUIPMENT: Food processor

In food processor, blend all ingredients with a pinch of salt and pepper until smooth. Place in storage container and drizzle a little extra olive oil over the top to keep.

Serves 6.

Chef Carol's comment: "Fresh, bright herb pesto, a versatile ingredient to keep on hand in your refrigerator."

Nutritional facts per serving: 144 calories; 15 g fat (92.4 percent calories from fat); 2 g protein; 1 g carbohydrate; trace dietary fiber; 54 mg cholesterol; 94 mg sodium.

Mayan Gold Perfect Meal Chocolate Smoothie

4 scoops Garden of Life Perfect Meal Chocolate	2 cups plain full-fat kefir
2 cups ice water	1 cup ice cubes

1 cup organic fresh squeezed orange juice	3 tsp. orange zest
1 tsp. cinnamon	¼ tsp. nutmeg
Pinch chili powder	

Place all ingredients in blender; blend well. Serve immediately.

Serves 4.

Chef Carol's comment: "Delicious smoothies featuring Garden of Life Perfect Meal, influenced by flavors of the Incas."

Nutritional facts per serving: 184 calories; 5 g fat (14.7 percent calories from fat); 13 g protein; 19 g carbohydrate; trace dietary fiber; 30 mg cholesterol; 6 mg sodium.

Roasted Corn and Zucchini Sauté

4 ears sweet corn	4 Tbsp. Garden of Life Extra-Virgin Coconut Oil
½ cup chopped scallions	½ tsp. garlic, finely chopped
2 medium zucchini, diced	¼ tsp. ground cumin
¼ tsp. sea salt	⅛ tsp. black pepper
½ cup chopped fresh cilantro	

Rub corn with 2 tablespoons of coconut oil; roast in 400°F oven for 20 to 24 minutes, turning occasionally. Remove corn from oven and let cool. Cut corn from cob, yielding about 2 cups corn. Heat remaining oil in a 12-inch heavy skillet over moderate heat until hot, but not smoking; then cook scallions, stirring occasionally, until softened, about 3 minutes. Add garlic and cook, stirring for 1 minute.

Add corn, zucchini, cumin, salt and pepper, and cook, stirring occasionally until zucchini is tender, 4–6 minutes. Stir in cilantro and season with salt and pepper.

Serves 4.

Chef Carol's comment: "Quick and easy, roasting the corn makes all the flavor difference."

Nutritional facts per serving: 136 calories; 10 g fat (59.3 percent calories from fat); 3 g protein; 13 g carbohydrate; 2 g dietary fiber; 0 mg cholesterol; 101 mg sodium.

Southwest Chopped Chicken Salad With Whole-Grain Mustard Balsamic Dressing

4 single chicken breasts	2 Tbsp. Garden of Life Extra-Virgin Coconut Oil
½ cup balsamic vinegar	½ cup corn kernels
1½ cups black beans	¾ cup celery, diced
2 cups cherry tomatoes, halved	¼ cup green onions, minced
3 Tbsp. cilantro, rough chopped	3 Tbsp. peppadew, finely chopped
2 cups romaine lettuce, shredded	1 jalapeño chili pepper, finely diced

BEFORE BEGINNING: Peppadew is a pepper native to South Africa; it's available pickled in supermarkets across the United States.

Sauté chicken breasts in a little coconut oil over medium high heat. When almost cooked through, add balsamic vinegar to pan; allow to reduce to a syrupy consistency, turning chicken often. Remove to plate and allow to cool. Cube chicken. Toss together remaining ingredients and chicken. Serve with whole-grain balsamic dressing on the side.

For the Whole-grain Mustard Balsamic Dressing, whisk 3 tablespoons lemon juice, 2 tablespoons whole-grain mustard, ½ cup olive oil, and 1 teaspoon honey.

Serves 4.

Chef Carol's comment: "I fell in love with Tex-Mex flavors living in Texas, flavors that challenge and wake up the palate, as in this chopped salad."

Nutritional facts per serving with the dressing: 509 calories; 25 g fat (83.7 percent calories from fat); 32 g protein; 43 g carbohydrate; 9 g dietary fiber; 62 mg cholesterol; 84 mg sodium.

Grilled Chicken and Pineapple Salad With Basil and Mint

Fresh mayonnaise dressing

4 egg yolks, raw or from three-minute hard-boiled eggs

3 Tbsp. Dijon mustard

Pinch sea salt

Pinch cayenne pepper

3 Tbsp. lemon juice

1 cup extra-virgin olive oil

2 Tbsp. Garden of Life Hawaiian Lehua Honey

Marinade

4 Tbsp. lemon juice

2 Tbsp. Dijon mustard

3 Tbsp. olive oil

2 Tbsp. Garden of Life Hawaiian Lehua Honey

1 Tbsp. seafood seasoning

8 chicken breasts, boned and skinned

¼ cup green onion, chopped

3 pineapples

1 red bell pepper

½ cup celery, diced

¼ cup basil leaf, julienned

3 Tbsp. mint, chopped

SPECIAL EQUIPMENT: Food processor

To make the mayonnaise: Place egg yolks, mustard, salt, cayenne pepper, and half the lemon juice in food processor. Blend just enough to combine ingredients; then, with machine running, add olive oil in slow stream. Add remaining lemon juice and honey. The mayonnaise will be very runny, as it is mayonnaise dressing. Pour in container and store in refrigerator until needed.

Combine all marinade ingredients and whisk together.

Butterfly the chicken breasts to allow for even cooking, cover in marinade, and refrigerate overnight. Halve the pineapples, with tops intact, and scoop out the flesh in two or three large chunks using a grapefruit knife or curved paring knife. Discard the core and cut remaining pieces in ½-inch chunks. Set aside scooped out pineapple halves for use later as serving bowls.

Heat grill on high, and grill chicken breasts. Allow to cool. Then cut into 1-inch pieces and dress with mayonnaise dressing. Lightly toss chicken pieces with pineapple chunks and remaining salad ingredients. Scoop evenly into pineapple boats and serve.

Serves 6.

Chef Carol's comment: "Grilling the chicken adds a new dimension to this flavorful salad with fresh mayonnaise. Presented in pineapple boats, it is perfect for summer outdoor entertaining."

Nutritional facts per serving: 556 calories; 37 g fat (59.1 percent calories from fat); 28 g protein; 30 g carbohydrate; 3 g dietary fiber; 184 mg cholesterol; 218 mg sodium.

Perfect Blender Chocolate Mocha Mousse

½ cup strong coffee, organic, fresh-brewed, and hot

2 oz. dark chocolate bar, 80 percent cacao, finely chopped

2 scoops Garden of Life Perfect Meal Chocolate

2 oz. Garden of Life Rainforest Cacao Chocolate Brazilian Nut and Coffee

1 tsp. stevia

1 envelope beef gelatin

3 egg whites

¾ cup heavy cream

½ cup ice water

Pour hot coffee in small bowl; sprinkle the gelatin over it. Stir to dissolve. Add chopped chocolate. Stir to dissolve; then allow to cool. Pour coffee and chocolate mixture into blender. Add egg whites and blend on high for two minutes.

With the blender running, slowly add the Perfect Meal, ice water, and stevia. Add ½ cup of the heavy cream and blend to a soft creamy texture; do not overwhip, as it will clot. Pour into individual ramekins, and allow to set in refrigerator to firm. Whip remaining cream. Top each ramekin with a spoonful, and then sprinkle with Rainforest Cacao.

Serves 4.

Chef Carol's comment: "I have a terrible sweet tooth, and this quick, easy, and very luxurious dessert is a great treat. Be sure to use good quality 80 percent cacao for full flavor."

Nutritional facts per serving: 269 calories; 16 g fat (70.5 percent calories from fat); 12 g protein; 20 g carbohydrate; 5 g dietary fiber; 11 mg cholesterol; 75 mg sodium.

Baked Herbed Eggplant With Tomatoes and Caramelized Onions

2 large eggplants (approximately 3 lbs.)

⅓ cup Garden of Life Extra-Virgin Coconut Oil, as needed

4 cloves garlic, minced

4 Tbsp. fresh parsley, finely chopped

½ cup crème fraîche

¼ cup Parmesan cheese (raw pecorino), grated

Pinch sea salt and fresh ground pepper

Sea salt, sprinkled

2 medium yellow onions, halved and sliced

15 oz. fresh tomato, red ripe, chopped

½ cup whole-milk yogurt

2 Tbsp. fresh dill, finely chopped

2 Tbsp. chives, snipped

Slice eggplant into ¾-inch rounds. Lay in a colander, and sprinkle liberally with salt. Allow to rest for 30 minutes until beads appear on the flesh. Rinse lightly and pat dry. (Salting the eggplant and allowing the bitter juices to degorge also allow less oil to be used in cooking. The eggplant will cook through properly in the baking process and soak up the wonderful flavors from the tomato and onions.)

While the eggplant is resting, heat a heavy-bottom pan over medium heat; add just enough coconut oil to lightly coat the bottom. Add onions and cook, stirring occasionally, scraping the bottom of the pan with a flat wooden spoon. (This is a patient process, but it's worth it as the onions begin to caramelize in their own natural sugars.)

Remove the onions to a plate and heat a ¼-inch depth of coconut oil in the pan. Fry the eggplant slices, a few at a time, turning until golden brown. Drain on kitchen paper. Heat a little more coconut oil in another pan and sauté the garlic for a few minutes. Add the tomatoes and simmer on low heat for 15 minutes. Season with salt and pepper. Reserving half the parsley, stir together the yogurt, crème fraîche, and herbs, and season to taste.

Preheat the oven to 350°F. Line the bottom of a medium ovenproof dish with a thin layer of tomatoes. Top with a layer of eggplant, followed by onions and eggplant again. Top with the remaining tomato sauce and finish off with the yogurt sauce. Sprinkle the cheese on top and bake for 20 to 25 minutes. Scatter remaining parsley and chives on top.

Serves 4.

Chef Carol's comment: "Rich and colorful, this fabulous dish is a wonderful accompaniment to fish or alone as a main dish with a side salad. Slowly caramelizing the onions is time consuming, but it imparts a rich flavor to this dish."

Nutritional facts per serving: 290 calories; 23 g fat (65.9 percent calories from fat); 6 g protein; 20 g carbohydrate; 6 g dietary fiber; 26 mg cholesterol; 105 mg sodium.

Herb-Crusted Rack of Lamb With Port Shallot Gravy

Gravy

12 small shallots	6 cloves garlic
¼ cup balsamic vinegar	1 tsp. raw sugar
3 Tbsp. extra-virgin olive oil	3 cups lamb stock
½ cup ruby port	

2 1¼ lb racks of lamb, French trimmed	
½ cup Dijon mustard	2 cloves garlic
2 cups yeast-free sourdough bread crumbs	½ cup fresh basil leaves
½ cup fresh parsley leaves	4 small sprigs rosemary
4 small sprigs thyme	½ cup grated pecorino cheese
¼ cup olive oil	Sea salt and pepper to taste

SPECIAL EQUIPMENT: Instant red meat thermometer, food processor, and stick immersion blender

Preheat oven to 425°F.

To prepare gravy: Combine shallots, garlic, balsamic vinegar, raw sugar, and 2 tablespoons olive oil in a shallow baking pan. Roast until shallots are caramelized, stirring a few times, about 20–30 minutes. In a pan, bring port and lamb stock to the boil; simmer until reduced by half, and season. Add caramelized shallots and garlic, and blend with a stick blender. Strain and set aside.

To prepare the lamb: In food processor, mince garlic, add sourdough crumbs and grated pecorino cheese. Then add herbs, using on/off turns. With machine running, slowly add olive oil, just enough to bind the mixture together. Season with a little salt and pepper. Brush lamb with Dijon mustard; then press the crumb mixture evenly over the lamb, keeping the bones clean to prevent them from burning. Arrange bone side down on a baking sheet and roast until meat thermometer inserted into center of lamb registers 135°F for medium rare, about 25 minutes. Let lamb rest for 15 minutes; then transfer to cutting board, and cut into individual or double chops. Serve with Port Shallot gravy.

Serves 6.

Chef Carol's comment: "For an elegant presentation, ask your butcher to 'French' the rack of lamb, which is trimming the fat from the end of the bones. With an herb crust and oven roasted, this dish has rich flavor and tender consistency, and is Jordan's favorite dish I have made to date!"

Nutritional facts per serving: 748 calories; 63 g fat (74.9 percent calories from fat); 29 g protein; 19 g carbohydrate; 1 g dietary fiber; 117 mg cholesterol; 568 mg sodium.

Butternut Orange Soup

2 Tbsp. clarified butter (ghee)	1 yellow onion, rough diced
2 medium carrots, rough chopped	2 celery ribs, chopped
4 cloves garlic, minced	1 tsp. nutmeg
3 tsp. cinnamon	2 large butternut squash, peeled, rough cubed
1 large sweet potato, peeled and cubed	4 cups fresh squeezed orange juice
½ gallon chicken stock	Sea salt and pepper, to taste
1 cup heavy cream	Chives or parsley, for garnish

Heat 1 tablespoon butter in large stockpot over medium heat, add the onions, and slow cook until caramelized. Add remaining butter, carrots, celery, and garlic; cook approximately 15 more minutes. Add spices, and cook a few minutes. Add butternut squash, sweet potato, and chicken stock. Simmer approximately 1 hour until all are tender. Purée soup, add orange juice, and adjust seasoning to taste. Serve, garnished with a swirl of cream and chopped chives or parsley.

Serves 4.

Chef Carol's comment: "Warming winter soup with a new twist."

Nutritional facts per serving: 400 calories; 28 g fat (62.8 percent calories from fat); 11 g protein; 27 g carbohydrate; 4 g dietary fiber; 34 mg cholesterol; 435 mg sodium.

Cardamom Poached Pear With Chocolate Glaze and Crème Fraîche

4 pears, slightly under ripe	1 cup pear juice
¼ cup white balsamic vinegar	4 pods cardamom
¼ cup Garden of Life Hawaiian Lehua Honey	4 oz. dark chocolate bar, 80 percent cacao, grated
½ cup crème fraîche	

Keeping the stalks intact, peel pears with a vegetable peeler. Set pears aside. Stir together pear juice, vinegar, cardamom, and honey in saucepan just big enough to hold the pears on their side. Bring the liquid to a boil; then add pears to the pan. Cover and reduce heat. Simmer, turning pears twice with a rubber spatula, until they are tender, about 8 minutes. Remove pears from pan; then stand up in individual serving dishes.

Whisk chocolate into sauce until melted. Pour over pears. Serve with crème fraîche on the side.

Serves 4.

Chef Carol's comment: "An elegant dinner party dessert, the chocolate melted in the poaching liquid makes for an instant sauce."

Nutritional facts per serving: 427 calories; 18 g fat (34.9 percent calories from fat); 3 g protein; 73 g carbohydrate; 7 g dietary fiber; 27 mg cholesterol; 25 mg sodium.

Beef Tenderloin Salad With Pomegranate and Avocado

Marinade and dressing

2 Tbsp. pomegranate syrup*

3 Tbsp. tamari soy sauce

1 Tbsp. Dijon mustard

Sea salt and pepper

½ cup pomegranate juice

½ cup extra-virgin olive oil

2 tsp. red pepper flakes

1 Tbsp. Garden of Life Extra-Virgin Coconut Oil

*Note: Pomegranate syrup can be bought at specialty stores. If you can't find it, boil down pomegranate juice and reduce it to about a third of the original volume.

1½ lbs. beef tenderloin steak, grass fed

Salad

3 cups lettuce, Mache

8 oz. spinach, baby leaves

½ cup spring onion, minced

1 cup sunflower sprouts

3 cups lettuce, spring mix

3 avocados, sliced

1 cup feta cheese

1½ cups pomegranate seeds

Combine all marinade ingredients and whisk together.

Heat grill or a grill pan to high heat. Season beef steaks with salt and pepper. Add coconut oil to pan, and grill beef steaks on high, 2–3 minutes per side, until still very rare in the middle. Remove to a plate, allow to cool, and slice thinly. Spoon just enough marinade over to coat; allow to marinate for several hours.

To assemble, toss salad leaves with just enough dressing to coat. Pile on serving plate, and place beef on top. Surround with avocado slices, and sprinkle feta, sprouts, and pomegranate seeds over the top.

Serves 6.

Chef Carol's comment: "A luxurious and beautiful salad; grass-fed beef steak in a tangy pomegranate marinade, thinly sliced and served with avocado and pomegranate jewels. The marinade 'cooks' the beef, so be sure not to overcook it when searing."

Nutritional facts per serving: 605 calories; 52 g fat (74.8 percent calories from fat); 21 g protein; 18 g carbohydrate; 4 g dietary fiber; 70 mg cholesterol; 626 mg sodium.

Fettuccine With Creamy Wild Mushroom Sauce

1 cup hot water

2 lbs. mushroom, variety

2 shallots, finely chopped

¼ cup dry white wine

1 cup crème fraîche

½ cup Parmesan cheese, grated

Sea salt and pepper to taste

¼ cup dried porcini mushroom

3 Tbsp. clarified butter (ghee)

2 cloves garlic, minced

½ cup chicken stock

12 oz. fettuccine (whole wheat, spelt, or sprouted pasta)

Chives, for garnish

Pour 1 cup hot water over porcini mushrooms and allow to soak for an hour. Remove mushrooms, and strain soaking liquid through cheesecloth to remove impurities. Set aside mushroom broth for use later. Finely mince porcini mushrooms.

Slice your other mushroom selection. Heat a large heavy bottomed pan over high heat. Add a little butter and sauté mushrooms in batches. Remove from pan and set aside.

Reduce heat and sauté shallots, garlic, and porcini mushrooms until softened. Turn heat up to medium high, add white wine and reduce down to a syrupy consistency. Add chicken stock and mushroom broth; simmer until reduced by half. Return mushrooms to the pan. Add crème fraîche, season, and allow to simmer gently for 10 minutes. In the meanwhile, cook pasta in salted water to tender. Drain pasta, then toss through the sauce. Serve topped with Parmesan and snipped chives.

Serves 4.

Chef Carol's comment: "The yacht I cooked for docked in Portland, Maine, one summer, and I discovered a fabulous market with the most gorgeous and exotic mushrooms I had ever seen! After provisioning, I went back onboard and created this pasta dish for very happy guests and crew. When selecting fresh mushrooms, they should be firm to the touch and not spongy. Look out for an exotic blend readily available at many markets, such as portabella, shitake, crimini, oyster, and maitake."

Nutritional facts per serving: 595 calories; 22 g fat (41.1 percent calories from fat); 20 g protein; 80 g carbohydrate; 5 g dietary fiber; 57 mg cholesterol; 427 mg sodium.

Appendix B

Perfect Snacks From Chef Mandy

OUR RECIPES FOR perfect snacks come from Mandilyn Canistelle, a graduate of Living Light Culinary Arts Institute in Fort Bragg, California, where she received her certification as a raw food chef and instructor. Mandy teaches raw culinary arts classes in Edmond, Oklahoma, where she's a mother of five. Currently, she can be seen on my weekly television series, *Extraordinary Health*, in a segment called, "Snack in a Minute," where Mandy shares recipes for quick raw snacks on the go.

Many of these recipes entail using a dehydrator, a small home appliance for drying fresh food yourself. They come in a variety of sizes and work by very gently heating the air and blowing throughout the food drying area. They generally cost a couple of hundred dollars and up.

For more information about Mandilyn Canistelle and her booklet, *Raw Fast Food*, go online to www.chefmandy.com.

Asian Nori Crackers

Asian Nori Crackers can be made from the leftover Sunny Sunflower Pâté (page 311) by adding chickpea miso paste and spreading the mixture onto Nori sea vegetable sheets. Below is the actual recipe.

2 cups sunflower seeds, soaked overnight	1 apple, chopped
½ red onion, chopped	3 stalks celery, chopped
6 organic dill pickles or a handful of fresh dill, chopped	¼ cup any chickpea miso paste
¼ cup whole dulse	2 Tbsp. lemon juice
2 Tbsp. dulse granules	2 tsp. wasabi
¼ cup any variety of miso paste	¼ cup Garden of Life Super Seed (optional)
1 package dried Nori sheets	2 cups sesame seeds

EQUIPMENT NEEDED: Dehydrator

Soak sunflower seeds for 8 hours in filtered water. Prepare ingredients. Process all ingredients, except for Nori sheets and sesame seeds, in food processor. Spread on Nori sheets, sprinkle with sesame seeds, and dehydrate at 105° until dry. Cut into desired shapes. Store in the freezer to keep on hand.

Makes 8–10 full sheets of Nori.

Avocado Rice Boats

Cauliflower, a member of the cruciferous family, is a vegetable that is often overlooked. It is an excellent source of fiber that helps to improve colon health.

Cauliflower rice

1 head cauliflower, chopped

1 tsp. Celtic Sea Salt

1 cup pine nuts

Boat ingredients

8 avocados, diced with reserved shells

4 tomatoes, seeded, and diced

4 ears of corn, kernelled

EQUIPMENT NEEDED: Food processor

Wash and chop cauliflower. Place rice ingredients in food processor and blend until mixture is slightly crumbly and slightly sticky. Prepare boat ingredients and toss with cauliflower rice. Fill each shell and serve on a large serving platter to accommodate eight to sixteen people. Only half of the meat of each avocado will be used in this recipe. The other half can be made into guacamole for another snack.

Serves 8–16.

Fruit Roll-Ups

Fruit roll-ups can be made from leftover fresh fruit smoothies by simply adding more fruit and agave to the mixture. Below is the actual recipe for fruit roll-ups, thicker and sweeter than a typical fruit smoothie.

1 cup fresh squeezed orange juice

2 fresh bananas

1 cup desired chopped fruit: peaches, nectarines, pineapple, blueberries, strawberries, mango, etc.

2 cups grapes

¼ cup agave

EQUIPMENT NEEDED: Vita-Mix blender

Prepare orange juice and fruit. Blend ingredients in a Vita-Mix blender until smooth and creamy. Pour nine small disks for each solid dehydrator sheet without spreading or smoothing them and dehydrate at 105° until completely dry. Flipping the roll-up is not necessary. Peel the roll-up from the solid sheet when completely dry. If roll-up does not peel easily, continue drying and check every 2 hours.

Fruit roll-ups can be rolled, or cookie cutouts can entertain children with dried sheets of fruit. Store in the freezer until ready to eat.

Makes 5 trays of roll-ups.

Easy Guacamole

The U.S. government recently revised its official nutrition guidelines to urge all of us to eat more avocados because the "good" fat in avocado helps to lower cholesterol levels. The avocado is also full of vitamin E, which is wonderful for the skin.

1 Tbsp. lime juice, from fresh lime

1 tsp. garlic powder

½ tsp. ground cumin

¼ tsp. celery seed (optional)

8 ripe avocados

1 tsp. onion powder

½ tsp. Celtic Sea Salt

EQUIPMENT NEEDED: Juicing gadget, bowl, and fork

Juice lime. Mash flesh of avocados, leaving some chunky bits to add texture. Combine remaining ingredients. Serve on a top a bed of organic mixed greens with flax chips or cut-up veggies.

Makes 1 pint.

Fresh Fruit Smoothies

One of the most popular fruits, the orange is a delightful snack or recipe ingredient. Oranges are known as an excellent source of vitamin C. In addition, they contain 170 different phytonutrients.

4 cups fresh squeezed orange juice	2 cups grapes
2 cups packaged frozen tropical fruit (pineapple, blueberries, and/or strawberries)	2 frozen bananas
Nutritious whole-food powders (optional choice is Garden of Life Perfect Meal)	

EQUIPMENT NEEDED: Vita-Mix blender

Peel and freeze bananas. Blend ingredients in a Vita-Mix until smooth and creamy. Serve in a tall glass with any desired fruit toppings.

Serves 8.

Key Lime Mousse

Limes are an excellent source of vitamin C and have antioxidant and anticancer properties. They help to build a strong immune system.

3 avocados	½ cup raw agave
½ cup lime juice	2 Tbsp. lime zest
Dash Celtic Sea Salt	3 kiwis
3 bananas	6 raspberries
6 lime wedges	

EQUIPMENT NEEDED: Vita-Mix blender

Process all ingredients—except kiwis, bananas, raspberries, and lime wedges—in a Vita-Mix. Serve in a small glass dessert bowl and garnish with fruit toppings.

Serves 6.

Key Lime Tart

Key Lime Tart can be made from the leftover Key Lime Mousse by adding extra-virgin coconut oil and creamy raw honey. Below is the actual recipe for this delicious dessert.

Crust

1 cup macadamia nuts	1 cup shredded coconut
2 Tbsp. agave	1 teaspoon Celtic Sea Salt

Mousse

3 avocados	¾ cup raw agave
½ cup lime juice	2 Tbsp. lime zest
2 Tbsp. Garden of Life Extra-Virgin Coconut Oil	1 Tbsp. creamy raw honey

Dash Celtic Sea Salt   Filtered water, small amount only if needed to blend

Toppings

8 kiwis   1 cup mixture of fruit compote (bananas, lime, strawberries)

EQUIPMENT NEEDED: Vita-Mix blender and food processor

To make the crust, grind macadamia nuts with the coconut in a food processor until crumbly. Add agave and salt while the machine is running. Do not overprocess to a mush state. Remove and press into small spring form tartlets.

To make the mousse, process all ingredients in a Vita-Mix blender. Pour the mixture into the tartlets and freeze until ready to serve.

When ready to serve, pop out of the spring form tart immediately from the freezer. Do not thaw. Serve on a white plate with layered kiwis and fruit compote.

Serves 8.

Oatmeal Raisin Cookies

Oatmeal Raisin Cookies can be made from the leftover Nutty Dates (below) by adding a ripe plantain or banana and whole oats or quinoa flakes. Dates are valuable for their tonic effect. Being easily digested, they are very useful for supplying energy and treating occasional constipation since the roughage stimulates sluggish bowels.

1 cup nuts (walnuts, pecans, and/or almonds)	1 cup macadamia nuts
1 cup coconut	1 cup dates, soaked
2 Tbsp. creamy raw honey	1 very ripe plantain or banana
1 cup raisins	1 tsp. cinnamon
½ tsp. Celtic Sea Salt	1 cup whole oats or quinoa flakes
¼ cup Garden of Life Goatein (optional)	

EQUIPMENT NEEDED: Food processor

Process walnuts, pecans, and/or almonds in food processor until crumbly. Remove to large mixing bowl. Process macadamia nuts and coconut until crumbly. Add to the nut mixture. Process dates, honey, and plantain (or banana) until creamy. Add to the nut mixture. Add remaining ingredients and mix well with hands until thoroughly blended. Drop by tablespoon onto a solid sheet and dehydrate at 105° until a crust forms. Flip and crust the bottom side. Cookies will have a moist, chewy, fresh-out-of-the-oven taste on the inside with a crust on the outside.

Serve on a wood plate surrounded with other dehydrated fruit, or they can be frozen or used for a quick, easy, satisfying snack later.

Makes 2 dozen.

Nutty Dates

Macadamias contain a significant amount of protein comprising all the essential amino acids.

1 cup nuts (walnuts, pecans, and/or almonds)	1 cup macadamia nuts
1 cup shredded coconut	1 cup pitted dates, soaked

2 Tbsp. creamy raw honey

1½ tsp. Celtic Sea Salt

1 tsp. cinnamon (optional)

1 cup raisins

1 Tbsp. orange zest (optional)

¼ cup Garden of Life Super Seed (optional)

Coating

1 cup sesame seeds

1 cup finely ground coconut

EQUIPMENT NEEDED: Food processor and zester

Process walnuts, pecans, and/or almonds in food processor until crumbly. Remove to large mixing bowl. Process macadamia nuts and coconut until crumbly. Add to the nut mixture. Process dates and honey until creamy. Add to the nut mixture. Add remaining ingredients and mix well with hands until thoroughly blended. Shape into small balls and roll in sesame seeds and/or finely ground coconut.

These little morsels are wonderful to freeze and take for a quick, easy, satisfying snack.

Makes 40–50.

Pastel Parfaits

They say money doesn't grow on trees? In some islands earlier in history, whole coconuts were used as currency for the purchase of goods. Coconuts are the fruit of the coconut palm.

Creamy Coconut Sauce

2 cups young Thai coconut meat, chopped

2 Tbsp. raw cashew butter

2 Tbsp. Garden of Life Extra-Virgin Coconut Oil

¼ tsp. Celtic Sea Salt

2 Tbsp. lemon juice

2 Tbsp. creamy raw honey

1 tsp. vanilla

Fruit toppings

1 cup chopped strawberries for bottom layer

1 cup chopped peaches for top layer

1 cup shredded coconut for garnish

1 cup chopped bananas for middle layer

1 cup cluster of blueberries to top

EQUIPMENT NEEDED: Juicing gadget, bowl, and fork

Open enough young Thai coconuts for approximately 2 cups chopped coconut meat. Reserve the coconut water, if needed, for blending. Juice lemons to get 2 tablespoons lemon juice. Process sauce ingredients in Vita-Mix blender until smooth and creamy. Layer parfaits with 2 tablespoons each of strawberries, bananas, and peaches. Drizzle ¼ cup of the cream sauce over fruit. Top with 2 tablespoons each of blueberries and shredded coconut. Serve parfaits in crystal goblets.

Serves 8.

Sherbet Sundaes

Sherbet Sundaes can be made by freezing the leftovers from the Pastel Parfait sauce. Below is an actual recipe for Sherbet Sundaes with all the toppings.

Sherbet

2 cups young Thai coconut meat, chopped

2 Tbsp. raw cashew butter

2 Tbsp. lemon juice

2 Tbsp. creamy raw honey

2 Tbsp. Garden of Life Extra-Virgin Coconut Oil

¼ tsp. Celtic Sea Salt

1 tsp. vanilla

4 bananas, peeled and frozen

Strawberry Agave Sauce

2 cups chopped strawberries

¼ cup agave

Toppings

A variety of chopped nuts

Medley of fresh berries

Shredded coconut

EQUIPMENT NEEDED: Vita-Mix blender, citrus juicer, any Twin Gear or Champion juicer

To make the sherbet, open enough young Thai coconuts for approximately 2 cups chopped coconut meat. Reserve the coconut water, if needed, for blending. Juice lemons to get 2 tablespoons lemon juice. Process sherbet ingredients, except for bananas, in a Vita-Mix blender until smooth and creamy. Freeze in ice cube trays. Run through a juicer with a blank screen with frozen bananas.

To make the strawberry agave sauce, blend ingredients in a Vita-Mix until smooth.

Serve sherbet in small dessert dishes with toppings and strawberry agave sauce.

Serves 8.

Sliced Apples With Cheese

Cheeses can be made from leftover dips and dressings. The Dilly Dip (page 312) makes a great cheese by simply adding nutritional yeast flakes, miso, flax meal, and turmeric to the dip recipe. Below is the actual recipe for a cheese. The dill has also been omitted from the recipe.

¼ cup golden flaxseeds or Garden of Life Super Seed

½ cup raw tahini

1 cup chopped celery

1 pitted date, soaked

2 Tbsp. chickpea miso

1 tsp. Celtic Sea Salt

¼ cup Garden of Life Goatein (optional)

2 Tbsp. lemon juice

2 zucchini, peeled and chopped

1 clove garlic, pressed

½ cup Kal nutritional yeast flakes

1 tsp. onion powder

1 tsp. turmeric

EQUIPMENT NEEDED: Vita-Mix blender, coffee grinder, and citrus juicer

Grind golden flax seeds in a coffee grinder to make flax meal, or use Super Seed. Juice lemons. Prepare vegetables. Blend ingredients, except flax meal, until smooth and creamy. Pulse flax meal at the end or add Super Seed. Pour small disks onto solid dehydrator sheets and dehydrate at 105° until dry.

Serve with an array of fresh cut-up apples.

Serves 8.

Sunny Sunflower Pâté

Sunflower seeds are an excellent natural source of vitamin E.

2 cups sunflower seeds, soaked 8 hrs.

½ red onion, chopped

6 organic dill pickles or a handful of fresh dill, chopped

1 apple, chopped

3 stalks celery, chopped

¼ cup chickpea miso paste

¼ cup whole dulse

2 Tbsp. dulse granules

2 Tbsp. lemon juice

2 tsp. wasabi (optional)

Garnish

Garden of Life Super Seed, sprinkled

1 cup alfalfa sprouts

24 lemon swirls, or 3 per person, made from cutting a lemon slice ¾ of the way through and twisting to sit on a plate

6 tomatoes, 3 large slices per person

2 cucumbers, sliced

EQUIPMENT NEEDED: Food processor

Soak sunflower seeds for eight hours in filtered water. Prepare and process ingredients in a food processor.

Serve 3 small scoops of Sunny Sunflower Pâté on each tomato with garnishes.

Serves 8.

Taco Lettuce Wraps

Walnuts are one of the best plant sources of protein and omega-3 fatty acids. They are rich in fiber, B vitamins, magnesium, and antioxidants such as vitamin E. Walnuts also aid in the lowering of LDL cholesterol.

Taco "meat"

2 cups walnuts, soaked

⅓ cup wheat-free tamari soy sauce

½ Tbsp. coriander powder

1 bunch cilantro

1 Tbsp. cumin powder

Taco wraps and toppings

1 head romaine lettuce

3 tomatoes, sliced

3 avocados, sliced

Celtic Sea Salt to taste

EQUIPMENT NEEDED: Food processor

In the afternoon of the day before, soak walnuts overnight in filtered water.

On the day of, process taco "meat" ingredients in a food processor until the mixture resembles ground taco meat. Stop to scrape sides. Remove and set aside. Wash and choose firm crispy lettuce leaves for taco wraps. Slice avocados and tomatoes. Fill lettuce cavities with taco "meat" and top with toppings.

Serve two tacos on a white salad plate with a favorite Mexican seasoning on top.

Serves 8.

Veggies With Dilly Dip

Tahini is made from sesame seed kernels. Not only are sesame seeds a good source of manganese and copper, but they are also an excellent source of calcium, magnesium, iron, phosphorous, vitamin B_1, zinc, and dietary fiber.

Dilly Dip

½ cup raw tahini

1 cup chopped celery

2 zucchini, peeled and chopped

1 clove garlic, pressed

2 Tbsp. lemon juice

1 tsp. onion powder

¾ cup fresh dill

2 pitted dates, soaked

1 tsp. Celtic Sea Salt

1 Tbsp. Garden of Life Goatein (optional)

Veggies

4 celery stalks, julienned

2 cucumbers, sliced

1 yellow squash, julienned

1 cup mushrooms, sliced

4 carrots, julienned

2 red bell peppers, circles

1 head broccoli spears

A handful of snow peas

EQUIPMENT NEEDED: Vita-Mix blender and citrus juicer

Juice lemons. Blend Dilly Dip ingredients, except fresh dill, until smooth and creamy. Add dill and pulse until mixed throughout. Refrigerate for an hour to thicken and cool.

Serve with an array of fresh cut-up vegetables.

Serves 8.

Veggie Patties

Veggie patties can be made from the leftovers of Taco Lettuce Wraps (page 312) by adding a few ingredients. These make great raw meals to store in the freezer for a quick dinner to warm in the dehydrator and throw on a salad.

Taco "meat"

2 cups walnuts, soaked

⅓ cup wheat-free tamari soy sauce

½ Tbsp. coriander powder

½ cup flax meal

1 bunch cilantro

1 Tbsp. cumin powder

¼ cup first cold-pressed olive oil

2 Tbsp. Frontier Barbeque Seasoning

Marinated veggies

2 Tbsp. wheat-free tamari soy sauce

1 Tbsp. lemon juice

¼ cup cold-pressed olive oil

2 cups variety of chopped veggies (red bell pepper, Crimini mushrooms, red onions, and broccoli)

Toppings

1 head green leaf lettuce leaves

1 slice cheese (per person)

3 red onion rings (per person)

3 slices of small cucumbers (per person)

1 radish flower for garnish (per person)

3 slices of colored bell peppers (per person)

2 Tbsp. sprouts (per person)

1 large slice of tomato (per person)

1 dollop of guacamole (per person; see recipe on page 307)

EQUIPMENT NEEDED: Food processor

Soak walnuts in filtered water for 8 hours. Combine marinated veggie ingredients and let set in refrigerator for 4 hours.

Process "meat" ingredients in a food processor until the mixture resembles ground taco meat. Remove and mix with the veggies. Form into patties and dehydrate at 105° for 4 hours. Flip for 2–4 more hours. Patties will be moist inside and have a crust on the outside.

Serve on a white dinner plate with all the toppings.

Serves 8.

Shiitake Chow Mein

The Orient is known for healthy low-fat dishes. This one is no exception. If noodles symbolize long lifespan in the Orient, then this raw version rivals not only the classic one in taste but also in promoting longevity filled with live nutrients, enzymes, and fiber.

Noodles

2 parsnips, spiralized

1 zucchini, spiralized

½ cup julienne jicama

2 carrots, spiralized

1 cup Mung bean sprouts

Shiitake

2 cups sliced Shiitake mushrooms

2 Tbsp. Spice Hunter poultry grill/broil

Fresh ground pepper, to taste (optional)

2 Tbsp. Spice Hunter poultry seasoning

Celtic Sea Salt, to taste (optional)

Oriental Dressing

1 green onion, chopped

2 Tbsp. minced scallion

2 Tbsp. wheat-free tamari soy sauce

1 Tbsp. Garden of Life Hawaiian Lehua Honey

2 Tbsp. toasted sesame oil

3 sprigs cilantro leaves

1 Tbsp. minced cilantro

1½ Tbsp. lemon juice

1 tsp. minced ginger

1 Tbsp. raw sesame oil

Seed garnish

2 Tbsp. hulled sesame or hemp seeds

2 Tbsp. Garden of Life Super Seed

EQUIPMENT NEEDED: Vita-Mix, chef knife, peeler or paring knife, spiralizer, shredder or kitchen shears

To make noodles, spiralize, combine, and cut long noodles; then set aside in mixing bowl. To make Shiitake, combine ingredients and toss with noodles. To make the dressing, blend ingredients in a Vita-Mix and coat the noodles.

Serve on a bowl of noodles garnished with hemp seeds, sesame seeds, and Super Seed.

Serves 8.

Vietnamese Spring Rolls

Vietnamese Spring Rolls are fun to create and a beautiful way to present a salad.

Vegetable filling

2 cups leftover Shiitake Chow Mein

4 cups Mung bean sprouts

1 small bunch cilantro

3 green onions, slivered

1 cup fresh mint leaves

2 heads Napa cabbage

Mock chicken filling

2 cups sliced shitake mushrooms

2 Tbsp. Spice Hunter poultry grill and broil

Fresh ground pepper, to taste

2 Tbsp. Spice Hunter poultry seasoning

Celtic Sea Salt, to taste

Other ingredients

8 Vietnamese wrappers

1 cup Tahini Ginger Sauce (below)

1 cup leftover Oriental Dressing (above)

Equipment: Chef knife, spiralizer, or shredder

Prepare vegetable ingredients and create an assembly line for quick stacking. Dip wrapper in a tray of filtered water. Lay the wrapper on a flat clean surface. Lay two Napa leaves on the bottom half of the rice wrapper. Layer ingredients inside the leaves. Fold in the sides and tightly roll the wrapper, being careful not to rip the wrapper. Slant cut the roll and stack the two halves on top of one another.

Serve stacked on top of each other with a side of Oriental Dressing and Tahini Ginger Sauce.

Serves 8.

Tahini Ginger Sauce

Tahini is a source of calcium, protein, B vitamins, and essential fatty acids, which help to maintain healthy skin. It is a wonderful alternative to peanut butter.

½ cup raw tahini

2 Tbsp. lemon juice

2 Tbsp. Garden of Life Hawaiian Lehua Honey

1 Tbsp. minced ginger

¼ cup filtered water

2 cloves garlic, pressed

2 Tbsp. wheat-free tamari soy sauce

2 Tbsp. Perfect Meal (optional)

EQUIPMENT NEEDED: Vita-Mix blender

Blend all ingredients until smooth. Add more filtered water, if needed.

Dip Vietnamese Spring Rolls into this sauce that rivals the classic peanut sauce.

Serves 8.

Clean Green Sweep

Green smoothies are an excellent meal choice because they provide healthy carbohydrates, vitamins, minerals, phytochemicals, and chlorophyll. They are also an excellent source of fiber. Favorite nutritious powders can be added for cleansing and extra nutrition.

Green Smoothie Base

2 bananas, peeled and frozen

2 cups fresh pineapple

1 cup green chard

2 cups green grapes

1 small cucumber, chopped

Crushed ice, as needed

Garden of Life Products

1 scoop DetoxiFiber

4 packets of Green Tea

EQUIPMENT NEEDED: Vita-Mix blender

Peel and freeze bananas the night before. Blend all ingredients in a Vita-Mix until smooth and creamy.

Serve in a tall glass with a straw.

Serves 8.

Garden of Life Bread

Garden of Life Bread can be made from leftover Clean Green Sweep.

2 cups Clean Green Sweep   ¼ cup Garden of Life Super Seed

EQUIPMENT NEEDED: Vita-Mix blender or fork or spoon to mix

Mix or blend the ingredients until mixture is a batter texture. Spread a ¼-inch thick layer of batter on solid sheet and dehydrate at 105° for 4 hours. Flip and continue drying. Bread will be moist. Slice into sandwich slices and store in the freezer until ready to eat.

Serve with Garden of Life Green Tea and Jammin' Fruit Spread for the perfect snack.

Serves 8.

Apple Pear Sauce

An apple a day truly keeps the doctor away. Apples help weight control, provide insoluble and soluble fibre, and help relieve occasional constipation. The pectin in apples reduces cholesterol. This is a fresher, tastier applesauce to encourage eating apples.

2 cups apples, peeled and chopped   2 cups pears, peeled and chopped

1 banana, peeled and sliced   1 tsp. lemon juice

Cinnamon, sprinkled to taste   Garden of Life Super Seed, sprinkled

EQUIPMENT NEEDED: Vita-Mix blender or food processor

Process ingredients in food processor until desired texture is achieved. Refrigerate until ready to serve.

Sprinkle with cinnamon. Serve as a comfort healthy snack, especially in fall or winter.

Makes 1 quart.

Apple Spice Cake

Apple Spice Cake can be made from leftover Apple Pear Sauce.

Cake layers

2 cups Apple Pear Sauce   1 cup soaked and dried pecans, ground

6 dates, soaked, or ⅓ cup date paste   1 scoop Garden of Life Super Seed

1 Tbsp. cinnamon   1 Tbsp. vanilla

½ tsp. Celtic Sea Salt

Icing

2 cups pine nuts, soaked   2 pears, peeled and chopped

¼ cup Garden of Life Hawaiian Lehua Honey   2 Tbsp. Garden of Life Extra-Virgin Coconut Oil

Topping

1 cup pecans and walnuts, mixed, chopped   ¼ cup Garden of Life Hawaiian Lehua Honey

1½ tsp. cinnamon   ½ tsp. Celtic Sea Salt

Garnish

1 full slice of pear with stem and seeds (per person)   Cinnamon sprinkles (per person)

EQUIPMENT NEEDED: Vita-Mix blender or food processor

Blend cake layer ingredients until smooth. Spread 2 cups cake batter on a solid sheet and dehydrate at 105° for four hours. Flip and continue until dry.

Blend icing ingredients in Vita-Mix blender until smooth, reserving some for garnishing slices. Place in freezer to firm up while layers are drying. Assemble cake, alternating between cake layers and icing until 3 to 4 inches in height. Freeze and slice for a quick healthy dessert to serve.

Combine topping and place in freezer to firm. When ready to serve, remove cake and slice while frozen to reveal the beautiful layers.

Sprinkle Apple Spice Cake with topping, and garnish with a slice of pear and sprinkled cinnamon. Drizzle with reserved icing.

Serves 8.

Sunny Bunny

Sunny Bunny is the perfect juice to introduce any age to the world of juicing. Oranges and carrots are sweet and supply vitamin C, beta-carotene, and antioxidants.

16 carrots, peeled and chopped	8 oranges, juiced

EQUIPMENT NEEDED: Twin Gear juicer and/or citrus juicer

Push ingredients separately through juicer to extract the juice. Keep carrot pulp separate to make other recipes. Optional method would be to juice the oranges in a citrus juicer.

Serve fresh squeezed juice in an elegant glass and sip slowly.

Serves 8.

Salmon Pâté

Salmon Pâté may look like a lot of work, but this tasty treat is worth it. This recipe can be made from leftover Sunny Bunny for a new creation.

Flaxnaise

1 cup filtered water	¼ cup lemon juice
2 tsp. ground mustard powder	1 Tbsp. Garden of Life Hawaiian Lehua Honey
¼ cup golden flaxseeds, soaked, or ½ cup Garden of Life Super Seed	½ tsp. Celtic Sea Salt

Pâté

1½ cups carrot pulp	¾ cup Flaxnaise (from recipe above)
¾ cup minced onion	1 cup chopped dill
2 Tbsp. minced garlic	1 Tbsp. dulse

EQUIPMENT NEEDED: Vita-Mix blender

To make Flaxnaise, grind flaxseeds to a meal or use Garden of Life Super Seed. Blend soaked seeds with lemon juice in a Vita-Mix blender until whipped to a cream. Add filtered water, if needed, to prevent thickening. Texture should be smooth, not jelly like. Add remaining ingredients, and mix until blended.

To make pâté, prepare ingredients and combine in a mixing bowl. Refrigerate to chill.

Serve pâté with flax crackers or flat bread, wrapped in a romaine leaf or a Nori sheet.

Serves 8.

Salmon Sushi

Salmon Sushi can be made from leftover Salmon Pâté for a new creation.

Rolls

2 cups Salmon Pâté (page 317)

2 carrots, shredded or julienned

2 cups alfalfa sprouts, or any variety sprouts

2 mangos, julienned

2 red bell peppers, julienned

2 avocados, julienned

2 cucumbers, seeded and thinly sliced

8 Nori seaweed sheets

Condiments

Wheat-free tamari

Wasabi

Pickled ginger

EQUIPMENT NEEDED: Food processor

Prepare ingredients. To assemble rolls, lay one sheet of Nori, shiny side down. Layer ingredients stacked atop 2–3 rows, on one-third of the Nori sheet closest to you. To roll the sushi, grip the edge of the Nori sheet with your thumbs and forefingers. Press the filling back with your other fingers. Roll the front end of the Nori over the filling. Pull the Nori back with your fingers, giving the roll a tight squeeze, and continue rolling. Seal the edge with water and set seam side down. Cut the roll into 8 pieces with a sharp knife.

Serve sushi with condiments for a satisfying flavorful snack or light meal.

Serves 8.

Break-Fast Salad

This salad is a great way to break a liquid fast. Dressing is not needed or missed because it satisfies every taste bud. The salad can be eaten any time during the day and can even replace a typical breakfast. Keep prepared ingredients refrigerated for easy assembly.

2 green leaf lettuce leaves, shredded

1 carrot, shredded

1 stalk celery, diced

1 peach or persimmon, diced

2 bananas, diced

4 small radishes, diced

1 avocado, diced

Garden of Life Super Seed, sprinkled

1 slice red cabbage, shredded

1 tomato, diced

1 plum or pear, diced

¼ cup raisins

8 dates, diced

1 apple, shredded

½ cup walnuts, chopped

Garden of Life DetoxiFiber, sprinkled

EQUIPMENT NEEDED: Chef knife

Layer ingredients in listed order, going from left to right. Arrange salad to include all the ingredients for a colorful display on a white dinner plate. Sprinkle Super Seed and DetoxiFiber over the salad.

Serves 8.

Zucchini Bisque

This soup is a rich and creamy soup without the extra fat. Zucchini contains large amounts of folate, potassium, and magnesium.

6 zucchini, peeled and chopped

3 cloves garlic, pressed

¼ cup chickpea miso

6 stalks celery, chopped

¼ cup lemon juice, from fresh lemon

3 cups water, add to thin

Garnish

4 tomatoes, seeded and diced

Garden of Life Super Seed, sprinkled

Garden of Life Extra-Virgin Coconut Oil, drizzled

EQUIPMENT NEEDED: Citrus juicer and Vita-Mix blender

Juice lemon and prepare vegetables. Blend first six ingredients in Vita-Mix blender until smooth. Chill to refrigerate or warm on a stovetop to 100°, stirring constantly.

Serve soup with diced tomatoes and Garden of Life Extra-Virgin Coconut Oil and Super Seed.

Serves 8.

Bounty Bars

Bounty Bars can be made from leftover Break-Fast Salad for a new creation.

2 cups Break-Fast Salad (page 318)

1 cup soaked pitted dates or date paste

2 Tbsp. cinnamon

2 cups mixture of seeds, soaked (sesame, flax, sunflower, and pumpkin)

½ Tbsp. Celtic Sea Salt

1 cup raisins or other choice of dried fruit

4 packages of Garden of Life Rainforest Cacao Chocolate

EQUIPMENT NEEDED: Dehydrator with solid and mesh sheets, and metal spatula

To make date paste, process or mash pitted and soaked dates to form a paste. Mix everything in a large mixing bowl with hands. Spread 6 cups of the mixture onto a solid dehydrator sheet. Smooth with a metal spatula and score into bars. Dehydrate at 105° for four hours. Flip and continue until dry.

Store bars in freezer container and keep frozen until ready to snack.

Serves 8.

ALT

ALTs (avocado, lettuce, and tomatoes) are made with zucchini wraps.

Flaxnaise

¼ cup golden flaxseeds or ½ cup Garden of Life Super Seed

1 cup filtered water

2 tsp. ground mustard powder

¼ cup lemon juice

1 Tbsp. Garden of Life Hawaiian Lehua Honey

½ tsp. Celtic Sea Salt

Filling

2 avocados, sliced

1 cup alfalfa sprouts

Mrs. Dash seasoning, to taste

2 cups mixed greens

2 tomatoes, sliced

EQUIPMENT NEEDED: Dehydrator, coffee grinder, or Vita-Mix blender

Prepare filling ingredients. To make Flaxnaise, grind flaxseeds to a meal or use Garden of Life Super Seed. Blend ingredients in a Vita-Mix blender. Texture should be smooth and not a jelly texture. Add more filtered water to prevent thickening. Fill wraps with filling and drizzle immediately with Flaxnaise.

Serve wraps as a light meal or quick snack.

Serves 8.

Tomatillo Salsa

This unique low-fat salsa explodes with flavor, using only fresh vegetables and herbs. *Tomatillo* means "little tomato" in Spanish. They are rich in potassium and have only 11 calories. In addition, tomatillos contain vitamins C and A, calcium, and folic acid.

6 tomatillos, chopped	3 red peppers, chopped
1 yellow sweet onion, chopped	1 anise bulb, chopped
2 Tbsp. ginger, minced	1 clove garlic, minced
¼ cup mixture of freshly minced thyme, basil, rosemary, and sage	

EQUIPMENT NEEDED: Food processor or chef knife

Pulse-chop all ingredients in food processor to reach a fresh salsa texture. Alternate method: dice all ingredients and toss. Refrigerate to blend flavors. Serve with fresh corn chips in a wooden chip and dip bowl.

Makes 1 pint.

Kim-Chi

Kim-Chi is made from leftover Tomatillo Salsa. Fermented foods are full of live enzymes and healthy flora to help digestion.

1 large head of cabbage, shredded with several reserved outside leaves	½ cup mixture of freshly minced thyme, basil, rosemary, and sage
1 head broccoli, chopped	1 cup chopped dandelion greens
1–2 cups lemon juice	2 Tbsp. ginger, pressed
2 cups Tomatillo Salsa (above)	2 cloves garlic, minced
1 Tbsp. celery seed	4 carrots, chopped

EQUIPMENT NEEDED: Chef knife and/or food processor and citrus juicer

Slice cabbage, carrots, broccoli, and dandelion greens through a food processor using the slicing attachment. Juice lemons. Combine remaining ingredients and massage to wilt. Place slaw half way full in a clean glass jar(s). Cover slaw and juices with reserved cabbage leaves to prevent spoilage. Place a smaller jar full of water with a lid inside to weigh down the slaw. Be careful to completely cover the mixture with the juices to prevent spoilage. Cover with a clean food cloth and place in a dark area such as an unused oven. Allow to ferment for 3 to 7 days. Daily check slaw for liquid coverage. Slaw will expand. Refrigerate when desired fermentation has been achieved.

Serve on a wooden dish along side flax crackers and a raw soup for a simple lunch.

Serves 8.

Korean Flax Crackers

Korean Flax Crackers are made from leftover Kim-Chi with flaxseed added.

2 cups Kim-Chi (page 320)	2 cups flaxseeds, soaked
¼ cup Garden of Life Super Seed	1 tsp. Celtic Sea Salt

EQUIPMENT NEEDED: Chef knife, spatula, dehydrator, and solid and mesh sheet

Combine ingredients and spread 3 cups mixture onto a solid sheet. Dehydrate at 105° for four hours and flip. Continue drying until crispy. Korean Flax Crackers can be stored in the pantry or freezer.

Serves 8.

Appendix C

PWC Resource Guide

THIS RESOURCE SECTION contains contact information for manufacturers and distributors of products recommended for the Perfect Weight Canada program. To the best of our abilities, we are suggesting well-established companies whose health goals match up with ours, but our Canadian readers must note that I am not well-versed enough to suggest Canadian companies or vendors for this resource guide. In addition, we cannot be held responsible for any possible consequences relating to the eating or ingestion of foods and/or supplements.

You will note that products from Garden of Life are recommended. In the interest of full disclosure, Jordan Rubin founded this company following his illness when he had trouble finding the nutritional supplements and superfoods that his body needed. Using his knowledge gained from years of studying health and wellness, Jordan set out to create high-quality functional foods, nutritional supplements, and educational resources to help you on your road to optimal health. All other products are recommended without compensation.

We believe that no matter which company you choose to purchase from, you will be well served on your road to vibrant health. Keep in mind that if you don't find these foods, supplements, or products in your local supermarket, natural food store, or vitamin store, you can purchase them by mail order or through online retailers. Also, if you have any questions, many of these companies can be reached via e-mail, usually through the company's Web site or by typing info@ plus the company's Web site (example: info@gardenoflife.com).

The importance of shopping for locally grown organic fruits, vegetables, and dairy cannot be underestimated. Several Web sites are tremendous resources:

- www.localharvest.org
- www.eatwild.com
- www.realmilk.com

Breads and Other Grain Products

Food for Life Baking Co.
P. O. Box 1434
Corona, CA 92878
(800) 797-5090
www.foodforlife.com

Food for Life, makers of Ezekiel 4:9 breads, English muffins, and tortillas, is an excellent supplier of grain products. Easily digestible, well tolerated by many who suffer from digestive ailments and allergies, and high in protein and fibre, Food for Life products truly provide the bread of life.

French Meadow Bakery
2610 Lyndale Ave. South
Minneapolis, MN 55408
(877) NO-YEAST (669-3278)
www.frenchmeadow.com

Food for Life and French Meadow products are found in natural food stores and grocery stores nationwide.

Whole-Food Nutrition Bars

Perfect Weight America Bars by Garden of Life
(800) 622-8986
www.gardenoflife.com

Perfect Weight America Bars are made with organic foods such as chia seeds, raw honey, nuts, coconut oil, and high-quality protein. Perfect Weight America Bars contain fucoxanthin, which has been shown to support fat loss and increase metabolism, and they are high in fibre and protein.

Available in natural food stores and via mail-order catalogues and online retailers.

Living Foods Nutrition Bars by Garden of Life
(800) 622-8986
www.gardenoflife.com

Living Foods Nutrition Bars are made with organic foods such as sprouted grains and seeds, raw honey, dates, cultured vegetables, nuts, berries, green foods, and coconut. Living Foods Nutrition Bars contain beta glucans from soluble oat fibre, high-quality protein, live probiotics, antioxidants, and more.

Living Foods Nutrition Bars are great for all ages and support overall health by supporting healthy serum cholesterol and triglycerides, promoting maintenance of healthy blood sugar levels, supporting healthy immune function, and aiding in maintenance of healthy body weight.

Available in natural food stores and via mail-order catalogues and online retailers.

Cacao/Trail Mix

Rainforest Cacao by Garden of Life
(800) 622-8986
www.gardenoflife.com

Rainforest Cacao Chocolate is all-natural, roasted cacao beans harvested from the Ecuadorian Amazon. These all-natural beans are treated with extreme care at the time of harvest and then undergo minimal processing to ensure they maintain their maximum nutritional values, which includes heart-healthy antioxidants.

Available in natural food stores and via mail-order catalogues and online retailers.

Meal Supplements

Perfect Meal by Garden of Life
(800) 622-8986
www.gardenoflife.com

Perfect Meal is a delicious and satisfying high-protein and high-fibre drink designed to be used as a meal supplement, available in two healthy and delicious flavours: creamy vanilla and milk chocolate. As part of a healthy diet and exercise program, Perfect Meal will help you successfully manage your weight by naturally curbing your appetite.

Available in natural food stores and via mail-order catalogues and online retailers.

Dairy Products

The following companies produce natural and organic milk, butter, cheese, cream, cottage cheese, yogurt, kefir, soft cheese, and buttermilk that are either available in natural food stores or by mail order.

Old Chatham Sheepherding Company
155 Shaker Museum Rd.
Old Chatham, NY 12136
(888) SHEEP-60 (743-3760)
www.blacksheepcheese.com

Old Chatham makes the finest quality sheep's milk yogurt and cheese. This is the yogurt favoured by the Rubin family. Available via mail order or in select natural food stores.

Amaltheia Dairy
3380 Penwell Bridge Rd.
Belgrade, MT 59714
(406) 388-5950
www.amaltheiadairy.com

Grade A goat's dairy kefir and cheeses. Available via mail order and in select natural food stores.

Destiny Dairy
27367 WCR 74
Eaton, CO 80615
(970) 454-9009
www.destinydairy.com

Organic goat's milk dairy of the highest quality. Easily digestible and rich in protein with probiotics and beneficial fatty acids. Offerings include yogurt smoothies, goat's milk, cheese, and ice cream. Available via mail order by calling or by ordering online at the Web address listed above.

Organic Pastures Dairy Co.
7221 South Jameson Ave.
Fresno, CA 93706
(877) RAW-MILK (729-6455)
www.organicpastures.com

Coconut Milk

Thai Kitchen Coconut Milk
Simply Asia Foods, Inc.
30315 Union City Blvd.
Union City, CA 94587
(800) 967-8424
www.thaikitchen.com

Thai Kitchen products are available in natural food stores.

Eggs

Gold Circle Farms
310 N. Harbor Blvd., Suite 205
Fullerton, CA 92832
(888) 599-4DHA (599-4342)
www.goldcirclefarms.com

DHA omega-3 eggs available in natural food stores and grocery stores.

Organic Valley
One Organic Way
La Farge, WI 54639
(888) 444-6455
www.organicvalley.coop

Certified organic high omega-3 eggs. Available in natural food stores and grocery stores.

Red Meats

Wyoming Natural Products Co.
P. O. Box 962
Newcastle, WY 82701
(800) 969-9946
www.wyomingnatural.com

Grass-fed beef available in select natural food stores and via mail order.

Maverick Ranch Natural Meats
5360 North Franklin St.
Denver, CO 80216
(800) 497-2624
www.maverickranch.com

Natural beef, chicken, lamb, and buffalo. Available in grocery stores.

Coleman Purely Natural Products
1767 Denver West Marriott Rd., Suite 200
Golden, CO 80401
(800) 442-8666
www.colemannatural.com

Naturally raised, hormone- and antibiotic-free beef products. Available in natural food stores.

Northstar Bison
1936 28th Ave.
Rice Lake, WI 54868
(888) 295-6332
www.northstarbison.com

One hundred percent grass-fed and finished bison meat.

Chicken

Oaklyn Plantation
1312 Oaklyn Rd.
Darlington, SC 29532
(843) 395-0793
www.freerangechicken.com

Free-range chickens and chicken feet (hormone- and antibiotic-free). Available via mail order.

Bell & Evans
154 W. Main St.
Fredericksburg, PA 17026
(717) 865-6626
www.bellandevans.com

Fresh and frozen natural poultry products. Available in natural food stores and grocery stores.

Deli Meat

Applegate Farms
750 Rt. 202 South, Suite 300
Bridgewater, NJ 08807
(866) 587-5858
www.applegatefarms.com

Packaged meats and deli slices (nitrate- and nitrite-free). Available in natural food stores and grocery stores.

Frozen Fish

Ecofish, Inc.
340 Central Ave.
Dover, NH 03820
(877) 214-3474
www.ecofish.com

Ocean-caught salmon, halibut, tuna, and other fish. Available in natural food stores and grocery stores.

Vital Choice Seafood
605 30th St.

Anacortes, WA 98221
(800) 608-4825
www.vitalchoice.com

Available in natural food stores.

Crown Prince
18581 Railroad Street
City of Industry, CA 91748
(626) 912-3700
www.crownprince.com

Canned sardines, salmon, tuna, and other fish. Available in natural food stores and grocery stores.

Sweeteners

Honey

Hawaiian Lehua Honey by Garden of Life
(800) 622-8986
www.gardenoflife.com

This certified organic honey comes from the island of Hawaii. Hawaiian Lehua Honey contains antioxidants, enzymes, vitamins, and minerals, providing all of the benefits that make honey a superfood from the hive. This raw, unheated honey is the original sweetener used for thousands of years and is a superb resource to sweeten smoothies, yogurt, tea, and coffee. This honey is also an important ingredient in many of the delicious recipes you'll find in this book.

Available in natural food stores and via mail-order catalogues and online retailers.

Salad Mixes (prewashed)

Earthbound Farm
1721 San Juan Highway
San Juan Bautista, CA 95045

(800) 690-3200
www.ebfarm.com

Fresh, packaged organic produce available in natural food and grocery stores.

Vegetables (including raw fermented)

Earthbound Farm
1721 San Juan Highway
San Juan Bautista, CA 95045
(800) 690-3200
www.ebfarm.com

Fresh, organic produce available in natural food and grocery stores.

Rejuvenative Foods
P. O. Box 8464
Santa Cruz, CA 95061
(800) 805-7957
www.rejuvenative.com

Rejuvenative Foods produces high-quality raw foods such as sauerkraut, kimchi, "live" salsas, nut and seed butters, chocolate spreads, raw oils, and more. Available in some grocery and health food stores, and online via mail order.

Frozen Fruits and Vegetables

Cascadian Farms
Small Planet Foods
P. O. Box 9452
Minneapolis, MN 55440
(800) 624-4123
www.cfarm.com

Frozen, packaged organic fruits and vegetables, including berries. Available in health food and grocery stores.

Protein Powder (from goat's milk)

Goatein by Garden of Life
(800) 622-8986
www.gardenoflife.com

Goatein, an exceptional goat's milk protein powder, is a source of eight essential amino acids crucial to good health. Easy to digest, Goatein is well tolerated by those who cannot digest cow's milk.

Available in natural food stores and via mail-order s and online retailers.

Extra-Virgin Coconut Oil

Extra-Virgin Coconut Oil by Garden of Life
(800) 622-8986
www.gardenoflife.com

Once thought to be a "bad" fat, coconut oil has been shown to be a stable, healthy saturated fat. In fact, extra-virgin coconut oil is one of the healthiest and most versatile unprocessed dietary oils in the world. Garden of Life Extra-Virgin Coconut Oil is an unprocessed culinary oil full of natural coconut flavour and aroma.

Available in natural food stores and via mail-order catalogues and online retailers.

Salad Dressings and Vinegars

Salad Dressings

Bragg Live Foods
Box 7
Santa Barbara, CA 93102
(800) 446-1990
www.bragg.com

Paul C. Bragg and his daughter Patricia have been health pioneers for decades. Bragg Organic Vinaigrette and Ginger & Sesame salad dressings bring you a healthy alternative with all the best of the Bragg tradition of healthy eating and living. Available in natural food stores, mail-order catalogues, and online retailers.

Apple-Cider, Organic Balsamic, or Other Vinegars

Bragg Live Foods
Box 7
Santa Barbara, CA 93102
(800) 446-1990
www.bragg.com

Apple-cider vinegar made from organically grown apples, as well as other natural products. Available in health food and grocery stores.

Nuts and Seeds

Living Nutz
P. O. Box 11413
Portland, ME 04104
(207) 780-1101
www.livingnutz.com

Variety of low-temperature-dried sprouted nuts available in select natural food stores and via mail order.

Nut and Seed Butters

Rejuvenative Foods
P. O. Box 8464
Santa Cruz, CA 95061
(800) 805-7957
www.rejuvenative.com

The highest-quality, best-tasting raw organic nut and seed butters, including those made from almond, sesame, pumpkin, cashew, and sunflower seeds.

Available in some grocery and health food stores, by mail order, or through online merchants.

Tea

Living Foods Teas by Garden of Life
(800) 622-8986
www.gardenoflife.com

Green and black tea delivered in convenient liquid-packs. Wellness Tea is great as hot or iced tea and comes in many flavours: unflavoured lemon green tea, and coffee-flavoured black tea. Living Foods Teas are loaded with antioxidants and the exciting compound epigallocatechin gallate (EGCG). Available with or without caffeine.

Available in natural food stores and via mail-order catalogues and online retailers.

Sea Salt

Celtic Sea Salt
The Grain & Salt Society
Four Celtic Dr.
Arden, NC 28704
(800) 867-7258
www.celticseasalt.com

Celtic Sea Salt (coarse and fine) is available in some health food stores and grocery stores.

Redmond RealSalt
475 West 910 South
Weber City, UT 84032
(800) FOR-SALT (367-7258)
www.realsalt.com

RealSalt is mined in central Utah and is available in health food and grocery stores.

Organic Spices

Simply Organic
Frontier Natural Products Co-op
P. O. Box 299
Norway, IA 52318
(800) 669-3275
www.frontiercoop.com

Packaged organic spices in glass jars.

Condiments

Spectrum Organic Products
5341 Old Redwood Hwy., Suite 400
Petaluma, CA 94954
(866) 972-6879
www.spectrumorganics.com

Healthy, organic omega-3 mayonnaise using expeller-pressed soy and flaxseed oils. Available in some health food stores and grocery stores.

Westbrae Natural Foods
4600 Sleepytime Drive
Boulder, CO 80301
(800) 434-4246
www.westbrae.com

Natural ketchup and mustard, available in some health food stores and grocery stores.

Flaxseed Oil

Barlean's Organic Oils
4936 Lake Terrell Rd.
Ferndale, WA 98248
(360) 384-0485
www.barleans.com

Organic high-lignan flaxseed oil and borage seed oil, as well as flaxseed fibre. Available at health food stores.

Organic Vegetable Oils

Garden of Life
(800) 622-8986
www.gardenoflife.com

High-quality organic oils, including extra-virgin olive oil. Available in natural food stores and via mail-order catalogues and online retailers.

Bionaturae
5 Tyler Drive
North Franklin, CT 06254
(860) 642-6996
www.bionaturae.com

Organic extra-virgin olive oil.

Bariani Olive Oil
1330 Waller St.
San Francisco, CA 94117
(415) 864-1917
www.barianioliveoil.com

Organic extra-virgin olive oil.

Raw Almond Oil, Evening Primrose Oil, Sunflower Oil, and Poppy Seed Oil

Raw Oils from Rejuvenative Foods
P. O. Box 8464
Santa Cruz, CA 95061
(800) 805-7957
www.rawoils.com

Organic Chocolate Spreads

Rejuvenative Foods
P. O. Box 8464
Santa Cruz, CA 95061
(800) 805-7957
www.rejuvenative.com

Healthy organic chocolate spreads, great for all ages.

Macaroons

Jennies Macaroons
Red Mill Farms, Inc.
209 South 5th Street
Brooklyn, NY 11211
(888) 294-1164
www.macaroonking.com

A personal favourite of the Rubin family, Jennies Macaroons coconut-rich macaroon treats are a wonderful dessert treat. Available in natural food stores or from online retailers.

Flaxseed Crackers

Glaser Organic Farms
19100 SW 137th Ave.
Miami, FL 33177
(305) 238-7747
www.glaserorganicfarms.com

Food Preparation/Utensils

Mercola.com
www.mercola.com

Provides food preparation tools such as juicers and convection ovens. Available online.

Vita-Mix Blender
8615 Usher Rd.
Cleveland, OH 44138
(800) 848-2649
www.vitamix.com

High-quality durable blender excellent for smoothies and soups. A must-have for every health-conscious family.

For more information on eating to live, visit www.BiblicalHealthInstitute.com.

Nutritional Supplements

Fucoxanthin Products

fücoTHIN by Garden of Life
(800) 622-8986
www.gardenoflife.com

fücoTHIN is a natural, whole food–based supplement that is made with a proprietary concentration of 5 percent fucoxanthin combined with pomegranate seed oil for a patent-pending formula that is naturally thermogenic. Available in natural food stores and via mail-order catalogues and online retailers.

sea-Thin by Specialty Nutrition Products, LLC
www.sea-thin.com

sea-Thin, a formulation of concentrated fucoxanthin made from strains of *undaria* (wakame) and *laminaria* (kombu) grown in unpolluted waters, is available at better pharmacies, grocery stores, and select price clubs.

Whole-Food Multivitamins

Living Multi by Garden of Life
(800) 622-8986
www.gardenoflife.com

Living Multi is a complete vitamin and mineral supplement that delivers superfoods to support your demanding nutritional needs. This comprehensive whole-food multi-nutrient formula contains fruits, vegetables, ocean plants, tonic mushrooms, botanicals, and ionic minerals including enzymes, antioxidants, amino acids, and homeostatic nutrient complexes. Living Multi is available in natural food stores, mail-order catalogues, and online retailers.

Omega-3 Cod Liver Oil

Olde World Icelandic Cod Liver Oil by
Garden of Life
(800) 622-8986
www.gardenoflife.com

Olde World Icelandic Cod Liver Oil is one of nature's richest sources of vitamins A and D, which can play an important role in supporting cardiovascular health. To ensure that its naturally occurring ingredients remain intact, Olde World Icelandic Cod Liver Oil is always harvested from the pure cold waters of Iceland and is cold-processed using traditional methods. Olde World Icelandic Cod Liver Oil is available in natural food stores, mail-order catalogues, and online merchants.

CODmega by Garden of Life
(800) 622-8986
www.gardenoflife.com

Don't like the taste of cod liver oil on your spoon? CODmega offers EPA and DHA omega-3 fatty acids as well as vitamins A and D in a new capsule form. Available in natural food stores, mail-order catalogues, and online merchants.

Green Food/Fibre Blend

Perfect Food by Garden of Life
(800) 622-8986
www.gardenoflife.com

Perfect Food is a green superfood containing organic ingredients, including cereal grass juices, microalgaes, vegetable juice concentrates, sprouts, and seeds. Perfect Food provides antioxidants, enzymes, chlorophyll, and trace minerals. Available in natural food stores and through online retailers.

Super Seed by Garden of Life
(800) 622-8986
www.gardenoflife.com

Super Seed is a whole-food fibre blend containing organic ingredients, including sprouted and fermented seeds, grains, and legumes. Super Seed is available in natural food stores, mail-order catalogues, and online retailers.

Probiotics and Enzymes

Primal Defense Ultra
(800) 622-8986
www.gardenoflife.com

Primal Defense Ultra contains probiotics and prebiotics in a blend that promotes overall wellness and is available in natural food stores, mail-order catalogues, and online retailers.

Ω-Zyme Ultra by Garden of Life
(800) 622-8986 www.gardenoflife.com

Ω-Zyme (pronounced omega-zyme) is a whole-food digestive enzyme blend that supports gastrointestinal health, carbohydrate digestion, and normal bowel function. Available in natural food stores, from mail-order catalogues, and through online retailers.

Digestive Complex by TriVita
TriVita, Inc.
P. O. Box 15700
Scottsdale, AZ 85267
(800) 991-7116
www.trivita.com

A digestive formula containing enzymes and probiotics to support digestion and elimination.

Antioxidant/Energy Formula with B Vitamins, Folic Acid, and Chromium

Clear Energy by Garden of Life
(800) 622-8986
www.gardenoflife.com

Clear Energy is designed to support overall health and wellness, manage stress and promote energy, and promote stamina and mental clarity as well as concentration. Clear Energy contains whole-food B vitamins to support healthy cardiovascular function, herbal adaptogens to manage stress, and extracts from beverages to promote cellular energy.

Available in natural food stores and via mail-order catalogues and online retailers.

Fitness Products

Functional Fitness DVD by Garden of Life
(800) 622-8986
www.gardenoflife.com

Experience the energizing, enjoyable world of functional fitness exercise. Functional exercise teaches you to train whole body movements, not just isolated muscles. Increase fitness, coordination, flexibility, and agility. Decrease your chances of injury during daily activity. Functional fitness is great for people of any age or skill level. This functional fitness video features fun and easy routines that can be performed anywhere and anytime. Call the toll-free number or visit the Web site for more information.

Kingdom Conditioning with Ron Kardashian
www.kingdomconditioning.com

Ron Kardashian has more than 12,000 hours of personal training under his belt and travels around the country as a much-in-demand speaker and trainer.

Russian Kettlebells
www.dragondoor.com

The Russians are coming! The Russians are coming! Pavel Tsatsouline and Dragon Door have spearheaded the kettlebell invasion of the United States. You can achieve power, strength, and conditioning by going to their Web site at www.dragondoor.com.

Institute of Human Performance
1950 NW Boca Raton Blvd.
Boca Raton, FL 33432
(561) 620-9556
www.ihpfit.com

The Institute of Human Performance in Boca Raton, Florida, is where fitness professionals from all over the world come to learn the latest training methods from Juan Carlos Santana and the IHP staff. Santana is one of the world's leading authorities on training and performance.

Perform Better
P. O. Box 8090
Cranston, RI 02920-0090
(888) 556-7464
www.performbetter.com

If you're looking to "get functional," go with the experts in functional training and rehabilitation done through stabilization, plyometric, speed and agility, and strength and conditioning exercises.

Optimum Performance Systems
1950 NW 2 Ave.
Boca Raton, Florida, 33432
(561) 393-3881
www.opsfit.com

Exercise videos, books, and programs for recreational, amateur, and professional athletes.

Mini Trampolines/Rebounders

Rebound Air
993 North 450 West
Springville, UT 84663
(888) 464-JUMP (5867)
www.reboundair.com

Supplier of rebounders, which are great for low-impact exercise.

Lympholine
Life Source International
1112 Montana Ave., Suite 125
Santa Monica, CA 90403
(310) 284-3565
www.lympholine.com

The Lympholine rebounder activates the lymphatic system to purify the body.

Needak Manufacturing
P. O. Box 776
O'Neill, NE 68763
(800) 232-5762
www.needak-rebounders.com

For more information on conditioning your body with exercise and body therapies, visit www.PerfectWeightCanada.com

Skin and Body Care

Aubrey Organics
4419 N. Manhattan Ave.
Tampa, FL 33614

(800) 282-7394
www.aubrey-organics.com

Aubrey Hampton, the founder of Aubrey Organics, has been formulating and manufacturing skin and body care products for thirty years. Aubrey produces hundreds of products, including skin care, hair care, soaps and cleansers, toothpaste, natural hair colour, and perfumes and colognes.

Cosmetics

Peacekeeper Cosmetics
50 Lexington Ave., #22G
New York, NY 10010
(866) 732-2336
www.iamapeacekeeper.com

In addition to using quality ingredients, the company donates all profits, after taxes, to support women's health advocacy and human rights issues.

Cleaning Supplies

PerfectClean Ultramicrofiber Mops, Wipes, and Dusters
SixWise.com
655 Deerfield Rd.
Suite 100, Box 123
Deerfield, IL 60015
www.SixWise.com

Indoor pollution has become one of the leading causes of disease. A main health risk is dust, which commonly contains over twenty toxins such as heavy metals, PCBs, viruses, bacteria, and allergens. Throw away your mops, sponges, and wipers that require the use of chemical cleaners and that only introduce more toxins into your environment while doing a remarkably poor job of eliminating dust and biological contaminants.

Instead, try the PerfectClean line of mops, wipes, and dusters are available exclusively at one of my favourite Web sites, www.SixWise.com. PerfectClean's innovative "ultramicrober" construction means that with just the use of water—no chemical cleaners required—the surfaces in your home will become clean down to the microscopic level, eliminating even the biological contaminants that no other cleaning tool or solution can touch. PerfectClean lasts for hundreds of uses, so it's also economical. PerfectClean products are available online at www.SixWise.com

Bi-O-Kleen Industries, Inc.
P. O. Box 820689
Vancouver, WA 98682
(800) 477-0188
www.biokleenhome.com

Try Turbo Plus Ceramic Laundry Discs and Flora Brite papaya enzyme laundry additive and whitener.

Orange TKO
3395 S. Jones Blvd. #221
Las Vegas, NV 89146
(800) 995-2463
www.tkoorange.com

All-purpose cleaner, stain remover, and odour remover made from organic orange oil.

Seventh Generation, Inc.
60 Lake Street
Burlington, VT 05401
(800) 456-1191
www.seventhgeneration.com

Air Purifiers

Pionair
HealthQuest Technologies, LLC
P. O. Box 400
Kathleen, GA 31047
(866) PIONAIR (746-6247)
www.pionair.net

The Pionair air purification system enhances the quality of air in the home and reduces harmful toxins such as yeasts, moulds, bacteria, and debris. Available in select health stores and via mail order.

Water Purifiers

New Wave Enviro Products
P. O. Box 4146
Englewood, CO 80155
(303) 221-3232
www.newwaveenviro.com

Water purifiers and shower filters remove harmful toxins, including chlorine.

Produce Wash

Veggie Wash
Beaumont Products
1560 Big Shanty Dr.
Kennesaw, GA 30144
(800) 451-7096
www.citrusmagic.com

Made 100 percent with natural ingredients derived from citrus fruit, corn, and coconut, Veggie Wash aids in the removal of pesticides, germs, and toxins from fruits and produce.

Paper Products

Seventh Generation
60 Lake Street
Burlington, VT 05401
(800) 456-1191
www.seventhgeneration.com

Unbleached paper towels, napkins, toilet paper, and tissue.

Notes

A Note to the Reader

1. University of Calgary, "Kansas City vs. Winnipeg: Quick Facts," http://www.ucalgary.ca/~dabrent/cbc/kanwin2.html (accessed September 24, 2007).

Introduction
The Perfect Weight Canada Campaign

1. MensHealth.com, "The Best and Worst Cities for Men 2007," http://www.menshealth.com/cda/article.do?site=MensHealth&channel=health&category=metrogrades&conitem=cf0e3adb5ef8f010VgnVCM10000013281eac____ (accessed August 13, 2007).
2. Erin McClam, "Smoking Rates Are Higher in Blue-Collar Cities," Ash.org, December 13, 2001, bhttp://no-smoking.org/dec01/12-14-01-3.html (accessed August 8, 2007).
3. Canadian Health Network, "How Healthy Are Canada's Communities?" Public Health Agency of Canada, http://www.canadian-health-network.ca/servlet/ContentServer?cid =1057876015677&pagename=CHN-RCS%2FCHNResource%2FCHNResourcePageTemplate&lang=En&c=CHNResource (accessed September 24, 2007).
4. Carol Sorgen, "Fad Diets: Weight Loss Magic or Myth?" FOXNews.com, August 31, 2006, http://www.foxnews.com/story/0,2933,211597,00.html?sPage=fnc.health/nutrition (accessed August 8, 2007).
5. Chelsea Martinez, "Quitting All at Once," *Los Angeles Times*, June 18, 2007, http://www.latimes.com/features/health/la-he-capsule-18jun18,1,6491724.story?coll=la-headlines-health&ctrack=2&cset=true (accessed August 8, 2007).

Chapter 1
Globesity

1. Associated Press, "Obesity an 'International Scourge,'" CBSNews.com, September 3, 2006, http://www.cbsnews.com/stories/2006/09/03/health/main1962961.shtml (accessed August 8, 2007).
2. Dr. Joseph Mercola, "The Global Obesity Epidemic Is More Harmful than Malnutrition," Mercola.com, November 16, 2006, http://v.mercola.com/blogs/public_blog/The-Global-Obesity-Epidemic-is-More-Harmful-Than-Malnutrition-1810.aspx (accessed August 9, 2007).
3. Worldpress.org, "Obesity: A Worldwide Issue," October 24, 2004, http://www.worldpress.org/Africa/1961.cfm (accessed August 9, 2007).
4. Associated Press, "European Nations Sign Anti-Obesity Charter," CBSNews.com, November 15, 2006, http://www.cbsnews.com/stories/2006/11/16/world/main2188875.shtml (accessed August 9, 2007).

5. Yuri Kageyama, "'In-Your-Face' Food," *Chicago Sun-Times*, April 4, 20074, http://www.suntimes.com/business/325487,CST-FIN-japan04.article (accessed August 9, 2007).

6. Associated Press, "Obesity Is Going to Extremes, Study Reports," Arcog.com, October 14, 2003, http://aspdemo.arcog.com/?ArticleID=v2t1g388363B1Y3W3B2r2dli (accessed August 9, 2007).

7. Michael Tjepkema, "Adult Obesity in Canada: Measured Height and Weight," Statistics Canada, Catalogue no. 82-620-MWE, http://www.statcan.ca/english/research/82-620-MIE/2005001/pdf/aobesity.pdf (accessed September 24, 2007).

8. Reuters.com, "Study Predicts 75 Percent Overweight in US by 2015," July 19, 2007, http://www.reuters.com/article/health-SP-A/idUSN1841918320070719 (accessed August 9, 2007).

9. Elisabeth Kubler-Ross, *On Death and Dying* (New York: Scribner, 1997).

10. Abby Ellin, "Fat Studies Gain Weight in Class," *San Diego Union-Tribune*, December 10, 2006, http://www.signonsandiego.com/uniontrib/20061210/news_1c10fat.html (accessed August 21, 2007).

11. PRWeb.com, "U.S. Weight Loss Market to Reach $58 Billion in 2007," April 19, 2007, http://www.prweb.com/releases/2007/4/prweb520127.htm (accessed September 17, 2007).

12. Tani Shaw, "Celebrities Increase Popularity of Gastric Bypass Surgery," http://gastricbypasssurgeryresource.com/blog/gatric-bypass/celebrities-increase-popularity-of-gastric-bypass-surgery (accessed August 9, 2007); Associated Press, "Star Jones: I Had Gastric Bypass Surgery," USAToday.com, July 31, 2007, http://usatoday.com/life/television/2007-07-31-864625929_x.htm (accessed August 9, 2007).

13. Herb Weisbaum, "Finally, These Diet Pill Pushers Get Pushed Back," MSNBC.com, January 15, 2007, http://www.msnbc.msn.com/id/16491115 (accessed August 21, 2007).

14. NewsReleaseWire.com, "Passenger Obesity as a Contributing Factor in Commuter Airline Crashes," August 28, 2006, http://www.expertclick.com/NewsReleaseWire/default.cfm?Action=ReleaseDetail&ID=13628 (accessed August 9, 2007).

15. Beverly Beyette, "Airline Seats Getting Even Smaller," *Los Angeles Times*, March 30, 2007, http://www.newsday.com/travel/am-airlines01,0,7156934.story?coll=ny-travel-headlines (accessed August 9, 2007).

16. HarrisInteractive.com, "The High Correlation Between Obesity, Illness and Poor Health," January 11, 2005, http://www.harrisinteractive.com/news/allnewsbydate.asp?NewsID=880 (accessed September 17, 2007).

17. National Center for Health Statistics, "Americans Slightly Taller, Much Heavier Than Four Decades Ago," October 27, 2004, http://www.cdc.gov/nchs/pressroom/04news/americans.htm (accessed August 21, 2007).

18. Ibid.

19. Ibid.

20. Ibid.

21. Rob Stein, "Obesity Passing Smoking as Top Avoidable Cause of Death," *Washington Post*, March 10, 2004, A1, http://www.washingtonpost.com/ac2/wp-dyn/A43253-2004Mar9?language=printer (accessed August 9, 2007).

22. WebMD.com, "Weight Loss: Health Risks Associated with Obesity," http://www.webmd.com/cholesterol-management/obesity-health-risks (accessed August 9, 2007).

23. Statistics Canada, "Selected Leadings Causes of Death, by Sex," http://www40.statcan.ca/l01/cst01/health36.htm (accessed September 24, 2007).

24. Jane E. Brody, "Personal Health: Another Study Finds a Link Between Excess Weight and Cancer," *New York Times*, May 6, 2003, http://query.nytimes.com/gst/fullpage.html?sec=health&res=9403EFDE143CF935A35756C0A9659C8B63 (accessed August 21, 2007).

25. Harvard School of Public Health, "Volume I: Human Causes of Cancer," *Harvard Reports on Cancer Prevention*, in *Cancer Causes and Control* 7 (Supplement) (November 1996): http://www.hsph.harvard.edu/cancer/resources_materials/reports/HCCPreport_1.htm (accessed August 21, 2007).

26. Statistics Canada, "Selected Leadings Causes of Death, by Sex."

27. Alex Barnum, "Major Obesity Threat Seen for Life Expectancy," WorldHealth.net, http://www.worldhealth.net/p/286,6703.html (accessed August 21, 2007).

28. Statistics Canada, "Deaths," The Daily, December 20, 2006, http://www.statcan.ca/Daily/English/061220/d061220b.htm (accessed September 24, 2007).

29. S. J. Olshansky et al., "A Potential Decline in Life Expectancy in the United States in the 21st Century," *New England Journal of Medicine* 352(11) (2005): 1138–1145.

30. Barnum, "Major Obesity Threat Seen for Life Expectancy."

31. David Hawkins, MH, CNC, "Obesity and Weight Management," MotherEarthWorks.com, http://www.motherearthworks.com/articles/Conditions/obes.htm (accessed August 21, 2007).

32. Tjepkema, "Adult Obesity in Canada: Measured Height and Weight."

33. Alyssa Schwartz, "Canadians Short on Waist-Size Knowledge," Canada.com, http://www.canada.com/topics/bodyandhealth/story.html?id=41bc7b50-0128-40ab-b29b-97cd3bd11eef (accessed September 24, 2007).

34. Peter Kessler, "Phil Mickelson Interview," GolfOnline.com, March 2003, http://www.golfonline.com/golfonline/features/kessler/columnist/0,17742,468530,00.html (accessed August 10, 2007).

35. Peggy Peck, "High-Fat Diets Ups Dangerous 'Hidden' Fat," WebMD.com, March 31, 2003, http://www.webmd.com/diet/news/20030331/high-fat-diet-ups-dangerous-hidden-fat (accessed June 7, 2007).

36. Associated Press, "Thin People Might Be Fat on the Inside," MSNBC.com, May 11, 2007, http://www.msnbc.msn.com/id/18594089/ (accessed June 26, 2007).

37. Christian Nordqvist, "Dangerous Visceral Fat Builds Up If You Don't Exercise, Can Go Down If You Do," MedicalNewsToday.com, http://www.medicalnewstoday.com/healthnews.php?newsid=30641 (accessed June 11, 2007).

38. Pew Research Center, "In the Battle of the Bulge, More Soldiers Than Successes," Pew Research Center Publications, April 26, 2006, http://pewresearch.org/pubs/310/in-the-battle-of-the-bulge-more-soldiers-than-successes (accessed June 12, 2007).

Chapter 2
What Are You Failing For?

1. ScienceDaily.com, "Dieting Does Not Work, Researchers Report," http://www.sciencedaily.com/releases/2007/04/070404162428.htm (accessed August 22, 2007).

2. North Dakota State University Extension News, "Fad Diets Popular but Have Major-League Failure Rate," Agriculture Communication, July 8, 1999, http://www.ext.nodak.edu/extnews/newsrelease/1999/070899/04faddie.htm (accessed August 9, 2007).

3. Elaine Magee, "Your 'Hunger Hormones,'" MedicineNet.com, http://www.onhealth.com/script/main/art.asp?articlekey=55992 (accessed on April 16, 2007).

4. Gary Taubes, "What if It's All Been a Big Fat Lie?" *New York Times Magazine*, July 2, 2002, 22.

5. Leonard Pitts Jr., "Search for Ideal Body Takes Toll," LJWorld.com, February 6, 2003, http://www2.ljworld.com/news/2003/feb/06/search_for_ideal/ (accessed August 22, 2007).

6. CommonSenseMedia.org, "What's the Skinny on the Media and Weight?" September 26, 2006, http://www.commonsensemedia.org/news/press-releases.php?id=29 (accessed August 22, 2007); and Mark Hyman, MD, *Ultrametabolism: The Simple Plan for Automatic Weight Loss* (New York: Scribner, 2006), 14–15.

7. Hyman, *Ultrametabolism: The Simple Plan for Automatic Weight Loss,* 14–15.

8. E. J. Mundell, "Furor Over Anorexic Models Hits U.S. Fashion Week," *Washington Post*, February 2, 2007, http://www.washingtonpost.com/wp-dyn/content/article/2007/02/02/AR2007020200500.html (accessed August 10, 2007).

9. Domino's Pizza Press Release, "Domino's Pizza Gets Ready to Kick-off for the Big Game," PRNewswire, January 31, 2007, http://phx.corporate-ir.net/phoenix.zhtml?c=135383&p=irol-newsArticle&ID=956166&highlight= (accessed April 17, 2007).

10. Community-University Partnership for the Study of Children, Youth, and Families, "How Much Television Should Children Watch?" University of Alberta, http://www.cup.ualberta.ca/component/option,com_docman/task,doc_view/gid,41/Itemid,67/ (accessed September 24, 2007).

11. CommonSenseMedia.org, "What's the Skinny on the Media and Weight?"

12. Judith A. Shinogle, Maria F. Owings, and Lola Jean Kozak, "Gastric Bypass as Treatment for Obesity: Trends, Characteristics, and Complications," *Obesity Research* 13 (2005): 2202–2209.

13. Robin Blackstone, David Engstrom, and Lisa Rivera, "Patients in Despair: Weight Regain After a Primary Bariatric Surgery Procedure," BariatricTimes.com, April 2007, http://bariatrictimes.com/category/patients-in-despair/ (accessed August 22, 2007).

14. EmpowerFoods.com, "Self-Image," http://www.empowerfoods.com.au/news/?article_id=11 (accessed August 22, 2007).

Chapter 3
Eat for Your Perfect Weight

1. *Toledo: Treasures and Tradition* (Memphis, TN: Towery Publishing, Inc., 2001), 17.

2. Judy Sarles, "McAlister's Deli to Expand with Brentwood Franchise," *Nashville Business Journal*, February 3, 2006, http://nashville.bizjournals.com/nashville/stories/2006/02/06/story6.html (accessed August 22, 2007).

3. Canadian Organic Growers, "Quick Facts About Canada's Organic Sector," http://www.cog.ca/orgquickfacts.htm (accessed September 24, 2007).

4. Ibid.

5. Sasha Nemecek, "Does the World Need GM Foods? Interview With Margaret Mellon," *Scientific American*, March 27, 2001, as viewed at http://www.mindfully. org/GE/World-Need-GM-Mellon.htm (accessed August 24, 2007).

6. Rick Weiss, "Americans Fuzzy on Biotech Foods," *Los Angeles Times*, December 11, 2006, F9.

7. Andrew Adamson, "Genetically Modified Crops in Canada," EXN.ca, Discovery Channel's Canadian, May 19, 1999, http://www.exn.ca/Templates/Story. asp?ID=1999051953 (accessed September 24, 2007).

8. Elisabeth Leamy, "Secrets in Your Food," ABCNews.com, August 21, 2006, http://abcnews.go.com/gma/story?id=2337731&page=1 (accessed August 14, 2007).

9. Anne Macey, "Retail Sales of Certified Organic Food Products in Canada in 2006," Organic Agriculture Centre of Canada, Truro, Nova Scotia, May 2007, http://www.organicagcentre.ca/Docs/RetailSalesOrganic_Canada2006.pdf (accessed September 24, 2007).

10. WholeFoodMarkets.com, "Organic Foods Continue to Grow in Popularity According to Whole Foods Market Survey," October 21, 2004, http://www. wholefoodsmarket.com/cgi-bin/print10pt.cgi?url=/company/pr_10-21-04.html (accessed April 26, 2007).

11. Don Lee, "China's Additives on Menu in U.S." *Los Angeles Times*, May 18, 2007, A1.

12. Julian Dibbell, "The Fast Supper," *New York* magazine, October 24, 2006.

13. MayoClinic.com, "Exchange List: Fruits," http://www.mayoclinic.com/health/ diabetes-diet/DA00070 (accessed April 18, 2007)

14. WebMd.com, "Healthy Eating for Weight Loss," http://my.webmd.com/content/ article/46/2731_1670 (accessed August 15, 2007).

15. Brenda Watson, *The Fiber35 Diet* (New York: Free Press, 2007).

16. Continuum Health Partners, Inc., "Dietary Fibre and Bowel Function," http:// www.wehealny.org/healthinfo/dietaryfiber/fibercontentchart.html (accessed Jung 26, 2007).

17. Lavon J. Dunne, *Nutrition Almanac*, fifth edition (New York: McGraw-Hill, 2001), 5–6.

18. Hyman, *Ultrametabolism: The Simple Plan for Automatic Weight Loss*, 51.

19. Ibid., 70–71.

20. Jaye Lewis, "The Food Pyramid: Its History, Purpose, and Effectiveness," Health. LearningInfo.org, http://health.learninginfo.org/food-pyramid.htm (accessed April 20, 2007)

21. Hyman, *Ultrametabolism: The Simple Plan for Automatic Weight Loss*, 70.

22. William Wolcott, *The Metabolic Typing Diet* (New York: Broadway Books, 2002).

23. Anahad O'Connor, "The Claim: C.L.A. Supplements Can Help You Lose Weight," *New York Times*, May 29, 2007.

24. Thomas L. Halton and Frank B. Hu, "The Effects of High Protein Diets on Thermogenesis, Satiety and Weight Loss: A Critical Review," *Journal of the American College of Nutrition* 23, no. 5 (October 2004): 373–385, http://www. jacn.org/cgi/content/full/23/5/373 (accessed August 24, 2007).

25. Framingham Heart Study, "History of the Framingham Heart Study," http:// www.framinghamheartstudy.org/about/history.html (accessed August 24, 2007).

26. G. V. Mann, ed., *Coronary Heart Disease: The Dietary Sense and Nonsense* (London, England: Janus Publishing Company, 1993), in Christian B. Allan, PhD, and Wolfgang Lutz, MD, *Life Without Bread: How a Low-Carbohydrate Diet Can Save Your Life* (Chicago: Keats Publishing, 2000), 83.

27. Diana Schwarzbein, MD, *The Schwarzbein Principle: The Truth About Losing Weight, Being Healthy, and Feeling Younger* (Deerfield Beach, FL: HCI Publishing, 1999).

28. Ibid., 253.

29. Ibid., 254.

30. Judy Monchuk, "Fat Cat Calgary Set to Slim Down," *Toronto Star*, July 16, 2007, http://www.thestar.com/News/article/236288 (September 24, 2007).

31. Netfit.Co.Uk., "Food Combining," http://www.netfit.co.uk/fatcom.htm (accessed August 24, 2007).

32. Jennifer Tryon, "Black Market Milk," CTV News, December 18, 2002, http://www.ctv.ca/servlet/ArticleNews/story/CTVNews/1040267690309_44?hub=TopStories (accessed September 24, 2007).

33. CBC News, "Sugar Surprise," March 9, 2004, http://www.cbc.ca/consumers/market/files/food/sugar/ (accessed September 24, 2007).

34. Ann Louise Gittleman, MS, CNS, *How to Stay Young and Healthy in a Toxic World* (Chicago, IL: Keats Publishing, 1999), 19.

35. Ibid., 21.

36. Sally Squires, "High-Fructose Corn Syrup May Act More Like Fat Than Sugar in the Body," *Washington Post*, March 11, 2003, H1, and Dr. Joseph Mercola with Rachael Droege, "Six Reasons Why Corn Is Making You Fat," http://www.mercola.com/2004/apr/10/corn_fat.htm (accessed April 26, 2007).

37. Jerry Hirsch, "Food Prices Continue to Rise," *Los Angeles Times*, May 15, 2007.

38. Patricia King, "Blaming It on Corn Syrup," *Los Angeles Times*, March 24, 2003, F1.

39. George A. Bray, Samara Joy Nielsen, and Barry M. Popkin, "Consumption of High-Fructose Corn Syrup in Beverages May Play a Role in the Epidemic of Obesity," *American Journal of Clinical Nutrition* 79, no. 4 (April 2004): 537–543.

40. T. L. Davidson and S. E. Swithers, "A Pavlovian Approach to the Problem of Obesity," *International Journal of Obesity* 28, no. 7 (July 2004): 933–935.

41. Daniel Engber, "The Scarlet Batter: Why Our Aversion to Artificial Coloring Makes No Sense," Slate.com, March 14, 2007, http://www.slate.com/id/2161806/ (accessed April 26, 2007).

42. Michael Pollan, "Discover How Your Beef Is Really Raised," *New York Times*, March 31, 2002.

43. Ibid.

44. Marian Burros, "Veal to Love, Without the Guilt," *New York Times*, April 18, 2007.

45. Agriculture and Agri-Food Canada, "The Canadian Chicken Market," in *Profile of the Canadian Chicken Industry*, http://www.agr.ca/poultry/prindc6_e.htm (accessed September 24, 2007).

46. Burros, "Veal to Love, Without the Guilt."

47. Ibid.

48. Russ Parsons, "New Rite of Spring," *Los Angeles Times*, April 4, 2007, F1.

49. Mary Shomon, *The Thyroid Diet* (New York: HarperCollins, 2004).

Chapter 4
Drink for Your Perfect Weight

1. Jerry Adler, "Attack of the Diet Cokes," *Newsweek*, May 14, 2007.
2. Andrew Martin, "Want Vitamins and Minerals With That Soda?" HamptonRoads.com, March 14, 2007, http://content.hamptonroads.com/story.cfm?story=121056&ran=73351 (accessed August 27, 2007).
3. H. J. Roberts, *The Aspartame Problem*, Statement for Committee on Labor and Human Resources, U.S. Senate Hearing on NutraSweet—Health and Safety Concerns, November 3, 1987, 83–178 (Washington DC: U.S. Government Printing Office, 1988), 466–467.
4. "Study First to Confirm Drinking Water Could Help You Lose Weight," Children's Hospital and Research Center in Oakland, California, December 14, 2006, http://www.childrenshospitaloakland.org/about/press_releases/Waterweightloss.asp (accessed August 27, 2007).
5. Environmental Protection Agency, "130 Cities Exceed Lead Levels for Drinking Water," *Environmental News*, October 1992.
6. R. J. Ignelzi, "Flow Chart: Don't Count on Those 'Eight Glasses' to Determine Your Proper Fluid Intake," *San Diego Union-Tribune*, February 20, 2007, E1.
7. Salynn Boyles, "Drinking Water May Speed Weight Loss," WebMD, January 5, 2004, http://www.webmd.com/diet/news/20040105/drinking-water-may-speed-weight-loss (accessed June 13, 2007).
8. F. Batmanghelidj, MD, *Water: For Health, for Healing, for Life* (New York: Warner Books, 2003), 161, 225–226.
9. F. Batmanghelidj, MD, *Your Body's Many Cries for Water* (Vienna, VA: Global Health Solutions, Inc., 1997), 110–111.
10. Stephen Daniells, "Do Antioxidants Make Tea Healthier Than Water?" NutraIngredients-USA.com, August 28, 2006, http://www.nutraingredients-usa.com/news/ng.asp?n=70121-tea-polyphenols-antioxidants (accessed June 14, 2007).
11. Nubella.com, "Stressed Out? Try a Cup of Black Tea," http://nubella.com/content/view/2277/62/ (accessed August 15, 2007).
12. GreenTeaAndCLL.com, "Health Benefits of Green Tea—Fact of Fairytale?" May 18, 2007, http://greenteaandcll.com/2007/05/18/ (accessed June 14, 2007).
13. Siobhan Roth, "Kombucha Fermenting a Revolution in Health Drinks," *Pittsburgh Post-Gazette*, June 7, 2007.

Chapter 5
Snack for Your Perfect Weight

1. BBC News, "Chocolate Better Than Kissing," April 16, 2007, http://news.bbc.co.uk/1/hi/health/6558775.stm (accessed May 8, 2007).
2. CBC News Online, "Nuts About Chocolate: Facts and Statistics," February 12, 2004, http://www.cbc.ca/news/background/valentines/facts.html (September 24, 2007).
3. NutraIngredients-USA.com, "The Sum of Chocolate," December 20, 2005, http://www.nutraingredients-usa.com/news/ng.asp?n=64689-chocolate-cocoa-flavonoids (accessed August 27, 2007).

4. David Wolfe and Shazzie, *Naked Chocolate* (San Diego, CA: Maui Brothers Publishing, 2005), 6.
5. Ibid., 65.
6. Richard and Rachel Heller, *The Carbohydrate Addict's Diet* (New York: Signet, 2000), 96–97.

Chapter 6
Supplement for Your Perfect Weight

1. H. Maeda et al., "Fucoxanthin From Edible Seaweed, *Undaria Pinnatifida*, Shows Antiobesity Effect Through UCP1 Expression in White Adipose Tissues," *Biochemical and Biophysical Research Communications* 332, no. 2 (July 1, 2005): 392–397.
2. H. Maeda et al., "Fucoxanthin and Its Metabolite, Fucoxanthinol, Suppress Adipocyte Differentiation in 3T3-L1 Cells," *Internal Journal of Molecular Medicine* 18, no. 1 (July 2006): 147–152.
3. Medical Research News, "Brown Seaweed with Anti-Obesity Potential," September 12, 2006, http://www.news-medical.net/?id=20082 (accessed July 10, 2007).
4. Yorkshire-Forward.com, "Seaweed 'Fights Fat,' Scientists Reveal," September 12, 2006, http://www.yorkshire-forward.com/www/view.asp?content_id=4283&parent_id=263 (accessed July 10, 2007).
5. Joanne Englash, "Weight Loss Supplements: 5 Myths!" eDiets.com, http://www.ediets.com/news/article.cfm/1/cmi_2310883/cid_1/code_30174 (accessed July 27, 2007).
6. Hal Bodley, "Medical Examiner: Ephedra a Factor in Bechler Death," March 13, 2003, http://www.usatoday.com/sports/baseball/al/orioles/2003-03-13-bechler-exam_x.htm (accessed August 27, 2007).
7. Sally Fallon and Mary G. Enig, PhD, "Vitamin A Saga," Weston A. Price Foundation, http://www.westonaprice.org/basicnutrition/vitaminasaga.html (accessed September 18, 2007).

Chapter 8
Cleanse for Your Perfect Weight

1. S. Bengmark, "Ecological Control of the Gastrointestinal Tract. The Role of Probiotic Flora," *Gut* 42 (1998): 2–7.
2. Wikipedia.org, "Horace Fletcher," http://en.wikipedia.org/wiki/Horace_Fletcher (accessed August 28, 2007).
3. Claire Heald, "Going Ape," BBC News, January 11, 2007, http://news.bbc.co.uk/2/hi/uk_news/magazine/6248975.stm (accessed July 16, 2007).

Chapter 9
Get FIT for Your Perfect Weight

1. Charles Stuart Platkin, "Counting Steps With Pedometer Seems to Encourage Fitness," *Honolulu Advertiser*, March 24, 2004.

2. Alan Sears, MD, *PACE: Rediscover Your Native Fitness* (Wellington, FL: Wellness Research & Consulting, Inc., 2006), 7.

3. Jeannine Stein, "The Amish Paradox," *Los Angeles Times*, January 12, 2004.

4. Jay Groves, EdD, "The Digital Pedometer," Diabetes Exercise and Sports Association, http://www.diabetes-exercise.org/Docs/jay_groves_practioners_article.asp (accessed August 15, 2007).

5. C. A. Gillette, R. C. Bullough, and C. L. Melby, "Post Exercise Energy Expenditure in Response to Acute Aerobic or Resistive Exercise," *International Journal of Sport Nutrition* 4, no. 4 (1994): 347–360.

6. Peter Jaret, "A Healthy Mix of Rest and Motion," *New York Times*, May 3, 2007.

7. Ibid.

8. Larry Trivieri Jr., *Alternative Medicine: The Definitive Guide* (Berkeley, CA: Celestial Arts, 2002), 37–38.

9. PowerAthletesMag.com, "Exclusive Interview with the 'Evil Russian' Pavel Tsatsouline," *Girevik* magazine, issue 1, http://www.powerathletesmag.com/archives/Girevik/First/interview.htm (accessed August 29, 2007).

10. J. T. Salonon et al., "Physical Activity and Risk of Myocardial Infarction, Cerebral Stroke, and Death: A Longitudinal Study in Eastern Finland," *American Journal of Epidemiology* 115, no. 4 (1982): 526–537.

11. Michael F. Roizen, MD, and Mehmet C. Oz, MD, *YOU: The Owner's Manual* (New York: Harper Collins, 2005), 122.

12. Nanci Hellmich, "Sleep Loss May Equal Weight Gain," *USA Today*, December 6, 2004, http://www.usatoday.com/news/health/2004-12-06-sleep-weight-gain_x.htm (accessed August 29, 2007).

13. Milly Dawson, "The Quest for Sleep," *bp Magazine*, Spring 2006, as reprinted at National Alliance on Mental Illness, http://www.nami.org/template.cfm?template=/ContentManagement/ContentDisplay.cfm&ContentID=32467&lstid=275 (accessed September 18, 2007); and Jacob Teitelbaum, MD, "Getting Eight to Nine Hours of Sleep—the Foundation of Pain Relief," TalkAboutSleep.com, http://www.talkaboutsleep.com/sleep-disorders/2005/04/fibromyalgia-eight-hours.htm (accessed September 18, 2007).

14. Cara Williams, "You Snooze, You Lose; Sleep Patterns in Canada," *Canadian Social Trends*, Spring 2001, http://www.statcan.ca/english/freepub/11-008-XIE/2000004/articles/5558.pdf (accessed September 24, 2007).

Chapter 10
Reduce Toxins for Your Perfect Weight

1. DietJokes.co.uk, "The Dieter's Psalm," http://www.dietjokes.co.uk/jokes/074.php (accessed August 29, 2007).

2. Liz Lipski, PhD, CCN, "Basics of Nutrition and Healthy Eating," WomentoWomen.com, http://www.womentowomen.com/nutritionandweightloss/nutritionalbasics.asp (accessed August 29, 2007).

3. Kelly James-Enger, "Sweet Stuff: How Artificial Sweeteners May Affect Your Stomach," MSN.com, http://acidreflux.msn.com/article.aspx?aid=64&GT1=7338.

4. Don Colbert, *Toxic Relief* (Lake Mary, FL: Siloam, 1999, 2003), 15.

5. Theo Colborn, *Our Stolen Future*, "About Phthalates," http://www. ourstolenfuture.org/NewScience/oncompounds/phthalates/phthalates.htm#health (accessed September 18, 2007).
6. Aubrey-Organics.com, "Scents and Sensitivity," *Healthy Living* magazine, http:// www.aubrey-organics.com/about/articles/scents.cfm (accessed September 18, 2007).
7. American Lung Association, "Indoor Air Quality," http://www.lungusa.org/site/ apps/s/content.asp?c=dvLUK9O0E&b=34706&ct=67136 (accessed September 18, 2007).
8. Mindy Pennybacker, "Healthier Home Cleaning," *The Green Guide* magazine, September 8, 2003.

Chapter 11
Think for Your Perfect Weight

1. Heinz von Foerster, "On Constructing a Reality," Readings That Matter to Me, http://grace.evergreen.edu/~arunc/texts/cybernetics/heinz/constructing/ constructing.html (accessed September 18, 2007).
2. Sue Goetinck Ambrose, "A Cell Forgets," *Dallas Morning News*, reprinted in *San Diego Union-Tribune*, October 20, 2004, http://www.signonsandiego.com/ uniontrib/20041020/news_z1c20cell.html (accessed September 18, 2007).
3. Ibid.
4. TheHealingCodes.com, "Interview with Bruce Lipton, PhD, Cellular Biologist and Author of *The Biology of Belief*," http://thehealingcodes.com/lipton_interview. htm (accessed September 18, 2007).

Chapter 12
Take Weight Off the World

1. Agriculture and Agri-Food Canada, "Canada's Organic Industry," http://ats-sea. agr.gc.ca/supply/factsheets/3313_e.pdf (accessed September 24, 2007).
2. Elizabeth Weise, "Study: 90% of the Ocean's Edible Species May Be Gone by 2048," *USA Today*, http://www.usatoday.com/tech/science/discoveries/2006-11-02-overfishing-threat_x.htm (accessed August 29, 2007).
3. *In Pink* magazine, Decatur, Georgia, Premiere Issue, 2007.
4. Elizabeth Weise, "Panel Calls Chemical a 'Likely Carcinogen,'" *USA Today*, June 29, 2005, http://www.usatoday.com/news/health/2005-06-29-teflon-usat_x.htm (accessed September 18, 2007).

Index

Bell, Dr. Jimmy, 29
belly fat, 107
beta-carotene, 108, 114, 317
*Beyond the 120-Year Diet: How to Double
   Your Vital Years*, 51
Big 5, the, 163
big agriculture, 46
Big Sugar, 55
binge, 36–37, 190
biodegradable packaging, 201
Biology of Belief, The, 187
biotechnological crops 108
bishop's weed, 138
bison, 47, 80, 325
black mould, 179
Blank, Tim, 199–200
blindness, 22
Bling H₂O, 90
bloating, 66, 130, 175, 210
blood lipids, 115
blood pressure, 7, 22, 25, 28, 39, 61,
   83, 89, 107, 109–110, 135, 160, 170,
   207–209, 223
blood sugar, 22, 28, 33, 53, 56, 58–60,
   85, 98–100, 118, 123, 126, 160, 323
blurred vision, 160
body fat, 23, 25, 28–31, 34, 36, 57–58,
   61, 65, 107, 109, 112, 159, 162, 172,
   208–209
body frame, 25, 27, 30–31
body mass index (BMI), 17, 24–28,
   30–31, 208
bone density, 157, 167
Borschmann, MD, Michael, 92
botanicals, 114, 137, 180, 330
bowel(s), 23, 53, 90, 103, 117, 131, 136,
   138, 175, 187, 309, 331, 338
brain, 23, 30, 32–34, 41, 59, 88, 93–94,
   105, 115, 130, 172, 187
Brasco, MD, Joseph, 112, 136
Brigham and Women's Hospital at
   Harvard Medical School, 13–14
Bristol University, 180
broccoli extract, 137
Brown, Richard P., 108

buffalo, 57, 61, 71, 80, 84, 118, 229, 231,
   235, 247, 265, 271, 283, 294, 325
bulimia, 35
Bulwer, MD, Bernard, 13–14, 17, 23, 27,
   59, 63, 88, 94, 98, 112, 132, 160
Burkitt, Sir Dennis, 132

C

cacao, 98, 100, 102–104, 106, 207, 243,
   245, 247, 249, 251, 253, 255, 257–258,
   279, 281, 283, 285, 287–288, 290, 292,
   294, 301, 303, 319, 323
caffeine, 57, 77, 87, 89, 94, 110, 328
calcium, 52, 55–56, 74, 99, 312, 315, 320
caloric intake, 30, 53, 78
calorie restriction with optimal nutrition
   (CRON), 51
calorie(s), 9, 32–33, 35, 38–40, 42,
   46, 51–53, 56–57, 59, 74, 76, 78–79,
   83–84, 87, 89, 93–96, 99–100, 103,
   106, 109, 113, 126, 156, 159, 168, 172,
   174–176, 297–305, 320
Camellia sinensis, 94
cancer, 3, 9, 22–24, 39, 42, 56, 73, 88,
   95, 177–178, 187, 205
   of uterus, 22–23
   of gallbladder, 22
   of cervix, 22–23
   of ovary, 22
   of breast, 22–23
   of colon, 22–23
   of prostate, 22–23, 56
   of rectum, 23
   of esophagus, 23
   of stomach, 19, 23,
   of pancreas, 23
   of liver, 23
   of kidney, 23
canned tuna, 82, 119, 176, 229, 235, 241,
   247, 253, 258, 264, 270, 276, 283, 294
Carbohydrate Addict's Diet, The, 105
carbohydrates, 36, 50, 52–53, 55–60, 63,
   65–67, 89, 93, 98–99, 105, 114, 118,
   125–126, 130–131, 156, 161, 315
carbon dioxide, 158, 179

hemorrhoids, 132, 136
Hendricks, Trent, 201–202
Hennessey, Stephen, 203
hernia(s), 20, 166
high-fructose corn syrup, 46, 75–78, 86, 93, 100
high-fibre, 53–54, 98, 106, 118, 133–134, 324
high-sugar foods, 23
Hippocrates Health Institute, 195
Hokkaido University, 109
Holloway, John, 81
homogenized, 46, 74–75
honey, 10, 75, 96, 100, 106, 113, 123–125, 133–135, 144, 147–148, 153, 225, 229, 231, 234, 237, 240, 243, 246, 248, 252, 254, 256, 258, 260, 264, 266, 270, 274, 276, 278, 282, 284, 286, 288, 290, 292, 294, 300, 303, 308–310, 314–317, 319, 323, 326
hoodia, 96, 111
hormones, 30, 33–34, 60, 104, 110, 132, 205
household cleaners, 178
Humane Farming Association, 80
humectants, 175
hybrids, 201
hydrogenated, hydrogenation, 62–63, 73–74, 103, 120, 184,
hydrolyzed soy protein, 72–73
hydroponic gardening, hydroponic tower, 196, 199
hydroxycitric acid, 96
hygiene, 24
Hyman, MD, Mark, 56
hyperinsulinemia, 59
hypertension, 5, 23, 160, 209
hypoglycemia, 59, 160
hypothalamus, 33, 187–188

I

immune system, 98, 115, 187–188, 190, 308
impaired balance, 160
Imperial College, 29

incandescent light bulbs, 203
indoles, 67
industrial chemicals, 23–24
infrared sauna, 167–168
infection, 171
inflammation, 50, 62, 84, 109–110, 112, 118, 126, 157
insoluble fibre, 54, 316
Institute of Medicine, 92
Institute of Solar Energy, 108
Institute of Technology and Marine Sciences, 109
insulin, 23, 25, 28, 56, 59–62, 67, 85, 105–106, 118, 126, 168, 171
insulin resistance syndrome, 28
ionizing radiation, 51
iron, 99, 166, 312
irradiation, 47
isomalt, 175

J

James, Henry, 130
Jenny Craig, 19, 85, 182
Jensen, PhD, Bernard, 136
Joe Arrington Cancer Center, 4
Johns Hopkins Medical Institutions, 29
Johns Hopkins University, 18
Johnson, MD, Ben, 185
joint pain, 23
Journal of Applied Physiology, 160
junk food(s), 7, 10, 17, 38, 51, 104–105, 113, 126, 137, 170, 223

K

Kardashian, Ron, 158, 163, 165, 331–332
Keith, William, 12
kerosene, 178
kettlebell(s), 156, 158, 163, 165–166, 170, 172, 225, 227, 229, 231–232, 234, 236, 238, 240, 242, 244, 246, 248, 250, 252, 254, 256, 258, 260, 262, 264, 266, 268, 270, 272, 274, 276, 278, 280, 282, 284, 286, 288, 290, 292, 332
kidney(s), 23, 89–90, 92, 137, 175–176
killer fat, 6, 29, 170
King's College, 14, 94

One-A-Day WeightSmart, 19
Oprah, 21
organic cosmetics, 179–180
organic feed, 47
organic skin care, 178, 333
organic tea, 95
organic wine, 79
osteoarthritis, 22
overhead presses, 166
oxidizers, 65
oxygen, 57, 84, 89, 156, 158, 162, 167–168, 172

P

PACE: Rediscover Your Native Fitness, 157
pancreatitis, 79
parasites, 98, 136
partially hydrogenated, 63, 73–74, 103, 120
pasteurized, 74–75
pasture raised, 47
pathogens, 91
PCBs (polychlorinated biphenyls), 175, 333
pea hull fibre, 138
pear-shaped, 27–28
pediatrician, 116
peppermint leaf, 138
perfluorooctanoic acid (PFOA), 204
personal hydration program, 47
personal trainer(s), 158, 162–163, 171–173
Pescatore, MD, Fred, 111
pesticide(s), 23, 47, 57, 95, 98, 104, 132, 176, 198–199, 205, 334
petroleum-based surfactants, 178
petroleum-derived, 47, 178
Pew Research Center, 30
phenolics, 67
phenylethylamine (PEA), 103, 120, 138
phthalates, 175, 178
phytic acid, 99
phytochemicals, 67, 315
placebo, 58, 94, 109, 112
plastic(s), 67, 87, 90, 178–180, 203, 205, 207

PLU codes, 49
Poliquin, Charles, 163
Pollan, Michael, 80
polycarbonate, 90, 178, 180
polyols, 175
polyphenols, 94
polyunsaturated fats, 56, 61–62, 86, 115
polyvinylpyrrolidone, 179
pomegranate seed oil, 110, 112, 330
pork products, 70, 219
potassium, 52, 83, 178, 319–320
potassium nitrate, 178
potato types, 63, 65–66
power breathing, 189
prescription drugs, 14, 25
preservatives, 46, 50, 90, 92, 98–99, 117, 122, 175, 184
Price, Dr. Weston A., 95
probiotic(s), 12, 83, 95, 98, 114, 137, 323–324, 331
processed food(s), 15, 25, 46, 49, 62, 83, 86, 113, 119, 130–131, 135, 138, 217
processed ingredients, 98
Prosch Jr., MD, Gus, 25
protein, 36, 40, 52–53, 55–60, 63–66, 72–74, 79, 82–83, 98–100, 108–110, 114, 118, 120, 123, 126, 182, 198, 201, 225, 237, 243, 249, 260, 266, 278, 290, 297–305, 309, 312, 315, 323–324, 327, 339
psychological trauma, 187
purge, 37
pyridoxine hydrochloride, 114

Q

quadruple bypass heart surgery, 4

R

radiation, 39, 51, 177
Ramazanov, PhD, Zakir, 107–110, 112, 114
Rapadura, 125
raw food(s), raw foodist(s), 69, 104, 195, 306, 326
Raw Life, The, 195
rebounder (mini-trampoline), 158–159,

291–295, 298, 304, 312–315, 328
soy-based inks, 201
sparkling water, 96, 123
spine, 164
spirulina, 108, 114
Splenda, 78, 88
stability ball, 155–156, 158, 162, 164–
    165, 167, 170–172
stair stepper, 156, 162, 225, 227–229,
    231–232, 234, 236, 238, 240, 242,
    244, 246, 248, 250, 252, 254, 256, 258,
    260, 262, 264, 266, 268, 270, 272,
    274, 276, 278, 280, 282, 284, 286,
    288, 290, 292–293
Stanford University Medical School, 187
starch, 59
stationary bike(s), 156, 159–160, 225,
    227, 229, 231–232, 234, 236, 238, 240,
    242, 244, 246, 248, 250, 252, 254,
    256, 258, 260, 262, 264, 266, 268,
    270, 272, 274, 276, 278, 280, 282,
    284, 286, 288, 290, 292–293
Steinman, David, 205
steroids, 81
Stone Age diet, 113
strength-training equipment, 163, 172
stress, 1, 4–6, 9, 24, 39, 113, 129, 160,
    167, 181, 184, 187–190, 331
stroke(s), 3, 9, 22–23, 42, 209
Styrofoam, 178
subcutaneous fat, 29–31, 161
subscapula, 28
sucanat, 125
sucralose, 78, 88, 123, 175
sucrose, 75–76, 93, 100, 113
sugar(s), 8, 25, 35, 46, 52, 55–56, 59, 67,
    75–79, 85–86, 88, 90, 92–93, 95–97,
    99, 101, 113, 117, 121–123, 125, 135,
    139, 190, 207, 301–302
sugar alcohol(s), 123, 175
sugar cane syrup, 103–104
sugar-free, 78, 87, 89
sulfites, 101, 125
Sunett, 88
sunlight, 168

Sunlight Saunas, 167
suprailium, 28
sustainable food, 197, 202
sustainably caught (fish), 198, 205
Swaroop, Dr. Prabhakar, 175
Sweet One, 88
Sweet'N Low, 78, 88
systolic pressure, 208

T

T3 (thyroid hormone), 84
Take Control of Your Health, 57
Talanian, Jason L., 160
talk test, 157–158, 172
tap water, 91, 123
taste buds, 46, 52, 68, 89, 219
Taubes, Gary, 35
tea(s), 39, 94–96, 105, 107–108, 123,
    326, 328
  herbal, 94
  green, 89, 94–96, 110, 315–316, 328
  white, 94,
  black, 94–95
  oxidized, 94
  oolong, 67, 94–95
tendons, 167
thalamus, 33
thermogenesis, thermogenic, 94, 107,
    110–111, 330
thiamine mononitrate, 114
thigh, 4, 28–29, 168
Thornton, Jon, 135
thyroid, 69, 84, 110, 179, 186
Thyroid Diet, The, 84
*Tissue Cleansing Through Bowel
    Management*, 136
tobacco smoke, 23
Toledo, 2–5, 13, 45, 211–214, 218–219,
    223
Toledo Blade, 207
Toledo: Treasures and Traditions, 45
toothpaste, 175, 178, 333
toxic load, 78–79, 137, 178
Toxic Relief, 175
toxin-free, 6

Weight Watchers, 19, 85, 182
Weston A. Price Foundation, 95
wheat-grass smoothie, 10
white adipose tissue, 29, 109–110
white blood cells, 84
white flour, 73, 92
whole food, 101, 114, 125, 137, 150, 330
whole-food nutrition bars, 98–100, 106, 125, 225, 227, 229, 231, 233, 235, 237, 239–241, 243, 245, 249, 251, 254, 256, 258, 260–277, 279–280, 282, 284, 286, 288, 290, 292, 294, 323
whole-food selenium, 137
whole grains, 47, 52, 54–56, 58, 60, 69
whole milk, 35, 64, 74
whole-house filtration system, 91, 177
wild-caught fish, 23, 53, 62, 82, 85
Willet, MD, Walter, 55
Wilson, Carnie, 19
wind power, 201
Wolcott, William L., 57
Wolfe, David, 104
World Health Organization (WHO), 1, 16
wrinkles, 176

X
Xenadrine EFA, 19

Y
yarrow flower extract, 137
yeasts, 50, 98, 131, 136, 334
Your Doctor Can't Make You Healthy, 13–14
yo-yo dieting, 50, 113, 184
Yphantides, MD, Nick, 38–39

Z
zero trans fats, 63, 74
zinc, 81, 88, 99, 312
Zocor, 4
Zone, The, 19, 36